# PSYCHIATRIC MENTAL HEALTH CASE STUDIES AND CARE PLANS

**Kim A. Jakopac, MSN, RN**
*Department of Nursing and Allied Health Professions*
*Nursing Instructor*
*University of Louisiana at Lafayette*
*Lafayette, Louisiana*

**Sudha C. Patel, DNS, MA, RN**
*Department of Nursing and Allied Health Professions*
*Assistant Professor*
*University of Louisiana at Lafayette*
*Lafayette, Louisiana*

**JONES AND BARTLETT PUBLISHERS**
*Sudbury, Massachusetts*
BOSTON    TORONTO    LONDON    SINGAPORE

*World Headquarters*
Jones and Bartlett Publishers
40 Tall Pine Drive
Sudbury, MA 01776
978-443-5000
info@jbpub.com
www.jbpub.com

Jones and Bartlett Publishers Canada
6339 Ormindale Way
Mississauga, ON L5V 1J2
Canada

Jones and Bartlett Publishers International
Barb House, Barb Mews
London W6 7PA
United Kingdom

Jones and Bartlett's books and products are available through most bookstores and online booksellers. To contact Jones and Bartlett Publishers directly, call 800-832-0034, fax 978-443-8000, or visit our website www.jbpub.com.

Substantial discounts on bulk quantities of Jones and Bartlett's publications are available to corporations, professional associations, and other qualified organizations. For details and specific discount information, contact the special sales department at Jones and Bartlett via the above contact information or send an email to specialsales@jbpub.com.

The authors, editor, and publisher have made every effort to provide accurate information. However, they are not responsible for errors, omissions, or for any outcomes related to the use of the contents of this book and take no responsibility for the use of the products and procedures described. Treatments and side effects described in this book may not be applicable to all people; likewise, some people may require a dose or experience a side effect that is not described herein. Drugs and medical devices are discussed that may have limited availability controlled by the Food and Drug Administration (FDA) for use only in a research study or clinical trial. Research, clinical practice, and government regulations often change the accepted standard in this field. When consideration is being given to use of any drug in the clinical setting, the health care provider or reader is responsible for determining FDA status of the drug, reading the package insert, and reviewing prescribing information for the most up-to-date recommendations on dose, precautions, and contraindications, and determining the appropriate usage for the product. This is especially important in the case of drugs that are new or seldom used.

**Production Credits**

Publisher: Kevin Sullivan
Acquisitions Editor: Emily Ekle
Acquisitions Editor: Amy Sibley
Associate Editor: Patricia Donnelly
Editorial Assistant: Rachel Shuster
Supervising Production Editor: Carolyn F. Rogers
Associate Marketing Manager: Rebecca Wasley

V.P., Manufacturing and Inventory Control: Therese Connell
Composition: Cape Cod Compositors, Inc.
Cover Design: Scott Moden
Cover Image: © Lepro/ShutterStock, Inc.
Printing and Binding: Courier Stoughton
Cover Printing: Courier Stoughton

**Library of Congress Cataloging-in-Publication Data**
Jakopac, Kim A.
    Psychiatric mental health case studies and care plans / Kim A. Jakopac, Sudha C. Patel.
        p. ; cm.
    Includes bibliographical references and index.
    ISBN 978-0-7637-6038-0 (pbk.)
    1. Psychiatric nursing—Case studies.    2. Nursing care plans.    I. Patel, Sudha C.    II. Title.
    [DNLM: 1. Mental Disorders—diagnosis—Case Reports.    2. Mental Disorders—diagnosis—Problems and Exercises.
    3. Mental Disorders—nursing—Case Reports.    4. Mental Disorders—nursing—Problems and Exercises.    5. Nursing
    Diagnosis—Case Reports.    6. Nursing Diagnosis—Problems and Exercises.    7. Risk Assessment—Case Reports    8. Risk
    Assessment—Problems and Exercises.    WM 18.2 J25p 2009]
    RC440.J25 2009
    616.89'0231—dc22
                                                                                        2008044971

6048

Printed in the United States of America
12   11   10   09   08        10   9   8   7   6   5   4   3   2   1

# Contents

# Preface

This book will provide nursing students with comprehensive practice in using critical thinking skills and planning evidence-based nursing interventions that evolve from patient case studies and psychiatric concept diagrams as well as nursing care plans. As in all areas of nursing, students will continue to use the nursing process when completing the case studies. The case studies occur in the inpatient setting, but the psychiatric concept diagrams, nursing care plans, and other information can easily be adapted for an outpatient setting. When using the forms provided here, nursing students will be expected to "think outside the box" by adapting complex information to the patient scenario requirements. Students may think of additional nursing diagnoses than those presented in Part II.

The psychiatric/mental health nurse should be familiar with the psychiatric disorders identified and classified by the American Psychiatric Association (APA) in the *Diagnostic and Statistical Manual of Mental Disorders,* Fourth Edition, Text Revision (*DSM-IV-TR*) as well as the North American Nursing Diagnosis Association–International (NANDA–I) Taxonomy II nursing diagnoses. These are located in Appendix II of *Psychiatric Mental Health Nursing: An Introduction to Theory and Practice* (O'Brien, Kennedy, & Ballard, 2008, Jones and Bartlett, pp. 551–557).

## Acknowledgments

We wish to thank three individuals who graciously consented to review material for this book: Dr. Ardith Sudduth, Dr. Evelyn Wills, and Nancy Ortego, APRN.

We also wish to thank Emily Ekle and Tricia Donnelly for their encouragement throughout this process.

# PART I

# Case Studies

CHAPTER 1

# Psychiatric Concept Diagrams

Throughout this book you will be asked to construct psychiatric concept diagrams and nursing care plans related to the patient case scenarios provided here. Psychiatric concept diagrams are an important method that will assist you in many ways: identifying patient problems and prioritizing them; planning outcomes; planning and implementing interventions; and evaluating patient care. These diagrams provide a way to visualize relationships between patients' responses to their psychiatric and medical problems, and the nursing diagnoses assigned to each patient's responses. This process will give you a holistic clinical picture of what is happening with a patient, thus helping you plan and provide more complete nursing care.

A psychiatric concept diagram also demonstrates how providing care for one patient problem has a positive impact on the outcome of another problem. By prioritizing patient problems you can more accurately determine a patient's needs and thus plan as well as provide more effective care. You can use information from the psychiatric concept diagram to formulate care plans based on priority nursing diagnoses. The answers to the case scenario questions, including prioritized psychiatric concept diagrams and nursing care plans, are located in Part II of this book. Remember that patient care is a fluid process that changes as the patient responds to nursing care and prescribed treatment. You may need to revise psychiatric concept diagrams and nursing care plans and make additions as priorities change according to a patient's condition over time.

*Source:* Adapted from P. M. Schuster (2002). *Concept mapping: A critical-thinking approach to care planning.* Philadelphia, PA: F. A. Davis, pp. 1–16.

Your first step in using a psychiatric concept diagram is to complete the five areas shown in the large center oval: the chief complaint (CC), or reason for seeking treatment; Axis I, II, and III diagnoses; and assessments. Your assessments here will be more general than the specific clinical objective and subjective data in the nursing care plans that will be the result of your assessments. There is only enough space in the large center oval to include three Axes, but you will need to include information from Axes IV and V to complete a holistic psychiatric concept diagram.

In each of the smaller ovals you will place one nursing diagnosis that you have identified after analyzing the key problems from all of the patient's data. You will support each of your nursing diagnoses with clinical data later on in the nursing care plans since there is limited space in the smaller ovals. The subjective and objective data will include information from the patient's reported symptoms, mental status, and physical assessment; laboratory and other diagnostics test results; medications, treatments, psychotherapy, psychiatric and medical history; and Axes I–V. You will next draw arrows between the smaller concept ovals containing nursing diagnoses to indicate the relationships between the nursing diagnoses and the large center oval. You will also use arrows between the smaller ovals to indicate relationships between the individual nursing diagnoses.

The final step will be to prioritize your nursing diagnoses (examples 1, 2, 3, etc.) in order of actual or potential life-threatening consequences. Remember that patients are hospitalized because of the high risk to attempt suicide or potentially harm others. Another reason is that the professional nurse role includes anticipating potential problems, planning and acting to prevent problems from actually occurring, and intervening early when unable to prevent their occurrence. Therefore, certain "risk for" or "potential for" nursing diagnoses will be treated as actual diagnoses. Individual nursing care plans will be written for the highest priority nursing diagnoses. Patients who have many psychiatric disorders or have additional medical complications will make the prioritization of nursing diagnoses a challenge. You may need to add new nursing diagnoses and care plans as a case scenario unfolds depending on the directions. Additions or revisions may be placed in a different color to differentiate them from the additional care plan information. A blank psychiatric concept diagram and nursing care plan are provided here for your reference. These are followed by some completed examples.

Psychiatric Concept Diagram and Nursing Care Plan:

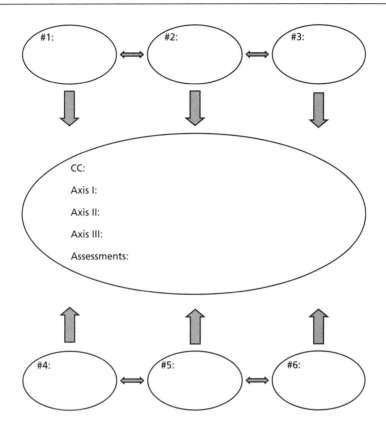

| Nursing Care Plan: |
| --- |
| **Nursing Diagnosis:** |
| **Outcomes** (include time frames): |

| **Assessment Data:** O = Objective, S = Subjective | **Evidence-Based Interventions:** | **Rationales:** | **Patient Responses:** |
| --- | --- | --- | --- |
|  |  |  |  |
| **Evaluation:** | | | |

Completed Psychiatric Concept Diagram and Nursing Care Plan for Nursing Diagnosis #1

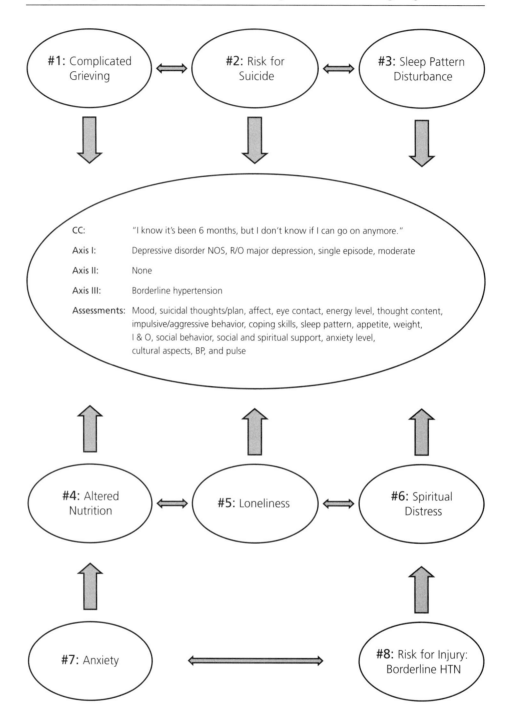

**Nursing Care Plan:** Depressive disorder NOS, R/O major depression, single episode, moderate.

**Nursing Diagnosis:** Complicated Grieving R/T difficulty moving through normal phases of grieving AEB statement "I know it's been 6 months, but I don't know if I can go on anymore."

**Outcomes** (include time frames): 1. Will agree to work with the nurse to realistically examine her current perceptions related to life without her spouse by the end of the second weekly visit. 2. Will verbalize hope that she will be able to go forward with her life by making decisions and engaging in activities by the third weekly visit.

| Assessment Data: O = Objective, S = Subjective | Evidence-Based Interventions: | Rationales: | Patient Responses:* |
|---|---|---|---|
| Sad, tearful affect (O) Fair eye contact (O) Psychomotor retardation (O) Decreased social activities (O) Sleeps only 4 hours/night (O) Eats two meals/day (O) Remains 5 lbs less than recommended weight range (O) Spouse died 6 months ago (O) States that she is unsure if she can go on anymore (S) Mood sad (S) | 1(a) Begin to establish rapport and therapeutic nurse/patient alliance that is the beginning of the therapeutic relationship. | 1(a) Developing a rapport with the client will assist in gaining the patient's cooperation in the future. According to Peplau, the therapeutic nurse/patient relationship is the foundation that must be established to initiate future work in the healing process (O'Brien, Kennedy, & Ballard, 2008). | 1(a) Met with primary nurse and agreed to meet with her during scheduled visits. |
| | (b) Use therapeutic communication techniques to facilitate client verbalizations of thoughts and feelings related to her life when her spouse was alive. | (b) Therapeutic communication techniques focus on the patient and help foster verbalization of thoughts and feelings, gather assessment information, and explore issues further as needed. | (b) Verbalized that she and her spouse "did everything together" and how much she misses him. |
| | (c) Assist patient to verbalize fears of living without her spouse. | (c) Verbalizing fears helps decrease feelings of powerlessness. | (c) Stated is afraid of continuing to feel lonely. Also stated that even though they did much together, her spouse took care of all the banking, paying of bills, car repairs, and maintenance of the house. |
| | (d) Help patient examine how realistic her fears are r/t living without her spouse. | (d) Realistic examination of fears helps empower the patient to begin to challenge inaccurate perceptions and move in a more positive psychological and emotional direction. | (d) Agreed that she is an intelligent human being and it may be possible for her to take on at least some of the responsibilities her spouse used to. |
| | (e) Explore ways of using fears to develop new areas of strength and coping | (e) Exploring ways to develop new areas of strength, coping skills, as | (e) States she is able to see the possibility of using her fear to motivate her to learn how |

*Patient responses are examples of what students would look for to decide whether their planned interventions were successful, needed more time, or needed to be changed. Responses will vary depending on the patient.

| Assessment Data:<br>O = Objective,<br>S = Subjective | Evidence-Based<br>Interventions: | Rationales: | Patient<br>Responses: |
|---|---|---|---|
| | skills and to improve problem-solving abilities. | well as problem-solving abilities promotes the healing process. It also helps ensure a positive outcome for this situation as well as assisting the patient to deal with future losses that may occur. | to develop a monthly budget and balance a checkbook. Agrees these are valuable skills to protect herself financially and to attain independence. Agrees that independence can be a valuable part of her general well-being. Completed a simple problem-solving exercise with the nurse's assistance. |
| | (f) Offer practical information, assistance, and solutions for actual needs and problems. | (f) During times of grief, many normal daily needs and responsibilities accumulate and contribute to the patient feeling overwhelmed. Practical assistance such as information on community resources and mobilizing family members or friends to help can decrease the patient's feelings of being overwhelmed. | (f) Identified need for assistance with lawn care and heavy housework. Accepted referral information for reputable landscaping and house-cleaning businesses in her area. Agreeable to suggestions of exploring possible assistance from extended family members and local religious organizations. |
| | (g) Monitor vital signs including BP at each visit. Refer for further medical evaluation if BP remains borderline high or increases and encourage a low sodium diet and appropriate exercise. | (g) The increased BP could be a physiological reaction to emotional distress. Further monitoring of vital signs by the nurse during treatment for grief can help determine if this is the reason or if there is a need for further medical evaluation and treatment. If the BP was dangerously high, this problem and its corresponding nursing diagnosis would become a priority nursing diagnosis —possibly even #1—due to possibility of being life threatening. Healthy lifestyle behaviors such as limiting dietary sodium and starting an exercise routine can also help reduce blood pressure as well as relieve emotional distress. | (g) Expresses gratitude for the nurse's care and concern of her total well-being. Verbalizes understanding and intent to follow a low sodium diet and appropriate exercise plan. Agrees to seek advice of medical physician for safe exercise routine if has not exercised in some time. Agreeable to future medical evaluation if needed. |

| Assessment Data: O = Objective, S = Subjective | Evidence-Based Interventions: | Rationales: | Patient Responses: |
|---|---|---|---|
| | 2(a) Express empathy for the patient's situation and convey hope that she can find meaning and purpose in her life even at a time like this in spite of still feeling sad and overwhelmed. | 2(a) Empathy helps the nurse focus on the patient's needs. It will help the patient feel emotionally supported and will promote the healing process. The instillation of hope also promotes healing and turns the patient's focus toward a more positive outcome for her situation. | 2(a) Accepts emotional support. States "maybe there is something still left for me to do in life even though my Henry isn't with me. I just assumed things would continue the way they were." Expresses continued belief in a "higher power." States she had not thought of being able to help someone else going through a similar experience. |
| | (b) Assist the patient to identify positive memories of her deceased spouse that she can turn to as needed. | (b) Realizing that she will always have good memories of her spouse helps the patient feel that the connection is not totally lost; a part of him will still be with her. | (b) Spoke of "many good times" that she and her spouse enjoyed together. Stated she now realizes her spouse will always be with her through these memories. |
| | (c) Assist the patient to identify what decisions must be made and tasks that must be done on a regular basis to maintain her living situation and meet financial obligations. | (c) This promotes a "here and now" focus with the patient to help keep her grounded in the present time which will help her to move forward more easily in the future. | (c) Reports that taxes on their home are late being paid and that her car is overdue for an oil change. Also mentioned needing to meet with their insurance agent regarding changes needing to be made with her life insurance policy. |
| | (d) Help the client make a schedule including day-to-day and week-to-week responsibilities. | (d) Making a schedule helps establish a routine that will help the client stay grounded in the present. | (d) Participated in preparing a daily and weekly written schedule. |
| | (e) Explore past social activities and the possibility of engaging in these on a more regular basis. Add these to the schedule developed in (d). | (e) Exploring past enjoyable social activities also helps to change the patient's focus and to open up the possibility of engaging in these again. Social support and activity will promote healing and moving forward with life. | (e) Identified playing cards and dancing with other couples as previously enjoyable social activities as well as involvement in a local church. Stated she might like to try volunteering at a local nursing home in the future, but she is hesitant to continue activities she and her spouse participated in as a couple. |
| | (f) Provide information on CBT and referral information for qualified therapists including APRNs. | (f) CBT is used to help clients examine and change their perceptions or beliefs, the emotions or | (f) Expressed interest in CBT and accepted contact information for qualified therapists. |

| Assessment Data: O = Objective, S = Subjective | Evidence-Based Interventions: | Rationales: | Patient Responses: |
|---|---|---|---|
| | (g) Discuss the benefit of community bereavement support groups and provide referral contact information. | feelings that accompany their perceptions, and the behavior that results from their perceptions and emotions.<br>(g) Support groups will help the client realize she isn't the only one who has suffered the same loss, provide a great benefit from individuals who have similar experiences, and promote the healing process. | (g) Stated unaware of such groups and eager to contact a group. |

**Evaluation:** 1. By the end of the 2nd weekly visit the patient stated she realizes her fear of not being able to take care of herself financially is unrealistic. She identifies this fear as possibly being the result of her spouse having "taken care of everything" the entire time they were married.
2. By the end of the 3rd weekly visit the client is able to talk about several positive memories of her spouse. Admits that her husband had more than adequate life insurance and their home is paid for. She has more than adequate financial income. Will continue to meet weekly with this client for 2 more weeks to work on the original planned outcomes and evaluate each week.

# References

Artinian, B. (1986). The research process in grounded theory. In W. C. Chenitz and J. M. Swanson (Eds.), *From practice to grounded theory: Qualitative research in nursing* (pp. 16–23). Menlo Park, CA: Addison-Wesley.

O'Brien, P. G., Kennedy, W. Z., & Ballard, K. A. (2008). *Psychiatric mental health nursing: An introduction to theory and practice.* Sudbury, MA: Jones and Bartlett.

Schuster, P. M. (2002). *Concept mapping: A critical-thinking approach to care planning.* Philadelphia, PA: F. A. Davis.

# CHAPTER 2

# Mood Disorders, Medical Disorders, and Substance Abuse

## *Major Depression and Suicide*

## Objectives

- Recognize signs and symptoms that meet *DSM-IV-TR* criteria for the diagnosis of a mood disorder.
- Apply knowledge of concepts of mood disorders when assessing a patient.
- Recognize risk factors and warning signs of suicide.
- Plan evidence-based nursing interventions to achieve patient-centered outcomes.

## Key Terms

| | |
|---|---|
| Affect | Mood |
| Anhedonia | Somatic |
| Depression | Unipolar |

The American Psychiatric Association (APA) recognizes two major types of mood disorders: major depression and bipolar disorder (Keltner, Schwecke, & Bostrom, 2007, p. 367). A person who has been diagnosed with bipolar disorder experiences symptoms of major depression at times and at other times experiences symptoms of mania. There are many etiologies of mood disorders including both biological and psychological factors. Mood disorders are treatable illnesses and may also be caused by a general medical condition that influences a person's mood and ability to think. Medication side effects may cause mood disturbances. In such cases, the symptoms are not due to alcohol or substance abuse.

In order for a person to be diagnosed with major depression or unipolar depression the symptoms must have occurred for a period of at least 2 weeks. If the symptoms have included suicidal thoughts, the person will meet the criteria for major depression at that moment, not after the required 2-week period. If suicidal thoughts are absent, a person must experience depressed mood and at least four other symptoms over a period of at least 2 weeks to meet criteria for a diagnosis of major depression. These other symptoms include an inability to experience pleasure (anhedonia), appetite disturbance, sleep disturbance, fatigue or loss of energy, psychomotor retardation or agitation, decreased ability to concentrate, feelings of worthlessness or inappropriate guilt, and somatic symptoms. Additionally, the person has problems functioning on a day to day basis, has problems with primary relationships, or has problems functioning at work or school (APA, 2000, pp. 375–376; Keltner, Schwecke, & Bostrom, 2007, pp. 369–370).

## Clinical Case Study

A 20-year-old college student has been coming to class late over the past month and is demonstrating poor academic performance. He looks disheveled and has decreased his social activities. His girlfriend of 2 years broke off the relationship approximately a month ago. He sought help at the college counseling center/student health office on the recommendation of his chemistry professor. The counselor has asked that he be evaluated further and recommended possible inpatient admission if indicated.

When speaking with him during your intake assessment, you observe him to be tearful and to have poor eye contact. He reports having insomnia, yet he stays in bed at least 12 hours "just lying there." He has difficulty getting out of bed in the morning, has a decreased appetite with a weight loss of 10 pounds, is disinterested in prior hobbies, declines offers of close friends to go out socially, experiences fatigue and memory disturbance, and he has difficulty concentrating. He admits he has not been able to study due to difficulty concentrating and memory problems and his academic performance is starting to become affected. You notice that his verbal responses to your questions are delayed and that he has psychomotor retardation. He is able to recall two out of three objects after 3 minutes and remembers the third object with verbal prompting. He denies abuse of alcohol, illegal substances, and prescription medications. He is oriented in five spheres and there is no evidence of psychosis on assessment. There is no history of previous suicide attempts, but when questioned regarding current suicidal ideation and plan he admitted to ideation only. The patient's current admission diagnoses are as follows:

Axis I: Major depression, single episode, severe, without psychotic features.

Axis II: None

Axis III: None

Axis IV: Loss of long-term relationship with girlfriend approximately 1 month ago, poor academic performance

Axis V: GAF = 25, past year = 90

Laboratory and diagnostic test results:

BAL/BAC = 0

UA = negative

Urine toxicology (UDS) = negative

# Questions

1. What symptoms does this patient have that meet criteria for major depression?
2. What suicide risk factors and warning signs can you identify? What additional factors and signs not included in the patient information would also be important to assess for that would increase the risk of suicide?
3. What passive risk factors and signs would you need to be aware of when a patient is depressed?

The student is admitted voluntarily to a mood disorder unit. He agrees to try medication if necessary as part of the treatment regimen. He also informs you that he has healthcare insurance coverage on his parents' plan since he is still a full-time student and under age 22. He has notified his parents regarding his admission and they are on their way to the hospital. He reports they are concerned about him and he feels guilty for causing them to worry about him.

4. What patient strengths can you identify?
5. Identify appropriate nursing diagnoses and develop a concept care map for this patient using the form provided in Chapter 1 and refer to the sample included in that chapter.
6. Prioritize the nursing diagnoses you have identified.
7. Choose three priority nursing diagnoses and write nursing care plans using the form provided. Nursing diagnoses should include what the problem is related to and evidence that supports the chosen nursing diagnoses. Support your nursing diagnoses with specific clinical data on the nursing care plans. Planned outcomes should be patient centered

and include specific time frames for evaluation. Nursing interventions should be evidence-based and include rationales.

  a. What collaborative interventions, including treatment, do you anticipate for this patient? Include these in your nursing care plans.

8. How will you evaluate the effectiveness of your nursing care? Add your evaluation to the nursing care plans.

9. The psychiatrist orders Lexapro/escitalopram 10 mg po daily. What information will you include when teaching the patient and his family regarding Lexapro/escitalopram?

10. The patient reports that the psychologist met with him and offered various types of psychotherapy including cognitive behavioral therapy (CBT) and interpersonal psychotherapy (IPT). How would each of these therapies help this patient?

You notice the patient becomes agitated and upset during a visit from a male friend. You approach them and ask if anything is wrong and offer assistance. The visitor responds that he thinks it is time for him to leave and the patient agrees. The patient remains agitated and upset even after the visitor leaves. Again you offer to help the patient: "I see that you're still upset and I'd like to help you. Tell me what you're feeling." The patient responds that he just found out that his girlfriend of 2 years had been seeing another man during the last few months they were together and is currently dating him since their breakup approximately 1 month ago. He also states that he feels like hurting himself. When you ask him if he can refrain from giving in to these feelings and impulses, he says, "no, I don't think I can."

11. How will this change in the patient's condition alter your nursing care? You have already identified the nursing diagnoses "Risk for Suicide" and "Ineffective Individual Coping" on your concept care map. Place the changes or additions to current care plans with the date initiated or add a care plan if indicated. You may also use a different color to indicate the additional information.

# Bipolar Disorder, Hyperthyroidism, and Marijuana Abuse

## Objectives

- Recognize signs and symptoms that meet *DSM-IV-TR* criteria for the diagnosis of a mood disorder.
- Apply knowledge of concepts of mood disorders.
- Identify priority patient-centered outcomes.
- Plan evidence-based nursing interventions.
- Assess the effect of a medical disorder on the patient's mood disorder.

## Key Terms

| | |
|---|---|
| Affect | Grandiose |
| Bipolar disorder | Hyperthyroidism |
| Delusion | Hypothyroidism |
| Depression | Mania |
| Flight of ideas (FOI) | Mood |

Accordingly the American Psychiatric Association (APA), bipolar I disorder consists of periods of depression and symptoms of mania that occur for a period of 1 week; bipolar II disorder—previously termed "hypomania"—has symptoms that last approximately 4 days and may be less intense than bipolar I symptoms. These symptoms include expansive, elevated, euphoric, or irritable mood and at least three of the following symptoms: decreased need for sleep, distractibility, excessive speech, racing thoughts or flight of ideas, grandiose (delusional) thinking, religious preoccupation, an increase in goal-directed activities, and excessive involvement in pleasurable activities that will result in problems later on (APA, 2000, pp. 388–389; Keltner, Schwecke, & Bostrom, 2007, pp. 396–396). In bipolar I disorder, and even in bipolar II, there are patients who experience impulsive behavior resulting in physical injury, attempted suicide or homicide attempts, sexually transmitted diseases, substance abuse, and financial hardship. Elevated vital signs may be present during the physical assessment. In addition, patients have problems functioning on a day-to-day basis as well as have problems with primary relationships or with work or school activities.

Thyroid disorders are very common in people who are also diagnosed with mood disorders. Because the symptoms overlap and one disorder influences the other, it is critical to diagnose and treat both thyroid and mood disorders. Symptoms of hypothyroidism are related to decreased metabolism, and they include fatigue and lethargy; decreased rate and force of cardiac contractions; anemia; somnolence; impaired memory; slow speech; decreased motivation and affect; muscle weakness; weight gain; constipation; decreased appetite; cold intolerance; loss of hair; and coarse skin. There is general slowing down of body processes and decreased deep tendon reflexes on physical examination (Lewis, Heitkemper, & Dirksen, 2004, pp. 1313, 1319–1320). Many of these symptoms are similar to those of major depression.

Symptoms of hyperthyroidism are related to increased metabolism and include nervousness, fatigue, or weakness preceded by increased energy levels, restlessness, irritability, and emotional lability. Patients are easily distracted, and they have decreased concentration; difficulty sleeping; heat intolerance; increased body temperature and blood pressure; palpitations, tachycardia, irregular heartbeat, and systolic heart murmurs; weight loss; warm, moist skin; diaphoresis; increased bowel movements; and manic behavior. There is a general speeding up of body processes as well as increased deep tendon reflexes on examination and fine tremors of the hands and tongue (Lewis, Heitkemper, & Dirksen, 2004, pp. 1311–1320; Thompson, McFarland, Hirsch, & Tucker, 2002, p. 773). Many of these symptoms are similar to those of bipolar disorder.

## Clinical Case Study

A 48-year-old, three times divorced female is brought to the emergency room by the police after being found at 4 a.m. walking in the middle of a highway against traffic. There were no signs of a struggle or evidence of rape. She was evicted from her apartment 2 weeks ago after refusing to pay the rent. Her children are in the legal custody of her first husband. She will be admitted involuntarily to an acute psychiatric unit.

She is dressed in a long, zebra-striped coat, red negligee, and dirty high-top sneakers. She has a strong body odor indicating poor hygiene. Her short, dyed, blond hair is matted to her scalp. Red lipstick is smeared crudely on her lips and cheeks, and some of her fake red fingernails are chipped and broken. Her speech is rapid, pressured, and loud. Her mood is labile and her affect at this time is very bright. She states that she was looking for her "movie agent" as the reason for walking on the highway at 4 a.m. She laughs off any suggestion that she may have been in danger, denies any need for treatment, and denies any substance abuse. She does admit to an undetermined amount of weight loss stating, "I'm too busy to bother eating." Her vitals signs are as follows: Temperature = 99.0°F, pulse = 100, respirations = 24, and blood pressure 140/90. Her skin is warm, moist, and pink in color, and she has no known allergies. Her current admission diagnoses are as follows:

Axis I: Bipolar I disorder, manic phase, recurrent, severe

Axis II: None

Axis III: Hyperthyroidism

Axis IV: Financial problems, homelessness, estrangement from primary support group (family), chronic/severe mental illness, problems with medication adherence

Axis V: GAF = 20, past year = unknown

During your nursing intake assessment, she frequently starts singing and getting in and out of her chair. Her conversation is difficult to follow due to not completing sentences and moving rapidly from topic to topic. She refuses to sign the consent form to allow any family members to be contacted. You ask if she is currently being prescribed any medications, and if so, which ones she is taking. She replies, "Well, I was supposed to take lithium, but I don't like it so I stopped taking it." She cannot remember when she stopped taking this medication and refuses to discuss with you the reasons she did not like to take it.

# Questions

1. Identify appropriate nursing diagnoses for this patient including the manic and depressed phases of bipolar I disorder. Develop a psychiatric concept diagram for this patient using the form provided in Chapter 1 and refer to the sample included in that section.

2. Prioritize the nursing diagnoses you have identified.

3. Choose three priority nursing diagnoses and write nursing care plans using the form provided. Nursing diagnoses should include what the problem is related to and evidence that supports the chosen nursing diagnoses. Support your nursing diagnoses with specific clinical data on the nursing care plans. Planned outcomes should be patient-centered and include specific time frames for evaluation. Nursing interventions should be evidence-based and include rationales.

   a. What collaborative interventions, including treatment, do you anticipate for this patient? Include these in your nursing care plans.

4. How will you evaluate the effectiveness of your nursing care? Add your evaluation to the nursing care plans.

5. What will you include in your teaching for this patient and her family regarding lithium/Eskalith therapy?

6. If the psychiatrist adds Depakote/valproic acid to the patient's treatment regimen, what would you need to monitor and teach the patient/family?

7. What symptoms does this patient have that meet criteria for the diagnosis of hyperthyroidism?

   a. Add a nursing diagnosis to your concept care map that addresses the client's diagnosis of hyperthryoidism.

8. How does hyperthyroidism affect the patient's mood?

9. What treatment do you anticipate being ordered for hyperthyroidism?

10. What additional patient teaching will you plan for her and her family?

11. There are also patients diagnosed with bipolar disorder who present with more depressed phases of the disorder and are diagnosed with hypothyroidism. What symptoms would you expect to see in a client who has hypothyroidism? How does hypothyroidism affect her mood?

    a. How would the treatment for hypothyroidism differ from the treatment for hyperthyroidism?

The following results of laboratory and diagnostic tests obtained in the ER are available:

CBC: RBCs = 4.5, Hgb = 12, Hct = 37%

Electrolytes: Na = 138, K = 4.0, Ca (total) = 9, Mg = 2

Glucose = 80

WBCs = 6

BUN = 12

Creatinine = 1.0

GFR = 125

Albumin = 2.8

Total protein = 5

TSH = 0.1

Total T3 = 225

T3 Uptake = 10

Total T4 = 60

Free T4 = 5

Free thyroxine index (FTI or T7) = 6

Lithium level = 0

BAL/BAC = 0

B-HCG = negative

RPR = pending

VDRL = pending

UA = pending

UDS/Urine toxicology = pending

CXR = bilateral views normal

EKG/ECG = normal sinus rhythm

12. What is the importance of a lithium level of 0 and the creatinine, BUN, and GFR being normal?

13. What is the purpose for ordering the BAL/BAC and the urine toxicology/UDS?

14. Why would it be important to know if the B-HCG, RPR, and VDRL were negative?

15. What will you do regarding her decreased albumin and total protein results?

The UA results showed no signs of infection, but the urine toxicology/urine drug screen (UDS) was positive for tetrahydrocannabinol (THC), indicating marijuana use.

16. What additional treatment and referrals do you anticipate this patient will need?

    a. What nursing diagnoses would be appropriate for a patient with substance use or abuse problems?

17. What discharge planning is appropriate for this patient?

    a. What type of housing situation?

    b. What referrals will be needed?

    c. What community resources would you suggest for this patient and family?

    d. What support groups would be beneficial for this patient and family?

# Psychotic and Medical Disorders: Schizophrenia and Hypertension

## Objectives

- Recognize signs and symptoms that meet *DSM-IV-TR* criteria for the diagnosis of schizophrenia versus schizoaffective disorder.
- Apply knowledge of concepts of psychotic disorders when assessing a client.
- Identify positive, negative, and cognitive signs and symptoms of schizophrenia.
- Plan evidence-based nursing interventions to achieve patient-centered outcomes.

## Key Terms

| | |
|---|---|
| Akasthesia | Extrapyramidal symptoms |
| Akinesia | Hallucination |
| Alogia | Negative signs |
| Aloofness | Neuroleptic |
| Antipsychotics | Neuroleptic malignant syndrome (NMS) |
| Apathy | Oculogyric crisis |
| Avolition | Opisthotonus |
| Cognitive signs | Positive signs |
| Delusion | Poverty of speech |
| Dystonia | Pseudoparkinsonism |

Psychotic

Schizoaffective disorder

Schizophrenia

Tardive dyskinesia

Torticollis

Psychotic disorders encompass a variety of signs and symptoms: alterations in thought processes or disorganized thought processes; cognitive misperceptions, various types of delusional thinking, hallucinations, unusual thought content, and bizarre or disorganized behavior; disorganized speech, impaired social skills, social withdrawal, decreased attention, and memory impairment; decreased motivation, decreased attention to self-care, anhedonia, flattening of the affect, or apathy. These disorders are easy to identify in patients and are typically what people think of when they hear the phrase "psychiatric disorders" or "mental illness." Schizophrenia is one of the most common psychotic disorders. More patients are being diagnosed with schizoaffective disorder as well.

A diagnosis of schizoaffective disorder is given to a patient who has had signs and symptoms of schizophrenia, has been diagnosed with schizophrenia and later develops signs and symptoms of a mood disorder that occur simultaneously with the symptoms of schizophrenia. The patient has periods when the signs and symptoms of the mood disorder become less prominent or decrease, but the signs and symptoms of schizophrenia remain prominent. There are two major subtypes of schizoaffective disorder: (1) bipolar type and (2) depressed type (O'Brien, Kennedy, & Ballard, 2008, p. 287). Patients diagnosed with schizoaffective disorder are prescribed treatment for both schizophrenia type symptoms and mood disorder symptoms. In the past schizoaffective disorder was regarded as a diagnosis of exclusion, but it is currently being diagnosed more frequently.

There are many causative etiologies of schizophrenia, most of which are neurobiological. They include genetics, brain structure abnormalities, and brain atrophy; imbalances of neurotransmitters (with the dopamine hypothesis being the oldest); abnormal programmed cell death; viral infections; lack of proper nutrition; decreased oxygen or exposure to environmental neurotoxins during the prenatal period; and the result of an interaction between a significant stressor (physical or psychological) and a genetic predisposition to develop schizophrenia (Sadock & Sadock, 2003, pp. 477, 479; Keltner, Schwecke, & Bostrom, 2007, pp. 350–351, 353). There is a high rate of genetic susceptibility in families of patients diagnosed with schizophrenia (Fontaine & Fletcher, 2003, pp. 406–407; Keltner, Schwecke, & Bostrom, 2007, p. 351). Psychological theories include poor ego development, poor ego boundaries, lack of nurturing early in life, inconsistent or chaotic family environment or problems with communication patterns within the family during the patient's early life (Keltner, Schwecke, & Bostrom, 2007, p. 353).

Although men and women are equally affected, men tend to have an earlier onset of symptoms that more often lead to a poorer prognosis because brain anatomical structure is frequently abnormal with more prominent negative symptoms. In later onset, brain anatomical structure is more likely to be normal leading to a better prognosis, but imbalances in neurotransmitters occur with more prominent positive symptoms (Sadock & Sadock, 2003, p. 489). Signs and symptoms of schizophrenia are usually divided into "positive" and "negative" categories (O'Brien, Kennedy, & Ballard, 2008, pp. 290–291). More recently there is mention of "cognitive" symptoms as well. Positive symptoms include delusional or bizarre thoughts as well as disorganized thoughts; hallucinations or abnormal perceptions; disorganized or bizarre behavior; inappropriate responses to situations' concrete thinking; belief in one's own special or magical abilities; and unusual speech patterns (i.e. loose association, disorganized speech, clanging, neologisms) that are not present in normal individuals. Negative symptoms are described as a decrease in normal functioning including flattened affect, alogia, avolition, anhedonia, anergia, poverty of speech, mutism, difficulty sustaining attention, decreased attention to ADLs, and social withdrawal (Keltner, Schwecke, & Bostrom, 2007, p. 343; O'Brien, Kennedy, & Ballard, 2008, pp. 290–291). Cognitive symptoms include problems with attention but also memory impairment and difficulty with problem-solving, abstract reasoning, judgment, and the ability to understand and respond appropriately to social cues (Varcarolis, Carson, & Shoemaker, 2006, p. 395).

In order for patients to be diagnosed with schizophrenia, their symptoms must be present for at least 6 months, but they should not be directly due to substance abuse or dependence. They should also cause significant problems or impairment in performance of social, occupational, or academic roles (APA, 2000, pp. 298, 312–313). Psychotic symptoms resembling schizophrenia may be caused by general medical conditions including neurological, neurodegenerative, and metabolic diseases; exposure to environmental toxins, steroid medications, and delirium. There are five subtypes of schizophrenia: (1) paranoid, (2) disorganized, (3) catatonic, (4) undifferentiated, and (5) residual. The paranoid and catatonic subtypes are the most easily identified due to the presence of paranoid delusions in the former and psychomotor disturbance in the later.

Hypertension is defined as elevated blood pressure of 140/90 or greater. A new category "prehypertension" has been identified and includes patients with a blood pressure ranging from 120/80 to 139/89. Patients who are diagnosed as having prehypertension typically are not prescribed medication, but they are treated with lifestyle behavior changes including smoking cessation, dietary modification, exercise, weight reduction, and stress reduction (www.american heartassociation.org).

# Clinical Case Study

A 42-year-old, obese male who recently tried to run away from an assisted living facility is admitted with a diagnosis of chronic paranoid schizophrenia and hypertension. He reports being followed by a midget with sharp pointed teeth who is trying to kill him. The midget is from another planet and travels in a spaceship. During your nursing intake assessment, he frequently looks over his right shoulder and mumbles to himself. Staff at the assisted living facility reported he became agitated and physically aggressive when they attempted to bring him back. They called the police and the patient was brought to the local hospital to be evaluated and was admitted involuntarily to the psychiatric unit. At this time he is cooperative, but frightened and paranoid. His affect is flat with poor eye contact. His current vital signs are as follows: temperature = 98.8°F, pulse = 96, respirations = 22, blood pressure = 168/90. He is 6 feet tall and weighs 250 pounds at admission. Over the past 22 years, he has smoked 1½ packs of cigarettes per day.

According to the assisted living facility staff, a new resident moved in 2 days ago. The patient has had the delusion of a midget from outer space trying to kill him for several years and a family history of schizophrenia. He has never been married and does not have children. There is no history of substance abuse, and the patient denies current substance abuse. He has no known allergies. In the past 2 days he has become more paranoid about staff and has needed more reminders from them to bathe and change his clothes. His current medications include Risperdal/risperidone 2 mg po bid, Ambien/zolpidem 10 mg po prn at bedtime for insomnia, and Coreg/carvedilol 25 mg po bid. It is documented in previous medical records that this patient had been treated with Haldol/haloperidol and Thorazine/chlorpromazine in the past. He received Ativan/lorazepam 2 mg IM and was briefly physically restrained in the emergency room prior to admission.

The patient's current admission diagnoses are as follows:

Axis I: Chronic paranoid schizophrenia, acute exacerbation

Axis II: None

Axis III: Hypertension

Axis IV: Admission of new resident to assisted living facility. Hurricane evacuee 1 year ago. Parents deceased. Has one brother living out of state who has not had contact with patient for several years.

Axis V: GAF = 30, past year = 50

Laboratory and diagnostic test results:

BAL/BAC = 0

UA = negative

Urine toxicology (UDS) = negative

The patient's admission orders include safety checks every 15 minutes.

CBC with differential, WBC, electrolytes, glucose, BUN, creatinine, GFR, HDL/HDL-C, LDL, triglycerides, total cholesterol/HDL ratio, RPR and VDRL; EKG/ECG and chest X-ray two views.

Risperdal 2 mg po tid, Coreg 25 mg po bid, Ambien 10 mg po hs prn insomnia, Zyprexa Zydis 5 mg prn agitation maximum dose 10 mg in 24 hours, Zyprex 5 mg IM prn agitation maximum dose 10 mg in 24 hours, Ativan 2 mg po every 6 hours prn anxiety maximum dose 4 mg in 24 hours, Ativan 2 mg IM every 6 hours prn anxiety maximum dose 4 mg in 24 hours, Catepres/clonidine 0.1 mg po prn for SBP greater than or equal to 170 or DBP greater than or equal to 100; notify physician.

Vital signs every shift; weigh every 3 days; and a low-sodium, low-fat diet. Medical consult to evaluate and manage hypertension.

# Questions

1. At this time should you place the patient in locked seclusion and physical restraints since the patient was physically aggressive with the assisted living facility staff, and in the emergency room had to be physically restrained briefly in addition to needing IM medication?

2. What signs and symptoms of chronic paranoid schizophrenia can you identify?

3. Identify appropriate nursing diagnoses for this patient. Prioritize them after you have identified them.

4. Choose three priority nursing diagnoses and write nursing care plans using the form provided. Nursing diagnoses should include what the problem is related to and evidence that supports the chosen nursing diagnoses. Support your nursing diagnoses with specific clinical data on the nursing care plans. Planned outcomes should be patient-centered and include specific time frames for evaluation. Nursing interventions should be evidence-based and include rationales.

   a. What collaborative interventions, including treatment, do you anticipate for this patient? Include these in your nursing care plans.

5. How will you evaluate the effectiveness of your nursing care? Add your evaluation to the nursing care plans.

The results of the patient's EKG/ECG and chest X-ray are normal, but the remaining laboratory test results are still pending.

6. On the 2nd day of admission the patient reports that his mouth "feels funny." He looks as if he is chewing gum or food. You ask him if he has gum or food in his mouth, but he denies this. Why would it be appropriate to perform an AIMS test at this time?

   a. The patient's mouth movements may be an adverse effect of which of the patient's medications?

      b. Discuss the various types of EPS.

      c. Why should you perform an AIMS test at this time?

      d. What medications may be used to treat EPS?

7. You notify the psychiatrist of the patient's mouth movements and the result of your AIMS test. The order from the psychiatrist reads as follows: "Cogentin 1 mg po now and follow with Cogentin 0.5 mg po tid." Why is the psychiatrist adding Cogentin/benztropine at this time?

      a. What side effects of Cogentin/benztropine will you teach the patient and need to be aware of yourself?

8. You receive the remaining results of the patient's laboratory and diagnostic tests:

      CBC: RBCs = 5, Hgb = 16, Hct = 46%

      Electrolytes: Na = 140, K = 4.2, Ca (total) = 9.6, Mg = 2.2

      Glucose = 108

      WBCs = 8

      BUN = 16

      Creatinine = 0.9

      GFR = 125

      ALT/SGPT = 10

      AST/SGOT = 20

      Total cholesterol = 200

      HDL/HDL-C = 35

      LDL = 130

      Triglycerides = 150

      Total cholesterol/HDL ratio = 4.2

      RPR = negative

      VDRL = negative

Are there any abnormal results? What is the significance of any abnormal results?

9. You are scheduled to attend a treatment team meeting. The psychiatrist discusses the possibility of changing the patient's regularly scheduled antipsychotic medication. He explains that the older, traditional antipsychotics are more likely than the newer, atypical or second generational antipychotics (SGAs) to cause extrapyramidal symptoms (EPS), neuroleptic malignant syndrome (NMS), cardiac arrhythmias, and orthostatic hypotension. However, there is still the possibility of EPS, NMS, and other serious adverse effects including blood dyscrasias, elevated liver enzymes, and increased risk for metabolic syndrome.

      a. What signs and symptoms should the nurse observe for that would indicate the patient is experiencing NMS?

b. What does the term "blood dyscrasias" mean? Why is this important?

c. Describe metabolic syndrome. Why is it important for the nurse to be aware of this syndrome in patients diagnosed with psychiatric illnesses?

d. Which atypical or SGAs are less likely to cause weight gain, increased glucose or cholesterol levels?

e. Which atypical or SGA antipsychotic medication should not be ordered if this patient had an abnormal EKG/ECG on admission?

10. Do you think this patient would benefit from psychotherapy and psychoeducation not only during admission but on an outpatient basis after discharge from the hospital? If so, what type of psychotherapy and psychoeducation would be appropriate?

a. How many days of partial hospitalization/day treatment would you recommend?

# Personality Disorders and Substance Abuse: Borderline Personality Disorder and Methamphetamine Abuse

## Objectives

- Recognize signs and symptoms that meet *DSM-IV-TR* criteria for the diagnosis of borderline personality disorder.
- Identify possible reasons patients engage in self-mutilation.
- Identify priority client-centered outcomes.
- Plan evidence-based nursing interventions to achieve patient-centered outcomes.

## Key Terms*

| | |
|---|---|
| Boundaries | Mindfulness |
| Cognitive distortion | Perception |
| Dialectical behavioral therapy | Personality |
| Dichotomous thinking | Personality traits |
| Dysphoria | Self-mutilation |
| Ego defense mechanisms | Splitting |

*Refer to the Key Terms in Chapter 6, which discusses the substance abuse/dependence.

The development of a person's personality is attributed to both genetic and environmental factors. The full expression of genetic tendencies is influenced by the environment in which a person is exposed to, including family and culture. From a humanistic viewpoint, personality is influenced by a natural inner capacity for self-fulfillment whereas psychoanalytic theory proposes that unconscious motivations and sexuality are strong influences on the development of personality. Erickson's psychosocial developmental theory is frequently used by nurses to understand personality development and stages of life.

Personality disorders occur when patterns of perceiving the self, others, and the environment become inflexible and maladaptive. There is also significant behavioral deviation compared to the expectations of the culture in which people with personality disorders live. The diagnosis of a personality disorder usually is not given before age 18 and is not due to another psychiatric/mental health disorder, substance abuse, medication or general medical condition. These disorders cause significant distress for the person because of how other people react to them. They themselves do not realize the problem lies within. Causative etiologies include psychosocial developmental problems of successfully completing a "separation-individuation process" (O'Brien, Kennedy, & Ballard, 2008, p. 441); environmental factors including emotional deprivation, inadequate nurturing or inconsistent parenting practices; childhood psychological trauma; and neurobiological factors including a possible deficit of the neurotransmitter serotonin. Psychopharmacological treatment has not been as effective for Axis II personality disorders as it has been for Axis I psychiatric disorders. Long-term psychotherapy, psychoeducation, and emotional support within healthy boundaries have been the most effective treatments for Axis II personality disorders.

There are several types of personality disorders, divided into groups known as clusters. The diagnoses in each cluster share similar characteristics, signs, and symptoms yet have distinct signs and symptoms of their own.

There are three distinct clusters:

- Cluster A includes paranoid, schizoid, and schizotypal personality disorders. The shared characteristics in this cluster include having a sense of distrust or suspiciousness of others, being detached from social relationships, and odd or eccentric behavior. There are no fixed delusions as in schizophrenia or schizoaffective disorders.

- Cluster B includes antisocial, borderline, histrionic, and narcissistic personality disorders. The shared characteristics in this cluster include being emotionally unstable or dramatic, and displaying erratic or extremely impulsive behavior. These patients also seem to require more personal attention than patients with other cluster disorders.

- Cluster C includes avoidant, dependent, and obsessive-compulsive personality disorders. The shared characteristics in this cluster include being anxious, fearful, or dependent on others; feelings of inadequacy; perfectionism; and having a need for control.

■ In addition to the three distinct clusters there is a diagnosis of personality disorder not otherwise specified (NOS). This diagnosis is used for those individuals who do not have enough signs and symptoms to meet criteria for a specific personality disorder or have mixed signs and symptoms that cause them significant distress.

*DSM-IV-TR* criteria for a diagnosis of borderline personality disorder include intense, unstable interpersonal relationships; alternating feelings about valuating and devaluating relationships; unstable image or sense of self; frantic efforts to avoid real or imagined abandonment; recurrent self-mutilation; suicidal threats, attempts, or gestures; chronic complaints of feeling empty inside; mood swings; intense anger or anger that is inappropriate to the situation; and impulsive behavior that may include overspending, provocative or hypersexual behavior, reckless driving, binge eating, and substance abuse. Some patients may experience temporary dissociative symptoms or paranoia. Patients with this disorder have great difficulty tolerating perceived or actual rejection or abandonment and will go to great lengths to prevent this. They will frequently use manipulative behavior to get what they think they need. They also may sabotage their own success in a relationship or career because they are afraid they will not be able to meet the expectations of the relationship or career position. They frequently engage in self-mutilation and sometimes go further than planned, leading to completed suicide. Patient behaviors demonstrate excessive use of the ego defense mechanism "projection" and cognitive distortions such as dichotomous thinking leading to a "splitting" phenomenon. These patients are very ill and provide unique challenges for any nurse working with them.

Methamphetamine is a CNS stimulant that is widely abused in urban, suburban, and rural communities in the United States. A person may use this substance only one time and become addicted. In addition to the usual problems associated with substance abuse/dependence, methamphetamine users may also be making the drug in homemade laboratories. Frequently burns and other serious injuries are sustained when explosions occur during the process of making methamphetamine. Dental caries, psychosis, and skin lesions secondary to picking at the skin while visually hallucinating that bugs are crawling on their skin or tactile hallucinations of crawling skin sensations, occur frequently in patients who abuse methamphetamine. There is no recommended detoxification treatment because the addiction is more psychological and not medically life threatening. Unfortunately there is no pharmacological treatment available to help maintain abstinence as there is for alcohol or opiate abuse/dependence. Although general supportive care is provided, there is no antidote available for methamphetamine overdose as there is for opiate, benzodiazepine, barbiturate, and alcohol overdose. (See Chapter 6 for additional information on substance abuse/dependence.)

# Clinical Case Study

A 26-year-old female with a history of self-mutilation has been treated in a local outpatient community mental health clinic for the past 2 years. She was admitted 4 days ago to a psychiatric/mental health unit after a fight with her boyfriend resulting in the patient cutting herself. The patient revealed she has been using methamphetamine for the past year. She has no known allergies.

Axis I: Methamphetamine abuse

Axis II: Borderline personality disorder

Axis III: None

Axis IV: Problems with primary support person/boyfriend, financial problems, current legal charges for drug possession and hearing scheduled 1 week from admission date; history of sexual and physical abuse as a child; healthcare insurance coverage recently terminated due to inability to pay premium

Axis V: GAF = 45, past year = 60

The admission laboratory and diagnostic tests are normal except for the UDS, which is positive for amphetamines. The BAL is 0 and there is no evidence of pregnancy or STDs. The patient is ordered every 15 minute safety checks, milieu therapy, psychotherapy including DBT, OT, AT, Prozac/fluoxetine 20 mg po daily, Ativan/lorazepam 1 mg po every 6 hours prn anxiety, maximum dose 4 mg in 24 hours and Ativan 1 mg IM every 6 hours prn anxiety, maximum dose 4 mg in 24 hours.

As the day-shift nurse assigned to care for this patient, you are performing a morning assessment. During this time, the patient states, "you know, nobody around here seems to understand me. They all think I'm crazy or they're just tired of seeing me. But I think you're different, yeah, you're somebody I can talk to. I'll bet you're the only one around here who could ever understand me. Do you think we could get together sometime after they let me out of here? You know, maybe get a cup of coffee or go to the mall?"

# Questions

1. How would you respond therapeutically to a patient who states that you are the only person she can talk to at the clinic?

2. How would you respond therapeutically to the patient's request to meet after she is discharged and go for a cup of coffee or to the mall?

The patient is very angry with your therapeutic response. She states, "You're just like all the rest of them! You come in here all nice and smiling like you're my friend and then stab me in the back!" Her voice volume increases to the point of yelling. The psychologist comes out of his office and walks to the day room to provide assistance. Other patients in the day room look up to see what is happening. Upon seeing the psychologist, the patient suddenly becomes calm, smiles sweetly, and says to the psychologist, "Oh there you are! You're my true friend. The only true friend I have here." The psychologist tells her that he will be ready to see her in 5 minutes, but she needs to remain calm. After the psychologist leaves, the patient stares angrily at you, but says nothing for a few minutes. She then says, "If nobody here cares about me, I might as well kill myself!"

3. The difference in the patient's behavioral response toward the nurse and psychologist would best be explained by what type of cognitive distortion?

4. What signs and symptoms of borderline personality disorder can you identify for this patient?

5. Explain how you would handle the patient's statement, "If nobody here cares about me, I might as well kill myself!"

6. What signs and symptoms of methamphetamine abuse would you assess this client for?

7. Identify appropriate nursing diagnoses for this patient. Develop a psychiatric concept diagram for this patient using the form provided in Chapter 1 and refer to the sample included in that section.

    a. Prioritize the nursing diagnoses you have identified.

8. Choose three priority nursing diagnoses and write nursing care plans using the form provided. Nursing diagnoses should include what the problem is related to and evidence that supports the chosen nursing diagnoses. Support your nursing diagnoses with specific clinical data on the nursing care plans. Planned outcomes should be patient-centered and include specific time frames for evaluation. Nursing interventions should be evidence-based and include rationales.

    a. What collaborative interventions, including treatment, do you anticipate for this client? Include these in your nursing care plans.

9. How will you evaluate the effectiveness of your nursing care? Add your evaluation to the nursing care plans.

10. What are some healthy ways that you could deal with your feelings related to this patient?

# CHAPTER 5

# Eating Disorders: Anorexia Nervosa

## Objectives

- Recognize signs and symptoms that meet *DSM-IV-TR* criteria for the diagnosis of anorexia nervosa.
- Recognize the differences between anorexia nervosa and bulimia nervosa.
- Identify factors important in the assessment of anorexia nervosa.
- Identify priority client-centered outcomes.
- Plan evidence-based nursing interventions to achieve patient-centered outcomes.

## Key Terms

| | |
|---|---|
| Anorexia nervosa | Cognitive distortion |
| Binge eating | Compensatory behaviors |
| Body mass index (BMI) | Ego-dystonic |
| Boundaries | Ego-syntonic |
| Bulimia nervosa | Enmeshed |

Although the causative etiologies of eating disorders include the interaction of multiple factors such as sociocultural, biological, cognitive, behavioral, and psychodynamic issues as well as family dynamics, eating disorders are a phenomenon of Western culture. There has been a tendency in the past to blame the families of origin as the major cause of eating disorders, but more current thinking looks at the interaction of multiple factors and the influence of culture.

In Western culture there is an exaggerated emphasis on physical attractiveness, specifically body thinness, that is continually perpetuated by the media. Other cultures or ethnic groups that have adopted Western culture and values also take on this exaggerated emphasis. On a continuum of disturbances in eating behaviors, obesity certainly is linked to health problems such as cardiovascular diseases that can lead to death. At the opposite end of the continuum, anorexia nervosa (AN) also causes serious health problems such as electrolyte disturbances and cardiac problems, and it can be fatal. The annual mortality rate for females diagnosed with AN is estimated to be 12 times greater than the mortality rate of females ages 15 to 24 years of all other causes. According to the National Institute of Mental Health (NIMH), mortality rates may be as high as 20% (O'Brien, Kennedy, & Ballard, 2008, p. 391). Death usually occurs due to the effects of starvation, cardiac arrhythmias, or suicide.

According to *DSM-IV-TR* criteria for AN and both subtypes (restricting and binge eating/purging), AN involves an intense fear of becoming fat or gaining weight even though such patients are significantly underweight. They refuse to maintain even a minimum normal body weight for their height and have a body weight of less than 85% of their ideal weight or body mass index (BMI) of less than or equal to 17.5 kg/ht in meters squared. The pursuit of thinness becomes relentless and there is strong denial of the seriousness of the weight loss. There is a disturbance in the perception of their appearance, the way in which they experience their body shape or weight, and an overvaluing of their body weight or shape while disregarding other aspects of the self. Females frequently experience a disturbance in their menses as evidenced by amenorrhea, the loss of at least three consecutive menstrual cycles (APA, 2000, pp. 583–584, 589).

Common characteristics of individuals with eating disorders include a sense of personal ineffectiveness or control over their lives, anxiety, perfectionism, obsessiveness, sensitivity to criticism, and an intense desire to please others. They often have a family member with an eating disorder and a history of sexual abuse. Not all patients with AN have a history of sexual abuse, but this is true of a high percentage of patients. Cognitive distortions are prevalent in patients with eating disorders. These distortions are ego-syntonic in patients with AN and anorexia is viewed as a solution rather than a problem. Lying, being secretive, and manipulating others are used as protective measures. Compensatory behaviors include restricting food intake and over exercising. If these measures are not successful, the patient may engage in abusing over the counter (OTC) diuretics, diet pills, and laxatives. Some families of these patients may be described as enmeshed, having difficulty communicating, and a general emphasis on perfection.

The causative etiologies of bulimia nervosa (BN) are similar to AN, but occur a little later in adolescence or young adulthood. Initially the individual is usually overweight. According to *DSM-IV-TR* criteria for BN and both subtypes (purging and nonpurging), patients engage in recurrent episodes of binge eating of a larger than normal amount of food during a specific amount of time with the binge eating followed by purging. The binge-purge episodes are accompanied by a sense of a lack of control over the eating. Patients engage in recurrent compensatory behaviors including self-induced vomiting, enemas, abusing OTC laxatives and diuretics, fasting, and overexercising. The episodes of binge eating and purging occur at least twice a week for at least 3 consecutive months and do not occur exclusively during episodes of AN. Additionally, patients' perception and evaluation of themselves is overly influenced by their body weight and shape (APA, 2000, pp. 589–590, 594). The binging and purging activities become self-reinforcing and addictive. Patients with BN share some common characteristics with those diagnosed with AN. Lying, being secretive, and manipulating others are also used as protective measures. However, in BN the cognitive distortions and behaviors engaged in are ego-dystonic. Ambivalence toward themselves exists as well as low self-esteem, feelings of unworthiness of being nurtured, unavailability of nurturing, use of food to nurture themselves, and use of binging and purging as a way to psychologically numb themselves from intense emotions or psychological trauma. The families of some patients may be described as emotionally distant, less nurturing, uninvolved, in conflict, chaotic, or disorganized.

Although the majority of individuals affected are female, males are also affected by eating disorders. According to a survey of 1,620 college students including Caucasian and African American women and men at the University of Michigan, 17.4% of women and 10.4% of men reported that an eating disorder behavior interfered with their academic performance. Members of sororities as well as athletes were at risk for developing eating disorders. Males are less often identified because their eating disorder behaviors are camouflaged by athletic training activities and eating disorders are viewed as "female" disorders. There are patients who also have Axis II personality disorders in addition to Axis I eating disorders. These patients require treatment tailored to their complex needs.

## Clinical Case Study

An 18-year-old female high school senior is complaining of fatigue, dizziness, and abnormal menses. She makes an appointment with her primary care provider (PCP) at her mother's insistence. The PCP orders laboratory and diagnostics tests after obtaining a complete history and performing a physical examination. The following laboratory and diagnostic tests were ordered to be obtained at the hospital outpatient department immediately after the visit with the PCP and results are to be called to the PCP:

CBC with differential, MCV, MCH, MCHC, WBC, electrolytes, glucose, albumin, total protein, BUN, creatinine, GFR, TSH, T3, T4, UA, UDS/urine toxicology, BAL/BAC, B-HCG, RPR, CXR, and ECG/EKG.

During the physical examination, the PCP notes the client to be extremely thin, to have poor skin turgor, and to be less than 85% of her ideal body weight/BMI of less than 17.5 kg/ht. When gently confronted, the client admits to restricting her intake of food to 600 calories a day and exercising at least 3 hours a day. She states that she recently started taking over the counter (OTC) diet pills and diuretics to lose weight because she thinks she is too fat. She feels in control of her life as long as she controls her weight, but denies any use of alcohol, illegal drugs, prescription pain pills, prescription amphetamines, or herbal supplements. She does admit to drinking at least 3 large cups of Starbucks coffee per day alternating with water.

The results of the laboratory and diagnostic tests are as follows:

CBC: RBCs = 3.2, Hgb = 11, Hct = 34% , MCV = 70, MCH = 20, MCHC = 28

Electrolytes: Na = 148, K = 2.8, Ca (total) = 10.8, Mg = 2.8

Glucose = 64

WBCs = 6

BUN = 4.5

Creatinine = 1.0

GFR = 90

Albumin = 2.4

Total protein = 4.8

TSH = 2.0

Total T3 = 125

T3 Uptake = 1.0

Total T4 = 60

Free T4 = 1.0

BAL/BAC = 0

B-HCG = negative

RPR = negative

UA = negative

UDS/urine toxicology = + for amphetamines

CXR = bilateral views normal (normal/absence of pathology)

EKG/ECG = irregular rate, bradycardia, flattened T wave

The patient and her mother are notified by the PCP to go directly to the hospital for the patient to be admitted to a telemetry unit. The admission diagnosis is hypokalemia, dehydration, malnutrition, and rule out anorexia nervosa. The patient is ordered intravenous fluids and intravenous potassium replacement, cardiac monitoring, I & O, regular diet, and a psychiatric consult.

# Questions

1. Identify the abnormal laboratory and diagnostic test results as well as the meaning related to the patient's diagnoses.

Upon assessment by the psychiatric nurse practitioner and psychiatrist, it is recommended that the patient be transferred to the psychiatric/mental health unit as a voluntary admission for further treatment when medically stable. The patient denies suicidal ideation or plan at this time and is able to contract verbally to notify any staff member if she has suicidal ideations or plans. The patient and her mother agree to the recommendation for transfer. The result of the patient's repeated CBC with differential, MCV, MCH, MCHC, electrolyte panel, serum glucose, total protein, albumin, GFR, and ECG/EKG are obtained before the patient is transferred:

CBC: RBCs = 3.2, Hgb = 11, Hct = 34% , MCV = 70, MCH = 20, MCHC = 28

Na = 143, K = 3.2, Ca (total) = 9.0, Mg = 2.0

Glucose = 80

GFR = 125

Albumin = 2.4

Total protein = 4.8

ECG/EKG = normal sinus rhythm

The patient is transferred to the psychiatric/mental health unit with the following diagnosis:

Axis I: Anorexia nervosa

Axis II: None

Axis III: Malnutrition, resolving; hypokalemia and dehydration, resolved

Axis IV: Problems in primary support relationships, academic and social issues

Axis V: GAF = 50, past year = 70

Admission orders include the following: therapeutic milieu therapy, safety checks every 15 minutes; vital signs every 4 hours for the first 72 hours of admission, nutrition stabilization contract; 1500 calorie regular diet; 1500 cc fluid intake per day, I & O; weigh twice per week before breakfast in a hospital gown facing away from the scale; constant observation during all meals and snacks, constant observation and restriction of use of the bathroom for at least 1 hour after all meals and snacks; Prozac/fluoxetine 60 mg po daily, K-Dur 20 mEq po daily; multivitamin with iron 1 tablet po daily; individual and group psychotherapy including CBT and IPT and individual and group psychoeducation; daily completion of a food diary; and contact social worker to schedule a family session in 1 week.

2. What is the purpose of the nutrition stabilization contract?

3. Why is the patient weighed only twice per week in a hospital gown and facing away from the scale?

4. What is the purpose of constantly observing the patient during meals and snacks? Why is constant observation and restricting the use of the bathroom necessary for at least 1 hour after all meals and snacks?

5. How will the food diary be used in this patient's treatment?

6. Identify appropriate nursing diagnoses and develop a concept care map for this patient using the form provided in Chapter 1. Refer to the sample included in that chapter.

7. Prioritize the nursing diagnoses you have identified.

8. Choose three priority nursing diagnoses and write nursing care plans using the form provided. Nursing diagnoses should include what the problem is related to and evidence that supports the chosen nursing diagnoses. Support your nursing diagnoses with specific clinical data on the nursing care plans. Planned outcomes should be patient-centered and include specific time frames for evaluation. Nursing interventions should be evidence-based and include rationales.

   a. What collaborative interventions, including treatment, do you anticipate for this patient? Include these in your nursing care plans.

9. How will you evaluate the effectiveness of your nursing care? Add your evaluation to the nursing care plans.

10. What support group information would you provide for this patient and her family?

11. What outpatient treatment do you anticipate as being part of the discharge plan for this patient and her family?

# Substance Abuse/Dependence: Alcohol Dependence and Opiate Abuse

## Objectives

- Recognize signs and symptoms that meet *DSM-IV-TR* criteria for the diagnosis of substance abuse and substance dependence disorders.
- Identify signs and symptoms of withdrawal from alcohol and opiates.
- Identify priority patient-centered outcomes.
- Plan evidence-based nursing interventions to achieve patient-centered outcomes.
- Discuss the benefits of 12-step programs for the individual, families, and communities.

## Key Terms

| | |
|---|---|
| Abstinence | Manipulation |
| Addiction | Recovery |
| Blackouts | Relapse |
| Codependency | Substance abuse |
| Cravings | Substance dependence |
| Delirium tremens | Synergistic effect |
| Denial | Tolerance |
| Detoxification | Wernicke-Korsakoff syndrome |
| Intoxication | Withdrawal |

People have abused psychoactive (mind-altering) substances including alcohol for centuries. Legally prescribed medications (i.e., opiate analgesics, stimulants prescribed for ADHD) have also become "substances" of abuse. The term "polysubstance abuse" refers to abusing more than one substance simultaneously or at different times. Anyone who abuses substances runs the risk of becoming dependent on them. The numbers of causative etiologies are almost as varied as the number of substances abused. The multiple factors involved include genetics or an inherited tendency for an increased risk to abuse or become dependent on substances; exposure to substances via family members or friends; peer pressure; maladaptive coping in response to multiple stressors; unstable family environments during childhood; lack of tolerance to frustration; lack of successes in life; tendency to take risks; low self-esteem; attempts to self-medicate; and sociocultural values. Adolescents who experiment with and abuse substances before age 15 have an increased risk of abusing or becoming dependent on substances as adults and are less likely to seek treatment (NIH, 2006, pp. 1–2). Stereotypes of homeless, weak-willed philanderers do not provide an accurate picture of people who abuse substances. People from all walks of life and socioeconomic backgrounds can be found among this patient population. An increasing number of professionals from many areas of expertise have wrestled with these problems. Unfortunately, healthcare professionals including nurses and physicians are not immune to substance abuse or dependence. Individual states have specific guidelines for treating impaired professionals (Keltner, Schwecke, & Bostrom, 2007, p. 531).

The tremendous negative impact upon the individual who uses or is dependent upon substances is compounded by the additional negative impact on families, communities, and society as a whole. Decreased occupational productivity, unemployment, decreased gross national product revenue, increased healthcare costs, accidents and other injuries; increased violence and domestic abuse, increased crime rates, STDs, teen pregnancies, academic failure, homelessness, and even death can be attributed to substance abuse or dependence. Substance abuse and mental health are critical indicators of health identified by *Healthy People 2010* as important in the development of healthy communities by improving the health of individuals in communities (Alters & Schiff, 2004, p. 164; Pender, Murdaugh, & Parsons, 2006, pp. 6, 116–117).

The American Psychiatric Association (APA) views substance abuse and substance dependence as medically treatable diseases and two distinct disorders. Criteria for a diagnosis of substance abuse includes the use of a substance, including alcohol, over a period of at least 1 year as an unhealthy coping strategy that results in failure to meet responsibilities or obligations; legal problems; recurrent social or interpersonal problems; or recurrent problems at work or school. The person continues to use the substance even during physically hazardous activity such as driving, boating, or operating machinery. There are no signs or symptoms of physical withdrawal, tolerance, or psychological dependence in substance abuse (APA, 2000, pp. 196, 198–199).

Substance dependence (addiction) includes the criteria for substance abuse and additional factors. There is excessive, continued use regardless of health consequences, significant impairment in major areas of life including failure to meet responsibilities or obligations; legal problems; recurrent social or interpersonal problems; or recurrent problems at work or school. The person becomes preoccupied by obtaining substances and a compulsion to use substances regardless of having to forfeit personal time with family or friends, and any attempts to stop using without professional treatment are unsuccessful. The person develops a tolerance to the amount of substance used, which results in a need to increase the amount in order to obtain the same effect. Physical and/or psychological withdrawal signs and symptoms develop when the person abstains from use, which leads to using the substance to avoid experiencing withdrawal (APA, 2000, pp. 196–198).

Treatment programs for substance abuse and dependence may be socially based, medically based, or both. Services are provided in inpatient or outpatient settings. Social programs focus on nonpharmacological or behavioral treatment methods such as individual, group, and family counseling; 12-step approaches; cognitive behavioral therapy (CBT); rational emotive behavior therapy (REBT); exploring reasons for using substances and identifying triggers to use them; education; and relapse prevention strategies including ways to deal with cravings. Medically based programs focus on the use of pharmacological and other necessary treatment methods for withdrawal signs and symptoms, malnutrition, dehydration, serious medical complications including delirium tremens (DTs) and cardiovascular responses, and detoxification. A patient may be discharged from a medically based program to a social program for continued treatment and rehabilitation. If a patient has a dual diagnosis, both the substance abuse/dependence disorder and other mental health disorder are treated. Community support groups led by laypersons including 12-step programs such as Alcoholics Anonymous (AA) or Narcotics Anonymous (NA) are of tremendous benefit for providing support and help in maintaining sobriety or abstinence from any substances. Al-Anon and Alateen are community support groups for families. New medications to help patients maintain abstinence from alcohol and opiates have provided better treatment options and increased success. Decreased funding and fewer available opportunities to remove the patient from an environment that continues to reinforce substance use have decreased the availability of programs and the success of treatment.

# Clinical Case Study

For the past month a 30-year-old male computer program specialist has been attending weekly counseling sessions provided by his company's employee assistance program to help deal with his divorce that occurred 6 months ago. He has shared custody of their two young children. During the last session, he admitted that his drinking has "gotten out of hand." The counselor uses the

CAGE test to assess him further. He answers "yes" to three out of four questions and agrees to seek help in a social treatment-based outpatient program.

During the initial intake assessment at the outpatient program, he admits to drinking heavily on a daily basis over "several years" and to abusing Oxy-Contin that was prescribed for him 2 years ago following knee surgery. The social worker performing the initial intake assessment advises him that the safest treatment option at this time would be an inpatient detoxification program, followed after that with a long-term rehabilitation program either as an inpatient or outpatient. After discussing these options with his employer, he agrees to try going to an inpatient detoxification program. The social worker calls and arranges for someone to meet him at the emergency room (ER) for medical clearance and subsequent voluntary admission to the substance disorders unit. The patient's EKG/ECG and chest X-ray obtained in the ER were both normal. The patient has no known allergies.

# Questions

1. Why is it important during your nursing intake assessment to ask the patient again about the type and amount of alcohol/substances usually used and what he currently is using?

2. What other information would be important to obtain at this time in addition to the type and amount of alcohol/substances used regularly?

During your nursing intake assessment, he states that he is here for "help with my drinking." He admits to drinking a fifth of vodka daily for the past year and taking eight 10 mg tablets of OxyContin/oxycodone daily for the past $1\frac{1}{2}$ years that he buys "off the street." Prior to a year ago, he drank half of a fifth of vodka daily for at least 1 year and increased his drinking as his marriage "was falling apart." He also stated that he smoked marijuana in college but denies any use for the past 5 years. He also denies any current or past use of IV drugs, tobacco products, OTC medication, herbals, steroids, supplements, or treatment for any other psychiatric or medical illnesses. When questioned about unsafe sex practices, he denied this type of activity and declined an offer for HIV testing. He states he last drank 4 hours ago and last took OxyContin/oxycodone approximately 6 hours ago. You notify the admitting psychiatrist of the information you have obtained and this matches what he told the psychiatrist. The psychiatrist documents a Clinical Institute Withdrawal Assessment (CIWA-AR) score of 22.

The patient is admitted with the following diagnoses and orders:

Axis I: Alcohol Dependence, opiate abuse; polysubstance abuse

Axis II: Deferred

Axis III: Chronic pain secondary to right knee injury in MVA $2^1/_2$ years ago; right knee surgical repair 2 years ago

Axis IV: Divorced 6 months ago

Axis V: GAF = 45, past year = 60

Librium/chlordiazepoxide 50 mg po every 6 hours, Librium/chlordiazepoxide 25 mg po every 8 hours prn breakthrough withdrawal symptoms: temperature of 100°F or greater, pulse of 100 or greater, respirations of 24 or greater, blood pressure greater than 140/90, or tremulousness; thiamine 100 mg IM now and follow with 100 mg po every day, folic acid 1 mg po every day, MVI 1 tab po every day, Catepres/clonidine TTS patch 0.3 mg every 3 days, Catepres/clonidine 0.1 mg po prn for SBP greater than or equal to 170 or DBP greater than or equal to 100 and notify physician; Ultram/tramadol 50 mg every 6 hours po prn knee pain alternating doses with ibuprofen, 600 mg po every 6 hours prn knee pain alternate doses with Ultram; 30 cc po every 8 hours prn indigestion, Imodium 4 mg po ¥1 prn diarrhea, then 2 mg po prn diarrhea maximum dose 16 mg in 24 hours; Tylenol 650 mg po every 4 hours prn headache.

Consult pain specialist.

Consult physical therapy for evaluation of right knee.

Vital signs every hour × 4; if stable, then every 2 hours × 4; if stable then every 4 hours × 72 hours.

Safety checks every 15 minutes.

Monitor I & O every shift.

Push fluids

Daily weight

Seizure precautions

Regular diet

Individual and group psychotherapy

Individual and group addictions counseling

Milieu therapy

Laboratory and diagnostic tests ordered at this time include the following: EKG/ECG, chest X-ray, CBC with differential, MCV, MCH, WBC, electrolytes, BUN, creatinine, GFR, ALT/SGPT, AST/SGOT, total cholesterol, HDL/HDL-C, LDL, triglycerides, total cholesterol/HDL ratio, TSH, IgM, anti-HBc, HBsAg, and anti-HCV.

  3. Why did the Psychiatrist order Librium/chlordiazepoxide for this patient?

     a. What medications other than Librium/chlordiazepoxide may also be used for this purpose?

4. What signs and symptoms of alcohol withdrawal will you need to assess this patient for?

    a. When would you expect to see early signs and symptoms of withdrawal?

    b. When would you anticipate the patient could begin to experience DTs?

5. What signs and symptoms of opiate withdrawal will you need to assess this patient for?

    a. Why does the patient have an order for Catepres/clonidine?

6. Why did the psychiatrist order thiamine, folic acid, and MVI?

The results of the patient's laboratory and diagnostic test results are as follows:

EKG/ECR = NSR

Chest X-ray = negative

CBC: RBCs = 4.0, Hgb = 11.0, Hct = 36%, MCV = 100, MCH = 48

Electrolytes: Na+ = 140, K+ = 4.0, Ca+ = 9.0, Mg+ = 2.0, Cl = 99

Glucose = 140

BUN = 12

Creatinine = 0.9

GFR = 125

Total protein = 5.0

Albumin = 2.0

Globulin = 1.8

ALT/SGPT = 200

AST/SGOT = 400

BAL/BAC = 180

UDS = positive for alcohol and opiates

TSH = 2.3

Total cholesterol = 220

Triglycerides = 300

HDL = 25

LDL = 180

Total cholesterol/HDL ratio = 6.4

IgM anti-HBc = negative

HBsAg = negative

Anti-HCV = negative

7. What is the significance of the results of the RBCs, Hgb, Hct, MCV, MCH, ALT/SGPT, AST/SGOT, the IgM, anti-HBc, HBsAg, and Anti-HCV?

8. What topics would you include in a health promotion psychoeducation group for this patient and others with the same diagnoses? Address the results of the patient's total cholesterol, HDL/HDL-C, LDL, triglycerides, total cholesterol/HDL ratio, IgM, anti-HBc, HBsAg, and anti-HCV laboratory tests.

9. Identify appropriate nursing diagnoses for this patient. Develop a psychiatric care diagram for this patient using the form provided in Chapter 1 and refer to the sample included in that section.

   a. Prioritize the nursing diagnoses you have identified.

10. Choose three priority nursing diagnoses and write nursing care plans using the form provided. Nursing diagnoses should include what the problem is related to and evidence that supports the chosen nursing diagnoses. Support your nursing diagnoses with specific clinical data on the nursing care plans. Planned outcomes should be patient-centered and include specific time frames for evaluation. Nursing interventions should be evidence-based and include rationales.

    a. What collaborative interventions, including treatment, do you anticipate for this patient? Include these in your nursing care plans.

11. How will you evaluate the effectiveness of your nursing care? Add your evaluation to the nursing care plans.

12. How will 12-step programs benefit this patient, his family, and his community?

On the 2nd day of admission, the patient states that he wishes to be discharged from the program: "My problem isn't that bad. I think I can take it from here. Besides, my kids are scheduled to stay with me this weekend and they'll be disappointed if they can't. Surely you can understand why I need to leave." You know that as a voluntary patient he is legally able to request to be discharged, but it is not in his best interest medically or psychologically since his detoxification treatment is not completed.

13. What type of behavior is the patient displaying?

14. What would your response be to this patient's request and statements? What are your legal and ethical nursing responsibilities in this type of situation?

# Anxiety and Medical Disorders: Post-Traumatic Stress Disorder and Type II Diabetes Mellitus

## Objectives

- Recognize signs and symptoms that meet *DSM-IV-TR* criteria for the diagnosis of post-traumatic stress disorder (PTSD).
- Assess the effect of a medical disorder on the patient's mental status.
- Identify priority patient-centered outcomes.
- Plan evidence-based nursing interventions.

## Key Terms

| | |
|---|---|
| Anxiety | Emotional numbing |
| Depersonalization | Fear |
| Derealization | Flashbacks |
| Desensitization | Flooding |
| Detachment | Hyperarousal |
| Dissociation | Trauma |

According to the American Psychiatric Association (APA), post-traumatic stress disorder (PTSD) may develop as a response to a personally experienced or witnessed extremely traumatic event. The traumatic event is something that does not occur within the accepted range of human experience; is sudden and unexpected; and involves threatened or actual death. This intense fear of threatened or imminent death causes an intense reaction in the victim or person witnessing the event. A similar type of reaction may also occur in people who learn of an unexpected or violent death of a loved one or the diagnosis of a loved one with a life-threatening illness (APA, 2000, p. 463). Common examples of traumatic events include violent physical, personal/sexual assault; being kidnapped or taken hostage; military combat; terrorist attack; torture; incarceration; natural or manmade disasters; motor vehicle accidents; and being diagnosed with a life-threatening illness. In the future, the criteria for a diagnosis of PTSD may include all persons who think or feel they may die regardless of the event triggering this reaction.

The signs and symptoms of PTSD may include depression, anxiety, dissociation or dissociative amnesia; derealization, nightmares or disturbing dreams; difficulty falling asleep; flashbacks; intrusive recollections of the event; avoidance of anything associated with the traumatic event; emotional numbing or absence of emotional responses; feelings of detachment; hyperarousal; poor concentration; and irritability or outbursts of anger. Patients may also feel that they may not live a normal life span because of the traumatic event. They also experience significant problems functioning in occupational, social, and academic areas. Signs and symptoms that occur within 1 month after the traumatic event are diagnosed as acute stress disorder (ASD). However, if the signs and symptoms occur after 1 month, the person is diagnosed with PTSD (APA, 2000, pp. 468–469). PTSD as well as ASD may cause serious, lifelong consequences. Early detection and treatment can offset these consequences and help the person affected achieve a better quality of life.

Diabetes mellitus (DM) is an endocrine system disorder characterized by abnormal insulin production, problems with insulin utilization, or both (Lewis, Heitkemper, Dirksen, O'Brien, & Bucher, 2007, p. 1253). DM can cause damage to multiple body systems resulting in increased risk of coronary artery disease (CAD), myocardial infarctions (MIs), cerebrovascular accidents (CVAs), renal disease, loss of vision, and amputations. Many patients with psychiatric disorders are also diagnosed with DM. This may be due to genetic predisposition, poor dietary habits, low income limiting food choices, infrequent exercise, and potential atypical antipsychotic medication side effects including increased serum glucose and cholesterol. DM is on the rise even in the general population without psychiatric disorders.

Type I insulin dependent juvenile onset DM is caused by the destruction of pancreatic beta cells that produce insulin, which leads to virtually no insulin production. Type II adult onset DM is the most common type, accounting for up to 90% of all cases. More recently Type II DM is being diagnosed in younger patients related in part to childhood obesity. In Type II DM, some insulin is still being produced by the pancreatic beta cells, but there is an insufficient quantity or it is poorly utilized by the body's tissues (Lewis, Heitkemper, Dirksen, et al., 2007, p. 1254). Type I DM is treated predominantly with subcutaneous insulin injections, diet, and exercise. In addition, insulin pump devices are being used more frequently than in the past. Type II DM is treated predominantly with various types of oral medications, diet, and exercise. During periods of stress (resulting from physical illness or psychological problems), a person with Type II DM may also require temporary subcutaneous insulin injections in addition to oral medication to control serum glucose levels. Patients with Type I DM may develop a life-threatening medical complication known as diabetic ketoacidosis (DKA) and those with Type II DM may develop a similar life-threatening medical complication known as hyperosmolar hyperglycemic syndrome (HHS). Both DKA and HHS result in hyperglycemia, osmotic diuresis, and dehydration.

# Clinical Case Study

A 26-year-old male who lives alone is creating a disturbance in the duplex building where he lives. An Iraq war veteran, he has had increasing difficulty sleeping lately and he has been out in the yard every night for the past week, dressed in camouflage, carrying a gun, and looking for people who may be trying to harm him or others living in the duplex. A male neighbor who works the evening shift came home late one evening to discover him prowling around the yard. The neighbor cautiously approaches him and asks if anything is wrong. He replies that he heard a noise and believes someone dangerous is hiding in the yard. As the neighbor begins to point out that the yard is well lit by floodlights and that there is not anyone there, the young man starts yelling and accusing him of helping the enemy forces. The neighbor again tries to state the facts, but the man pushes him down, runs past him into the duplex, and barricades himself in his half of the building. The neighbor is unsuccessful in trying to talk him into opening the door and resorts to calling the police.

When the police arrive, the man threatens to shoot them. The police and SWAT team evacuate the building and enter his home. They find him lying unconscious, but still breathing, on the floor of his living room. He is transported via ambulance to the local hospital emergency room (ER). All weapons are removed from the home by the police. In the ambulance, IVFs of 1000 cc 0.9% normal saline at 125 cc per hour and oxygen 40% via mask are started. The patient awakens, pulls off the oxygen mask, and attempts to dislodge the IV. When the paramedic tries to explain that he needs the IV and oxygen, he becomes physically combative, starts screaming, and verbally threatens to harm anyone who comes near him. This information is communicated to the local ER, and per the ER physician's orders he is given Ativan/lorazepam 2 mg and Haldol/haloperidol 5 mg IVP, and he is physically restrained.

The patient is calmer by the time the ambulance reaches the ER. He is irritable, but cooperates with having laboratory and diagnostic tests including an EKG/ECG and CT of the head. He has no known allergies. The following laboratory and diagnostic tests are abnormal:

Glucose = 420

HgA1C = 8.5

1. What treatment will the patient be given for the abnormal laboratory and diagnostic tests?

The patient is admitted to a telemetry unit for 2 days with the following diagnoses: hyperosmolar hyperglycemic syndrome (HHS), and uncontrolled Type II DM. The serum acetone level is 0. He receives a visit from a friend and fellow Iraq war veteran. This friend had tried to reach him when he did not come to their weekly support group meeting 2 weeks in a row. The friend also called the patient's neighbor when he could not reach him and was informed that the patient had been taken to the hospital. Additional information available from both the patient and his friend includes the patient's history of PTSD and Type II DM, which were diagnosed approximately a year ago. The patient has been offered treatment by his area Veterans Affairs Medical Center, but declined medication for treatment of PTSD. He sporadically attends psychotherapy sessions. He states that he regularly checks his blood sugar and takes Starlix/nateglinide 80 mg po tid before meals, but forgets to do this when experiencing flashbacks. He reports having increased flashbacks and nightmares for the past 2 weeks after watching CNN coverage on television of the current situation in Iraq. He estimates that the last time he checked his blood sugar and took Starlix was approximately 2 weeks ago. He does not remember being out in the yard or barricading himself in his home. He reluctantly agrees to see the psychiatrist who was consulted.

2. What patient signs and symptoms meet criteria for a diagnosis of PTSD?

The patient has been ordered IVFs of 1000 cc 0.9% normal saline, regular insulin on a sliding scale starting at 151, CBGs every 1 hour for 4 hours; then change CBGs to ac and hs. The patient's telemetry reading has been NSR for 24 hours and the repeat EKG/ECG is also normal. The patient's laboratory tests are repeated with the following results:

K+ = 3.8

Glucose = 250

UA – Glucose = 80

The physician gives orders to change the IVFs to 1000 cc D5W at the same rate of 125 cc per hour and continues the orders for the insulin sliding scale, CBGs ac and hs. After the psychiatric consult has been completed, the psychiatrist recommends a short inpatient psychiatric admission to begin medication and continued psychotherapy if the patient is agreeable. The patient, realizing that his behavior would be grounds for an involuntary psychiatric hospital admission, agrees to be transferred to the medical-psychiatric inpatient unit on a voluntary admission. He also signs consents for psychiatric and medical records to be obtained from his area Veterans Affairs Medical Center.

3. Is it legal and safe to allow this patient to be admitted or transferred voluntarily to the medical-psychiatric unit?

   a. What would happen if the patient attempted to elope from the hospital?

The patient is transferred to the medical-psychiatric unit of the hospital with the following diagnoses:

Axis I: PTSD

Axis II: None

Axis III: Uncontrolled Type II DM, HHS resolving

Axis IV: Military combat during Iraq war, chronic medical illness

Axis V: GAF = 30; past year = unknown

His admission orders included the following:

Klonopin/clonazepam 0.5 mg po tid, Starlix/nateglinide 80 mg po tid before meals, Geodon/ziprasidone 20 mg po bid with food, Geodon/ziprasidone 10 mg IM prn agitation × 1. If not effective, call psychiatrist for further orders. Ativan/lorazepam 2 mg po q 6 hours prn anxiety, maximum dose 4 mg in 24 hours; Ativan/lorazepam 2 mg IVP q 6 hours prn anxiety, maximum dose 4 mg in 24 hours; Ativan/lorazepam 2 mg IM q 6 hours prn anxiety, maximum dose 4 mg in 24 hours.

IVFs: 1000 cc D5W at 125 cc per hour, vital signs every 4 hours, I & O every shift, weigh one time per week, 2000 calorie ADA diet, CBGs ac & hs. Regular insulin sliding scale with coverage starting at 151. If CBG greater than or equal to 400, obtain stat serum glucose and acetone and call medical physician with results; if less than or equal to 60, administer dextrose 50 mg IVP and call medical physician.

Safety checks every 15 minutes; individual and group psychotherapy; individual and group psychoeducation; milieu therapy, OT, AT. With patient consent, begin systematic desensitization psychotherapy and CBT.

Medical consult to evaluate and manage uncontrolled Type II DM.

4. Identify appropriate nursing diagnoses for this patient. Develop a psychiatric care diagram using the form provided in Chapter 1 and refer to the sample included in that section.

   a. Prioritize the nursing diagnoses you have identified.

5. Choose three priority nursing diagnoses and write nursing care plans using the form provided. Nursing diagnoses should include what the problem is related to and evidence that supports the chosen nursing diagnoses. Support your nursing diagnoses with specific clinical data on the nursing care plans. Planned outcomes should be patient-centered

and include specific time frames for evaluation. Nursing interventions should be evidence-based and include rationales.

   a. What collaborative interventions, including treatment, do you anticipate for this client? Include these in your nursing care plans.

6. How will you evaluate the effectiveness of your nursing care? Add your evaluation to the nursing care plans.

7. What teaching will you plan for this patient and his family? Include the neighbor who lives next door if the patient agrees.

8. Make a list of appropriate discharge referrals for this patient.

# CHAPTER 8

# Sexual and Gender Identity Disorders: Gender Identity Disorder

## Objectives

- Recognize signs and symptoms that meet *DSM-IV-TR* criteria for the diagnosis of gender identity disorder (GID).
- Identify priority patient-centered outcomes.
- Plan evidence-based nursing interventions.

## Key Terms

| | |
|---|---|
| Gender identity | Sexual orientation |
| Gender role | Transgender |
| Genetic identity | Transsexual |

The internal sense or perception of who a person is as a male or female forms the basis of gender identity. Sexual orientation describes the gender to whom a person is physically or erotically attracted. According to the American Psychiatric Association (APA), a diagnosis of gender identity disorder (GID) is made when there is a strong, continuous identification with the opposite gender, and a stated desire to be the opposite sex. Such individuals have typical reactions and feelings of the opposite sex; desire to live and be treated as the opposite sex; frequently attempt to pass for the opposite sex; are consistently uncomfortable with their own physical sex; believe they have been born the wrong sex; and are preoccupied with removing primary and secondary sex characteristics. In addition, the gender disturbances cause significant distress or problems performing in social, work, or other important roles in their lives (APA, 2000, p. 581).

# Clinical Case Study

A 22-year-old male wearing gender-neutral clothing is referred to a community mental health clinic by his family physician after requesting a sex change operation. The medical physician reports that there are no physical problems, including endocrine abnormalities, in the client's past or current medical history. He has no known allergies. After the initial assessment, the client* is diagnosed with the following:

Axis I: Gender identity disorder

Axis II: Deferred

Axis III: None

Axis IV: Problems with primary family support group; problems with social and occupational environments; difficulty sustaining employment

Axis V: GAF = 50, past year = unknown

During the behavioral and nursing intake assessment, the client tells the nurse that he has always felt uncomfortable being around men. He feels the most comfortable in the company of women and enjoys engaging in what would typically be described as "women's work." At age 12 he began secretly dressing in his younger sister's clothing. His father discovered him at age 16 wearing a dress belonging to his younger sister and kicked him out of the house. He has not seen his family since. He states that he then went to stay "with a friend." Over the past few years he has become increasingly convinced that he should have been "born a woman" and "God must have goofed up with me." At the end of the interview he admits to having difficulty with satisfying sexual experiences because of his gender problems.

1. What signs and symptoms of gender identity disorder can you identify?

2. Identify appropriate nursing diagnoses for this patient. Develop a psychiatric care diagram using the form provided in Chapter 1 and refer to the sample included in that section.

   a. Prioritize the nursing diagnoses you have identified.

3. Choose three priority nursing diagnoses and write nursing care plans using the form provided. Nursing diagnoses should include what the problem is related to and evidence that supports the chosen nursing

---

*When working with individuals in the outpatient setting, the individual is referred to as a "client" rather than a "patient."

diagnoses. Support your nursing diagnoses with specific clinical data on the nursing care plans. Planned outcomes should be patient-centered and include specific time frames for evaluation. Nursing interventions should be evidence-based and include rationales.

    a. What collaborative interventions, including treatment, do you anticipate for this patient? Include these in your nursing care plans.

4. How will you evaluate the effectiveness of your nursing care? Add your evaluation to the nursing care plans.

# Cognitive and Medical Disorders: Alzheimer's Dementia, Coronary Artery Disease, and Atrial Fibrillation

## Objectives

- Recognize signs and symptoms that meet *DSM-IV-TR* criteria for the diagnosis of Alzheimer's dementia.
- Identify priority patient-centered outcomes.
- Plan evidence-based nursing interventions.
- Assess the effect of medical problems on the patient's mental disorder.

## Key Terms

| | |
|---|---|
| Agnosia | Coronary artery disease (CAD) |
| Amnesia | Cognition |
| Aphasia | Delirium |
| Apraxia | Dementia |
| Atrial fibrillation | Sundowning |

Dementias are chronic, progressive, cognitive disorders occurring in people at least 60 years of age and associated with changes in brain structure and functioning. The cost in terms of human suffering, economic loss, and health-care resources are staggering for both patients and their families. There are numerous etiologies for dementias including genetic, neurogenerative, vascular, metabolic, toxic, and infectious causes. Prevention efforts have focused on early detection, regular physical exercise, keeping mentally active as one ages, and the use of NSAIDS, statins, B vitamins, and estrogen if not contraindicated (Keltner, Schwecke, & Bostrom, 2007). Because patients with major depression experience memory and concentration problems similar to early dementia, major depression should be ruled out because the treatment differs from the treatment for dementia, which will depend on the type and etiology.

There are many types of dementias, the most common of which include Alzheimer's and vascular (formerly multi-infarct) types. Alzheimer's type dementia involves a gradually decline in cognitive abilities and many times is a diagnosis of exclusion after other causalities have been ruled out. Alzheimer's dementia is a neurodegenerative disease thought to be caused by one of the following processes: a decrease in acetylcholine, increased oxidative stress resulting in increased free radicals, the formation of beta-amyloid plaques and neurofibrillary tangles secondary to abnormal DNA or the loss of connections between neurons (Lewis, Heitkemper, Dirksen, O'Brien, & Bucher, 2007, p. 1565). According to the American Psychiatric Association (APA), the early onset subtype occurs at 65 years of age or younger and the late onset subtype occurs after 65 years of age (APA, 2000, p. 155).

The signs and symptoms of Alzheimer's dementia include multiple cognitive deficits such as impairment in memory, concentration, and orientation that appear gradually and progress slowly. Changes in mood and personality may be seen in even early stages of the disease process. Agnosia, apraxia, aphasia, and amnesia also occur. The person has increased difficulty remembering words or following a plot in a story or television program and begins to withdraw from former activities that were pleasurable. Some patients experience visual or auditory hallucinations and paranoid delusions. Many patients exhibit sundowning, wandering, incontinence of bladder and bowel, and self-care deficits in all major areas. There are also disturbances in the area of executive functioning including problems with organizing, planning, sequencing, and abstracting (APA, 2000, p. 157). Patients experience significant problems in occupational or social functioning representing a change from their previous level of functioning. The signs and symptoms of Alzheimer's dementia are not due to other CNS disorders, systems conditions, vitamin deficiencies, alcohol or other substance abuse, and delirium or other Axis I disorders (i.e., schizophrenia, major depressive disorders). Additional subtypes occur with or without behavioral disturbance. Behavioral disturbances include behaviors such as wandering or agitation (APA, 2000, p. 157).

Atrial fibrillation is a very common dysrhythmia that may occur intermittently or chronically. It usually occurs in patients who have underlying cardiac disease. It may also occur secondary to electrolyte disturbances, alcohol intoxication, caffeine use, or stress. Atrial fibrillation often results in decreased cardiac output, and there is a danger of thrombi formation in the atria due to blood stasis (Lewis, Heitkemper, Dirksen, O'Brien, & Bucher, 2007, p. 852).

Decreased cardiac output results in less blood supply and oxygen available for the brain and other vital organs, which will also have an impact on a patient's cognitive function.

# Clinical Case Study

A 64-year-old divorced resident of a personal care home who was diagnosed with Alzheimer's dementia a year ago has been wandering away from the facility causing increased concern for his personal safety. He has also demonstrated a gradual decline in ADLs and sundowning behavior over the past 4 months. There have been several new residents admitted due to recent expansion of the facility. The patient's additional medical-surgical history includes CAD and chronic atrial fibrillation diagnosed approximately 3 years ago. He has no known allergies. There is a psychiatric family history of Alzheimer's dementia. After speaking with the resident and his family, both the medical physician and psychiatrist agree to an inpatient admission to evaluate for further progression of Alzheimer's dementia and change in placement needs. The patient's daughter has control of the resident's finances, but no one in the family has been specifically designated to make decisions involving medical care. The patient is admitted to an acute geriatric psychiatric unit with the following diagnoses and orders:

Axis I: Alzheimer's dementia, early onset, with behavioral disturbance

Axis II: None

Axis III: CAD, chronic atrial fibrillation

Axis IV: Change in personal care home environment related to several new residents and expansion of the facility

Axis V: GAF = 40, past year = 65

Continue Exelon/rivastigmine 6 mg po bid with meals, Lopresser/metoprolol 50 mg po bid, Lipitor/atorvastatin 60 mg po daily, and Coumadin/warfarin 5 mg po every day at 5 p.m.; hold dose and notify physician if INR greater than 3.

Start Namenda/memantine 5 mg po × 7 days; Vistaril/hydroxyzine 25 mg po every 6 hours prn anxiety or agitation; Vistaril/hydroxyzine 25 mg IM every 6 hours prn.

Laboratory and diagnostic tests ordered at this time include the following: EKG/ECG, chest X-ray, CBC with differential, WBC, electrolytes, BUN, creatinine, GFR, ALT/SGPT, AST/SGOT, total cholesterol, HDL/HDL-C, LDL, and triglycerides. Daily PT and INR. Call physician if results are abnormal. Safety checks every 15 minutes; vital signs every 4 hours; I & O every shift; weigh 2 × week; individual and group psychotherapy; individual and group psychoeducation; milieu therapy, OT, and AT.

During the admission assessment, the nurse notes the presence of agnosia, apraxia, amnesia, and some aphasia. The patient is able to remember only one object out of three after 5 minutes. The patient is alert but oriented to self and place only. There is memory impairment and problems with concentration. He frequently gets up out of his chair and slowly wanders around the room in which the admission intake interview is being conducted. Admission vitals signs: temperature = 99.0°F, pulse = 92, respirations = 20, and blood pressure = 130/80.

# Questions

1. What signs and symptoms of Alzheimer's dementia can you identify in this patient?

The results of the patient's laboratory and diagnostic tests are available and are normal except for the following:

EKG/ECG = atrial fibrillation, no change from previous EKG/ECG

PT = 60 (normal range 11–13; control range 11–22)

INR = 3.8 (normal range 2–3)

2. What action should the nurse take regarding the PT and INR results? Support your answers.

3. Identify appropriate nursing diagnoses for this patient. Develop a psychiatric care diagram using the form provided in Chapter 1 and refer to the sample included in that section.

   a. Prioritize the nursing diagnoses you have identified.

4. Choose three priority nursing diagnoses and write nursing care plans using the form provided. Nursing diagnoses should include what the problem is related to and evidence that supports the chosen nursing diagnoses. Support your nursing diagnoses with specific clinical data on the nursing care plans. Planned outcomes should be patient-centered and include specific time frames for evaluation. Nursing interventions should be evidence-based and include rationales.

   a. What collaborative interventions, including treatment, do you anticipate for this patient? Include these in your nursing care plans.

5. How will you evaluate the effectiveness of your nursing care? Add your evaluation to the nursing care plans.

6. What supportive resources can the nurse provide for the family of this patient?

CHAPTER 10

# Psychiatric Emergencies

## *Domestic Violence and Sexual Assault*

## Objectives

- Recognize signs and symptoms of domestic violence and abuse.

- Become familiar with the cycle of abuse and victimization.

- Apply knowledge of concepts of emergency treatment for victims of sexual assault.

- Plan evidence-based nursing interventions to achieve patient-centered outcomes.

## Key Terms

| | |
|---|---|
| Abuse | Incest |
| Assault | Perpetrator |
| Battering | Rape |
| Domestic violence | Recovery |
| Empowerment | Victim |

There are many causative theories that explain why violence has been increasing in our society. Taking on many forms, violence and abuse occur across all socioeconomic levels, genders, and age spans and can be categorized according to physical, sexual, emotional, psychological, and economic issues. All forms of violence, abuse, and sexual assault or rape involve core issues of a perpetrator exerting control and power over a victim. Even though mandatory reporting laws exist for healthcare professionals, it is still difficult to obtain accurate statistics on the number of abuse, domestic violence, and sexual assault or rape cases. Many victims are too ashamed, afraid, and traumatized to seek treatment or report what has happened to them. Of those who do seek treatment, many choose not to press legal charges due to fear of reprisal or the belief that what happened to them is a private matter (Townsend, 2008, p. 565). Many victims also erroneously believe that they are somehow at fault for what happened to them (O'Brien, Kennedy, & Ballard, 2008, pp. 118–119; Keltner, Schwecke, & Bostrom, 2007, p. 612). Unfortunately, many myths related to violence, abuse, and rape still abound, wrongfully placing the blame on the victim. Typically victims are socially isolated, have limited freedom, and have limited access to financial resources making it difficult to leave the perpetrator (Townsend, 2008, p. 565). Situations become even more difficult when there are children involved. Many healthcare professionals become frustrated when victims of violence and abuse return repeatedly for treatment. It is difficult to understand why they continue to tolerate the same situation rather than leave.

The cycle of violence includes four typical stages: (1) an escalation or tension-building stage, (2) a triggering event, (3) an acute or battering stage, and (4) a honeymoon or de-escalating stage (Townsend, 2008, p. 566; O'Brien, Kennedy, & Ballard, 2008, pp. 189–190; Varcarolis, Carson, & Shoemaker, 2006, p. 511). It is during the honeymoon phase when the perpetrator promises to change and says that the behavior will never happen again. The perpetrator then does something nice for the victim, which gives the victim the hope that the perpetrator will carry through on promises made. This behavior helps keep the victim in the relationship. There are many other reasons victims stay in destructive relationships, including finances, children, religion, fear of retaliation, and lack of supportive networks outside of the relationship. Victims temporarily leave a situation and return many times before leaving a final time. Nurses and other healthcare professionals need to be empathetic and supportive of these individuals rather than give in to frustration and blame or judge them.

## Clinical Case Study

A married 28-year-old mother of two young children is brought to a local hospital emergency room (ER) by her husband for treatment of fractured right arm. She has completed 2 years of college, but currently does not work so that she can care for her children. Her husband's employment requires that he travel for weeks at a time. During the initial part of the physical examination, she reports that her neighbor raped her 2 days ago before her husband came home from his last business trip. She also reports that this afternoon she tripped over some of the children's toys in the living room and that is how she broke her arm. As the nurse assists the physician, she notes several bruises in various stages of healing on the woman's extremities. It is documented in her record that the patient was treated in the ER 1 year ago for a fractured nose and facial contusions. At that time the patient stated she had fallen while chasing the neighbor's dog out of her flowerbeds. She also reported being clumsy. X-rays of the patient's right arm show a spiral fracture of the humerus. The patient guards her arm and winces with any movement. There is also evidence of vaginal trauma upon examination. She has no known allergies.

During the assessment, the husband insists on staying with the patient. The patient's affect is anxious, displays poor eye contact, and flinches when the husband stands close to her. When the physician asks the husband to step out of the examination area for the rest of the exam, he starts to become argumentative, but then complies with the request. The patient is visibly more relaxed after the husband leaves the area. The patient reports a history of major depression, but denies suicidal thoughts, plans, or any previous attempts.

# Questions

1. What potential signs and symptoms of domestic violence and abuse can you identify in this situation?

2. A sexual assault nurse examiner (SANE) is consulted for this patient and a sexual assault advocate is requested. What are the roles of the SANE and sexual assault advocate in this situation?

3. What legal and ethical responsibilities does the nurse in the ER have working with this patient?

4. Identify appropriate nursing diagnoses for this patient. Develop a psychiatric care diagram using the form provided in Chapter 1 and refer to the sample included in that section.

   a. Prioritize the nursing diagnoses you have identified.

5. Choose three priority nursing diagnoses and write nursing care plans using the form provided. Nursing diagnoses should include what the problem is related to and evidence that supports the chosen nursing diagnoses. Support your nursing diagnoses with specific clinical data on the nursing care plans. Planned outcomes should be patient-centered and include specific time frames for evaluation. Nursing interventions should be evidence-based and include rationales.

   a. What collaborative interventions, including treatment, do you anticipate for this patient? Include these in your nursing care plans.

6. How will you evaluate the effectiveness of your nursing care? Add your evaluation to the nursing care plans.

# Overdose: Mood Stabilizers, Benzodiazepine, and Muscle Relaxants

## Objectives

- Recognize signs and symptoms of overdoses.
- Apply knowledge of concepts of both mood and anxiety disorders.*
- Apply knowledge of concepts of emergency treatment for overdoses.
- Plan evidence-based nursing interventions to achieve patient-centered outcomes.

## Key Terms

| | |
|---|---|
| Bipolar disorder | Overdose |
| Generalized anxiety disorder | Toxicity |

An overdose of medications or any substances is not only a psychiatric emergency but also a medical emergency. Many overdoses are fatal, but early discovery and treatment can greatly reduce the fatality rate as well as any residual effects following the survival of an overdose. Unfortunately, many psychiatric patients overdose on the very medications that have been prescribed to treat their conditions and help them function as normally as possible. Precautions can be taken for patients at risk, such as prescribing smaller amounts of medications at one time and, when possible, prescribing medications with a safer side-effect profile. However, some patients save up medications to use in a future suicide attempt or during very stressful periods. Patients diagnosed with bipolar disorders are very impulsive during a manic phase and, therefore, are at greater risk for impulsively taking an overdose of medications, drugs, alcohol, or any other substances.

While many people at some time in their lives have experienced anxiety, generalized anxiety disorder (GAD) includes symptoms occurring over at least

---

*The student may need to review information in Chapters 2 and 7 regarding mood disorders.

a 6-month period that are excessive and significantly interfere with the person's ability to function socially, occupationally, or academically. Symptoms include restlessness, muscle tension, fatigue, difficulty concentrating, irritability, and sleep disturbance. The symptoms are not due to another Axis I disorder, medical condition, or substance abuse. The individuals affected are aware that their reaction to situations is irrational and excessive, but they are unable to control their responses. GAD may also be accompanied by panic attacks. This disorder may be secondary to a general medical condition such as hyperthyroidism and may occur as early as childhood (APA, 2000, pp. 472, 476).

Emergency care is both general and specific to the medication or substance ingested. The reasons for the overdose must be identified and preventive measures implemented to help prevent future occurrences and risk of death.

# Clinical Case Study

Kate, a 26-year-old female, returns home after work to find Nina, her 24-year-old female roommate, who has a history of bipolar I disorder and generalized anxiety disorder, displaying manic behavior, which began at least 2 days ago but has now been increasing. An argument erupts between the roommates over Nina's behavior. During the argument, Nina alternates between yelling and crying. She runs into the bathroom and locks the door. Noticing that the medicine cabinet door is slightly open, she opens it wider and quickly pulls out several bottles of medication. She impulsively ingests her own medications and those of her roommate. These include Nina's prescribed Depakote/valproic acid, Eskalith/lithium/lithium carbonate, Ativan/lorazepam, Klonopin/clonazepam, and her roommate's Soma/carisoprodol. Concerned when Nina does not return, Kate unlocks the bathroom door with a spare key and discovers that Nina has overdosed. She calls 911 and also Nina's psychiatrist. Nina is taken to the local hospital emergency room (ER) for immediate treatment. She has no known allergies.

# Questions

1. What general and specific treatment for benzodiazepine (Ativan/lorazepam and Klonopin/clonazepam) overdose do you anticipate this patient will receive in the ER?

2. What specific treatment for Eskalith/lithium/lithium carbonate and Depakote/valproic acid overdose would be ordered for you to administer?

There is no available ICU bed at this time due to multiple trauma, cardiac, and other surgical patients needing ICU level care. The patient remains conscious and is kept in the ER on a telemetry monitor and 1:1 observation/constant observation (COs) until an ICU bed is available or she is medically cleared to be transferred to a psychiatric unit. She has been involuntarily committed to a hospital setting. The psychiatrist has written an order to transfer the patient to the psychiatric unit when she is medically stable. Even though the patient will be transferred to an ICU bed when available, she will need a comprehensive, holistic nursing care plan formulated and initiated within the first 8 hours of admission.

3. Identify appropriate nursing diagnoses for this patient. Develop a psychiatric care diagram using the form provided in Chapter 1 and refer to the sample included in that section.

    a. Prioritize the nursing diagnoses you have identified.

4. Choose three priority nursing diagnoses and write nursing care plans using the form provided. Nursing diagnoses should include what the problem is related to and evidence that supports the chosen nursing diagnoses. Support your nursing diagnoses with specific clinical data on the nursing care plans. Planned outcomes should be patient-centered and include specific time frames for evaluation. Nursing interventions should be evidence-based and include rationales.

    a. What collaborative interventions, including treatment, do you anticipate for this patient? Include these in your nursing care plans.

5. How will you evaluate the effectiveness of your nursing care? Add your evaluation to the nursing care plans.

# *Adverse Medication Effects:*
# *Serotonin Syndrome*

## Objectives

- Recognize signs and symptoms of serotonin syndrome.
- Apply knowledge of concepts of mood disorders.
- Apply knowledge of concepts of emergency treatment of serotonin syndrome.
- Plan evidence-based nursing interventions to achieve patient-centered outcomes.

## Key Terms

| | |
|---|---|
| Mood disorders | Selective serotonin-norepinephrine reuptake inhibiters (SNRIs) |
| Serotonin syndrome | Selective serotonin reuptake inhibitors (SSRIs) |

Serotonin syndrome is a potentially serious adverse reaction caused by the synergistic action of two or more medications or substances resulting in increased levels of serotonin or increased action of the amount of serotonin already available. This syndrome is usually associated with selective serotonin reuptake inhibiters (SSRIs) or serotonin-norepinephrine reuptake inhibitors (SNRIs). SSRIs are used (in addition to a mood stabilizer, but not alone) in the treatment of major depression, the depressed phase of bipolar disorder, anxiety disorders, eating disorders, and some types of chronic pain secondary to neuropathy or myalgia. SNRIs are also used (in addition to a mood stabilizer, but not alone) in the treatment of major depression, the depressed phase of bipolar disorder, and some types of chronic pain secondary to neuropathy. Many patients use over the counter (OTC) herbal products or supplements that also increase the levels of serotonin or increase the action of the amount of serotonin already available.

The most common OTC herbal supplement used to elevate mood is Saint-John's-wort. Tryptophan is a common OTC supplement used to promote sleep. Combining SSRIs with Saint-John's-wort or tryptophan may cause serotonin syndrome. This syndrome may also occur when combining SSRIs or SNRIs with other medications including monoamine oxidase inhibitors (MAOIs), Eskalith/lithium/lithium carbonate, Buspar/buspirone, Ritalin/methylphenidate, Elavil/amitriptyline, Aventyl/Pamelor/nortriptyline, Tofranil/imipramine, Anafranil/clomipramine, Sinequan/doxepin, Desyrel/trazodone, Demerol/mepheridine, and Dextromethorphan (McKenry, Tessier, & Hogan, 2006, p. 406).

Due to the potentially serious outcomes, resulting from serotonin syndrome, it is important that nurses recognize the symptoms as early as possible so that treatment may begin immediately. These will include the following: restlessness, agitation, altered mental status including confusion or hypomania, hyperreflexia, tremor, seizures, muscle rigidity, fever as high as 107°F, fluctuating blood pressure, tachycardia, increased respirations, shivering or shaking chills, ataxia, headache, coma, nausea, and abdominal cramping or diarrhea (Townsend, 2008, p. 193; Keltner, Schwecke, & Bostrom, 2007, p. 239; Stuart & Laraia, 2005, p. 592; Fontaine & Fletcher, 2003, p. 193). Serotonin syndrome may occur as early as 2 to 72 hours after starting to take more than one medication or supplement than affects serotonin or several weeks later (McKenry, Tessier, & Hogan, 2006, p. 406).

# Clinical Case Study

A 24-year-old female is brought to the emergency room with a fever of 103°F, shaking chills, difficulty walking, and muscle rigidity. The patient has been prescribed Zoloft/sertraline 100 mg po daily and 50 mg po at bedtime for at least 3 months. She has no known allergies.

1. List examples of medications classified as follows:

    a. Selective serotonin reuptake inhibitors

    b. Serotonin-norepinephrine reuptake inhibitors

    c. Monoamine oxidase inhibitors

During the nursing assessment, the patient admits to also taking Saint-John's-wort on a daily basis for the past 2 weeks.

2. What signs and symptoms of serotonin syndrome can you identify at this time?

    a. What other signs and symptoms of serotonin syndrome would you assess this patient for?

3. What is the standard treatment for serotonin syndrome?

The patient is admitted to a medical-psychiatric unit with the following diagnoses:

Axis I: Major depression, recurrent, moderate

Axis II: None

Axis III: Serotonin syndrome

Axis IV: Job stress

Axis V: GAF = 60, past year = 70

The patient's primary care physician (PCP) is notified of her admission and a consult is requested for her admission history and physical. Upon examination, she is noted to have an unsteady gait and a moderate amount of muscle rigidity. Her admission orders include the following: discontinue Zoloft/ sertraline. Obtain a UA, UDS, and B-HCG. Notify physician if B-HCG is positive. Vital signs every 1 hour for 4 hours, then every 2 hours for 4 hours, then every 4 hours for 72 hours. Monitor every 15 minutes. Start IV 0.9% normal saline at 125 cc per hour, Inderol/propranolol 10 mg qid, hold if SBP less than 100 and DBP less than 60; and Cogentin/benztropine 1 mg IVP every 8 hours, maximum dose 4 mg in 24 hours. Tylenol/acetaminophen 650 mg po prn every 4 hours for temperature of 100°F or greater, maximum dose 4000 mg in 24 hours. Ativan/lorazepam 1 mg IVP prn every 4 hours for seizure activity, maximum dose of 6 mg in 24 hours. Cooling blanket for temperature greater than 104°F.

If symptoms increase or patient experiences difficulty breathing, notify physician and start Dantrium/dantrolene sodium 1 mg/kg IVP for severe muscle rigidity or hyperthermia—oral temperature greater than 104°F; may repeat dose up to a maximum of 10 mg in 24 hours; administer 2 liters of oxygen via nasal cannula and transfer to ICU.

4. Identify appropriate nursing diagnoses and develop a concept care map for this patient using the form provided in Chapter 1. Refer to the sample included in that chapter.

5. Prioritize the nursing diagnoses you have identified.

6. Choose three priority nursing diagnoses and write nursing care plans using the form provided. Nursing diagnoses should include what the problem is related to and evidence that supports the chosen nursing diagnoses. Support your nursing diagnoses with specific clinical data on the nursing care plans. Planned outcomes should be patient-centered and include specific time frames for evaluation. Nursing interventions should be evidence-based and include rationales.

   a. What collaborative interventions, including treatment, do you anticipate for this patient? Include these in your nursing care plans.

7. How will you evaluate the effectiveness of your nursing care? Add your evaluation to the nursing care plans.

# Adverse Medication Effects: Neuroleptic Malignant Syndrome

## Objectives

- Recognize signs and symptoms of neuroleptic malignant syndrome (NMS).
- Apply knowledge of concepts of schizophrenia.
- Apply knowledge of concepts of emergency treatment of neuroleptic malignant syndrome (NMS).
- Plan evidence-based nursing interventions to achieve patient-centered outcomes.

## Key Terms

| | |
|---|---|
| Antipsychotics | Neuroleptic malignant syndrome |
| Atypical antipsychotics | Traditional |
| Neuroleptics | Undifferentiated schizophrenia |

Neuroleptic malignant syndrome (NMS) is a potentially fatal adverse reaction to neuroleptic (antipsychotic) medication. It is usually associated with traditional (conventional) antipsychotic medication. NMS can also occur, although less frequently, with atypical or second generation atypical (SGA) antipsychotics. Patients receiving atypical antipsychotic medications have developed NMS, but the condition has gone undetected in early stages because it is expected to occur more often in patients receiving traditional (conventional) antipsychotics. Antipsychotics medications are used to treat schizophrenia and other psychotic disorders. The Food and Drug Administration (FDA) recently approved the use of atypical antipsychotics or SGAs for the treatment of mood disorders. Many times patients who are psychotic are either unable to report symptoms or do so in ways that are difficult for nurses to understand.

Due to the potentially fatal outcome, it is critical that nurses recognize NMS as early as possible so that treatment may begin immediately. Signs and symptoms of NMS include the following: muscular rigidity; difficulty breathing; increased or labile blood pressure, pulse, and respirations; fever as high as 108°F, elevated CPK, WBC, and liver function tests; diaphoresis; dysphagia; salivation; hyperreflexia; tremors; rhabomyolsis; altered levels of consciousness, confusion, and muteness (O'Brien, Kennedy, & Ballard, 2008; Keltner, Schwecke, & Bostrom, 2007; Fontaine, 2009).

## Clinical Case Study

A 40-year-old male with a history of chronic undifferentiated schizophrenia is brought to the emergency room (ER) by the police after finding him running around in a field and wearing very little clothing. He physically resisted getting into the police car before being brought to the ER. He has not been taking his medication. He tells the triage nurse he is from another planet and there is a force field around him. As the CNA tries to put him in a hospital gown, he pushes her to the floor and strikes her in the face. The patient is ordered and given an IM medication cocktail of Haldol/haloperidol 5 mg, Ativan/lorazepam 2 mg, and Benadryl/diphenhydramine 50 mg. Before being admitted to the psychiatric unit as an involuntary admission, he is given an oral dose of Haldol/haloperidol 5 mg. The patient has no known allergies. His admission orders include Haldol/haloperidol 5 mg po tid.

## Questions

1. What would be examples of traditional (conventional) antipsychotics (neuroleptics)?
2. What would be examples of atypical antipsychotics (SGAs)?
3. What medication did the patient receive that can cause NMS?

On the 3rd day of admission the patient complains of muscle spasms, difficulty breathing, and difficulty remembering where his room is. The nurse assigned to the patient obtains his vital signs: oral temperature = 105°F, pulse = 100, respirations = 24 and irregular, pulse oximetry of 89%, and blood pressure = 160/96. The patient has significant muscle rigidity, +3 deep tendon reflexes, and diaphoresis. The nurse notifies the psychiatrist and receives orders for stat laboratory tests. The patient's CPK = 1000, ALT/SGPT = 100, AST/SGOT = 80, = 120, Creatinine = 0.8, BUN = 20, WBCs = 15.

4. What signs and symptoms of NMS can you identify in this patient?

5. What standard treatment for NMS would you anticipate being ordered?

6. Identify appropriate nursing diagnoses and develop a concept care map for this patient using the form provided in Chapter 1. Refer to the sample included in that chapter.

7. Prioritize the nursing diagnoses you have identified.

8. Choose three priority nursing diagnoses and write nursing care plans using the form provided. Nursing diagnoses should include what the problem is related to and evidence that supports the chosen nursing diagnoses. Support your nursing diagnoses with specific clinical data on the nursing care plans. Planned outcomes should be patient-centered and include specific time frames for evaluation. Nursing interventions should be evidence-based and include rationales.

   a. What collaborative interventions, including treatment, do you anticipate for this patient? Include these in your nursing care plans.

9. How will you evaluate the effectiveness of your nursing care? Add your evaluation to the nursing care plans.

# Adverse Medication Effects: Hypertensive Crisis

## Objectives

- Recognize signs and symptoms of hypertensive crisis.
- Apply knowledge of concepts of emergency treatment of hypertensive crisis related to medication and dietary interactions.
- Plan evidence-based nursing interventions to achieve patient-centered outcomes.

## Key Terms

| | |
|---|---|
| Hypertensive crisis | MAOIs |
| Major depression | Tyramine |

Hypertensive crisis can be a serious, life-threatening adverse reaction caused by the synergistic action of certain antidepressant medications used to treat resistant major depression, monoamine oxidase inhibitors (MAOIs), and dietary substances containing the amino acid tyramine. Many medications interact with MAOIs, therefore, a 14-day period is recommended between stopping the MAOI and introducing another psychotropic medication. Patients are also advised to notify all healthcare professionals they are receiving treatment due to many interactions between MAOIs and medications commonly used in the medical-surgical setting.

Due to the increased risk for CVA, MI, or death due to circulatory collapse or intercranial bleeding, it is important that nurses recognize hypertensive crisis as early as possible so that treatment may begin immediately. Signs and symptoms of hypertensive crisis include the following: stiff or sore neck, occipital headache described by some as throbbing, sudden increase in blood pressure, tachycardia or bradycardia, chest pain, nosebleed, photophobia, dilated pupils, nausea, diaphoresis, and vomiting. Additionally, patients may also have an elevated temperature and cold, clammy skin. Symptoms usually occur suddenly (Keltner, Schwecke, & Bostram, 2007, p. 249; Bezchlibnyk-Butler & Jeffries, 2005, p. 51; Fontaine & Fletcher, 2003, p. 193).

# Clinical Case Study

A 28-year-old male is brought to the emergency room (ER) of a local general hospital after dining with friends. The patient started complaining of a stiff neck and severe, throbbing occipital headache that began suddenly at the end of the meal. His vital signs at this time are as follows: temperature = 99.2°F, pulse = 108, respirations = 22, blood pressure = 190/104. The friend accompanying the patient states that the patient has been taking medication for at least 1 year for depression and believes there may be a medication bottle in the pocket of his jacket. You discover a bottle with the following directions on the label: Nardil 15 mg po tid. He has no known allergies.

# Questions

1. What signs and symptoms of hypertensive crisis can you identify at this time?
   a. What information on dietary restrictions should be included when planning teaching for patients prescribed MAOIs?
2. What is the standard treatment for hypertensive crisis?

After receiving emergency treatment in the ER, the patient is admitted to a 23 hour observation bed with the following diagnoses:

Axis I: Major depression, moderate, recurrent

Axis II: None

Axis III: Hypertensive crisis

Axis IV: Financial problems

Axis V: GAF = 65, past year = 70

3. Identify appropriate nursing diagnoses and develop a concept care map for this patient using the form provided in Chapter 1. Refer to the sample included in that chapter.
4. Prioritize the nursing diagnoses you have identified.
5. Choose three priority nursing diagnoses and write nursing care plans using the form provided. Nursing diagnoses should include what the problem is related to and evidence that supports the chosen nursing diagnoses. Support your nursing diagnoses with specific clinical data on the nursing care plans. Planned outcomes should be patient-centered

and include specific time frames for evaluation. Nursing interventions should be evidence-based and include rationales.

    a.  What collaborative interventions, including treatment, do you anticipate for this patient? Include these in your nursing care plans.

6.  How will you evaluate the effectiveness of your nursing care? Add your evaluation to the nursing care plans.

# PART II

# Answer Keys, Including Care Plans

# CHAPTER 2

# Mood Disorders, Medical Disorders, and Substance Abuse

## *Major Depression and Suicide*

### ANSWER KEY

## Question 1

Suicidal ideation, tearfulness/crying, difficulty sleeping, psychomotor retardation, social isolation, delayed verbal responses, difficulty concentrating, memory disturbance, poor academic performance, fatigue/decreased energy, disinterest in former hobbies, decreased appetite with a weight loss of 10 pounds, disheveled appearance, major psychological loss due to the breakup of a long-standing relationship with his girlfriend approximately 1 month ago.

## Question 2

Suicidal ideation, being a male versus being a female (males more often succeed at committing suicide), age (suicide is the 3rd leading case of death among those 15 to 24 years of age), significant psychological loss of girlfriend, tearfulness/crying, social isolation, poor academic performance, and the other signs and symptoms of major depression listed in the answer to question 1.

Additional risk factors and signs to assess include whether the patient had a plan, the lethality of the plan, access to the means to carry out the plan, whether the plan involved physical harm to others (if so "duty to warn" laws and ethics will apply), prior suicide attempts or gestures (gestures are nonlethal attempts), ability to at least verbally contract not to harm self; feelings of hopelessness, helplessness, or powerlessness; anxiety; anhedonia; substance abuse/dependence; impulse control problems, including a history of or current self-mutilation behavior; psychomotor agitation; writing a suicide note; multiple losses of any type (actual and perceived); presence of other psychiatric/mental health or physical problems; acute or chronic pain, the anniversary date of a major loss; limited or absent social support, or not immediately available (i.e., if attending college or lives a far distance away from family and friends); ability to accept offered emotional support and enter into a therapeutic alliance; insight into need for treatment; poor coping skills or usual coping strategies no longer effective; psychosocial difficulties including problems in major areas of life, including academic performance, occupation, relationships; primary support groups, legal, financial, housing; making a will when mood is depressed; degree of adherence to treatment regimen if there is a history of previous mental health treatment; and family history of mental health problems, suicide, or substance abuse/dependence.

# Question 3

Statements such as "Everybody would be better off without me," "I like to go to sleep and just not wake up," "It won't be long now," or "I won't have to worry about things much longer." Giving away personal or prized possessions, engaging in hazardous behavior (i.e., drinking and driving, reckless driving habits), and obsessed with ideas, conversation, music, movies, art, books, or poetry about death, dying, or suffering.

# Question 4

Seeking help, good insight, and judgment regarding need for treatment, cooperative, intelligent, supportive parents, financial resources including healthcare insurance coverage, and support for treatment from college counselor and chemistry professor. The patient's strengths are used to help increase the response to treatment and help him gain more individual control over his own situation. Having adequate health insurance provides payment for treatment and increases the probability that the patient will receive treatment needed. The more strengths the patient has, the greater chance of a successful outcome.

# Questions 5 and 6

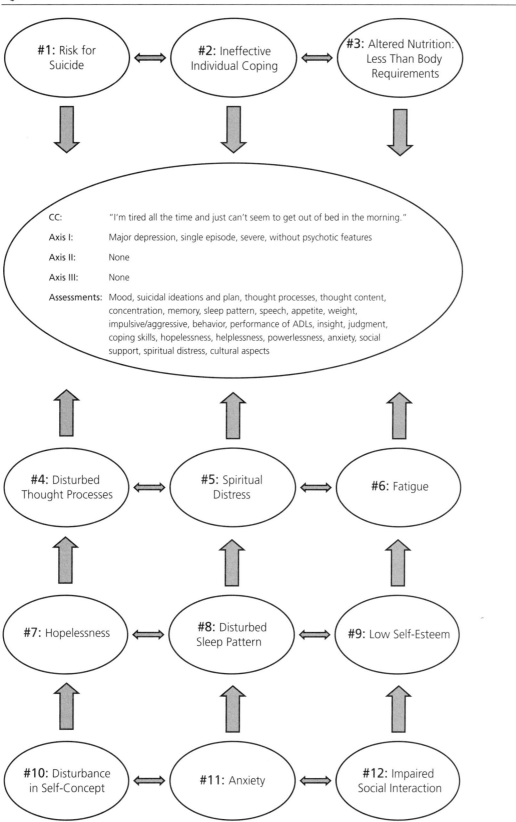

# Question 7 and 8

**Nursing Care Plan:** Major depression, single episode, severe, without psychotic features.
**Nursing Diagnosis:** Risk for Suicide r/t severe psychological loss AEB breakup of 2-year relationship with girlfriend approximately 1 month ago.
**Outcomes** (include time frames): 1. Will remain free from self-harm during the intake assessment process and throughout hospitalization. 2. Will verbally contract with staff not to harm self every shift and prn throughout hospitalization.

| Assessment Data: O = Objective, S = Subjective | Evidence-Based Interventions: | Rationales: | Patient Responses:* |
|---|---|---|---|
| Suicidal ideations without plan (S) Loss of long-term relationship (S) Tearful affect (O) Poor eye contact (O) Psychomotor retardation (O) Delayed verbal responses (O) Decreased appetite (S) 10-pound weight loss (O) Reports insomnia while lying in bed for 12 hours without sleeping (S) Fatigue (S) Decreased energy (S) Poor academic performance (O) Decreased concentration (S) Memory problems (S) Disheveled appearance (O) Decreased interest in hobbies (S) Social withdrawal (O) | 1(a) Begin to develop a rapport and a therapeutic nurse/patient alliance that is the beginning of the therapeutic nurse/patient relationship. | 1(a) Developing a rapport with the patient will assist in gaining the patient's trust and cooperation in the future. According to Peplau, the therapeutic nurse/patient relationship is the foundation that must be established to initiate future work in the healing process (Keltner, Schweke, & Bostrom, 2007; O'Brien, Kennedy, & Ballard, 2008). | 1(a) Actively seeks and accepts help. Expresses appreciation of any assistance available. |
| | (b) Continue to perform a suicide risk assessment and obtain a verbal no harm to self contract during the initial intake assessment process, every shift, and prn throughout hospitalization. | (b) There is still high risk for committing suicide due to his suicidal thoughts and the severity of his depression. A verbal behavior contract actively engages the patient as an active participant in his treatment and encourages personal responsibility for his behavior. It also demonstrates staff involvement. The patient's condition may change, making it necessary to obtain another contract earlier than the next scheduled shift. | (b) Verbally contracts to refrain from harming self and to tell staff if thoughts increase or thinks he may act upon thoughts. |
| | (c) Maintain an environment free from potentially harmful objects. (d) Initiate and maintain safety rounds or checks every 15 minutes. | (c) This decreases opportunities for the patient to harm himself. (d) This measure ensures the patient's location is known by staff, which | (c) Has not engaged in any harmful behavior to self. (d) Accepts safety checks and verbalizes understanding of reason they are ordered. |

*Patient responses are examples of what students would look for to decide whether their planned interventions were successful, needed more time, or needed to be changed. Responses will vary depending on the patient.

| Assessment Data: O = Objective, S = Subjective | Evidence-Based Interventions: | Rationales: | Patient Responses: |
|---|---|---|---|
| | (e) Maintain a calm, soothing environmental atmosphere. | helps maintain his safety. (e) The patient is experiencing difficulty concentrating. A noisy, distracting environment would be nontherapeutic and interfere with his treatment. A calm, soothing environment also decreases the potential for the patient becoming agitated. | States he feels safe on the unit. (e) Remains calm and states it is easier for him to think here on the unit versus being on campus. |
| | (f) Offer emotional support and therapeutic use of self. | (f) According to Peplau, this is very important not only to the start of the healing process but also to continuing this process (Keltner, Schwecke, & Bostrom, 2008). | (f) Accepts emotional support offered and the nurse's presence. |
| | (g) Use therapeutic communication techniques to facilitate patient verbal expression of feelings and establish realistic goals. | (g) This promotes a healthy expression of feelings versus unhealthy ways of hurting himself. It is also therapeutic for the patient to be an active participant in his treatment and work toward gaining or maintaining independence by establishing attainable goals. | (g) At first admitted to difficulty expressing his feelings but states it is becoming easier each time he meets with the nurse. Stated that his goals would include learning more about major depression and returning to college classes as soon as possible. |
| | (h) Administer scheduled Lexapro and prn medication if ordered. Reinforce need to take medication consistently no matter how he feels. | (h) Medication is used to treat existing neurochemical imbalances in the brain. It is most effective when combined with psychotherapy and psychoeducation. Lexapro is an SSRI antidepressant that is usually well tolerated due to a low side-effect profile. The SSRI antidepressants are physically safer than other antidepressant drug classes (i.e., tricyclics, SNRIs, or MAOIs) if the patient would try to overdose after discharge. Most patients do not like to take | (h) Adheres to treatment regimen. No prn medication ordered at this time. Verbalizes understanding of reason for being prescribed Prozac and intention to continue medication as ordered after discharge. |

*(continues)*

| Assessment Data: O = Objective, S = Subjective | Evidence-Based Interventions: | Rationales: | Patient Responses: |
|---|---|---|---|
| | | medication because of the side effects or because they do not believe they are ill and need medication. Failure to take medication or stopping medication on their own is a major cause of relapse and readmission. | |
| | (i) Perform a mental status exam every shift. | (i) The mental status exam includes areas such as thought processes, thought content including suicidal/homicidal ideations, speech, psychomotor activity, appearance, cognition, judgment, and insight. It can provide valuable information to determine whether the patient is improving. | (i) Admits to suicidal thoughts without a plan, decreased concentration, and memory problems. No evidence of delusional thinking or hallucinations noted. Psychomotor retardation and delayed verbal responses noted. |
| | (j) Administer the Hamilton Depression Scale to determine the severity of the patient's depressed mood upon admission and again prior to discharge from hospital. | (j) This is a reliable, research-based assessment tool used to assess the severity of a patient's depression. If the depression is primarily due to an imbalance in neurotransmitters, it will take a significant amount of time to notice an improvement; initial therapeutic effect of Prozac may be as long as 4–6 weeks for a full therapeutic effect. | (j) Hamilton Depression Scale score = 15. |
| | (k) Ask patient to rate his depression on a scale of 0–10 where 0 = none and 10 = extremely depressed. | (k) Using a scale helps quantify the patient's subjective feelings and provides a way to measure how depressed he feels. | (k) Rates his depression as a "5." |
| | (l) Plan psychoeducation groups on topics of diagnosis, medication, coping skills, problem solving, relapse prevention, and signs and symptoms of relapse. | (l) Psychoeducation is a very important part of both inpatient and outpatient treatment. Nurses provide psychoeducation in one-on-one and group settings as well as for families. | (l) Expresses interest in learning more about major depression and how he can help himself. Relieved to learn that major depression can be managed just like many other types of illnesses. |

| Assessment Data: O = Objective, S = Subjective | Evidence-Based Interventions: | Rationales: | Patient Responses: |
|---|---|---|---|
| | 2(a) Obtain a verbal no harm to self contract during the initial intake assessment process, every shift, and prn throughout hospitalization.<br>(b) Continue therapeutic use of self to strengthen therapeutic nurse/patient alliance. | 2(a) Refer to rationale for 1(b).<br><br>(b) This promotes and strengthens trust between the patient and nurse and also helps promote the healing process. | 2(a) Verbally contracts to refrain from harming self and to tell staff if thoughts increase or thinks he may act upon thoughts.<br><br>(b) Accepts nurse's presence and states he feels more comfortable now on the unit. |

**Evaluation:** 1. Remains free from self-harm although suicidal ideations are still present and Hamilton Depression Scale score indicates some degree of depression. Adheres to treatment regimen including medication.
2. Able to contract verbally to refrain from harming self and to contact staff if unable to do so. Continue care plan and evaluate plan every shift and prn if condition changes.

**Nursing Care Plan:** Major depression, single episode, severe, without psychotic features.
**Nursing Diagnosis:** Ineffective Individual Coping r/t situational crisis perceived as overwhelming AEB suicidal ideations without a plan, poor academic performance, social withdrawal, decreased interest in hobbies, insomnia, and disheveled appearance following loss of long-term relationship approximately 1 month ago.
**Outcomes** (include time frames): 1. Will try at least two positive coping strategies while hospitalized.
2. Will identify at least two positive coping strategies to continue using after discharge.

| Assessment Data: O = Objective, S = Subjective | Evidence-Based Interventions: | Rationales: | Patient Responses: |
|---|---|---|---|
| Suicidal ideations without plan (S) Poor academic performance (O) Social withdrawal (O) Disheveled appearance (O) Tearful (O) Poor eye contact (O) Decreased interest in hobbies (S) Insomnia (S) Lays in bed for 12 hours not sleeping (S) Fatigue (S) Decreased concentration (S) Decreased appetite (S) 10-pound weight loss (O) | 1(a) Accept temporary emotional dependency needs and provide emotional support. | 1(a) Normal reactions to loss, stress, anxiety, or crisis include temporary increased emotional dependency on others and psychological, even behavioral, regression to an earlier developmental stage. Accepting this and explaining this to patients will help increase their understanding of what is happening and that they are still valuable individuals worthy of help. | 1(a) States "I don't know what's wrong with me. I usually can handle things. I don't understand what's happening." |
| | (b) Assess quality and availability of support systems. | (b) The prognosis for this patient will be substantially better if he has a strong, available support system. | (b) States he knows his parents care about him and want to help him. They live 50 miles away from his college campus. |
| | (c) Assess coping skills, and spiritual practices used prior to breakup with girlfriend. | (c) Many people have adequate coping skills that are sometimes overwhelmed by the degree of situational stress. They can regain control of their response to situational losses or crises with proper support. | (c) States he used to get together with friends or play tennis, but this time he just couldn't bring himself to do this. Verbalized that he does not understand why he could not do these things this time. |
| | (d) Using simple terms, explain that sometimes there are situational and maturational crises that overwhelm a person's usual strategies and ability to cope. Also explain that if he has developed a biochemical imbalance in neurotransmitters he will be more easily overwhelmed. | (d) These explanations are based on psychosocial developmental, neurobiological, and stress theories of why people experience difficulty coping and may go on to develop psychiatric/mental health disorders. Use of simple terms helps the patient more easily understand and process information when anxious or stressed. | (d) Verbalized that this information gave him "some relief" and increased his understanding of what was happening to him. |

| Assessment Data:<br>O = Objective,<br>S = Subjective | Evidence-Based<br>Interventions: | Rationales: | Patient<br>Responses: |
|---|---|---|---|
| | (e) Assess level of anxiety and stress every shift and prn. | (e) The patient's ability to cope is also affected by his anxiety or stress level. As the patient's level of anxiety increases, the degree of impulsivity and potential for psychological/ emotional crisis also increases, which in turn increases the possibility of harming himself. If his mental state changes, he will have to be evaluated more frequently than just every shift. | (e) Suicidal ideations and sleep disturbance indicate a Stage +3 level of anxiety. |
| | (f) Teach relaxation techniques such as deep breathing, simple guided imagery, and simple meditation. Explore effect of music and aromatherapy. Give verbal praise and emotional support for any effort to try new skills. When patient has tried these methods, add progressive relaxation type exercises (i.e., tightening and then relaxing various muscle groups). Suggest daily journaling of feelings and thoughts. | (f) Relaxation techniques are health-coping strategies and help relieve anxiety and stress. These methods have been proven to be effective and are easy methods to learn and use on a daily basis. Verbal praise and emotional support will reinforce new behaviors. | (f) Today practiced deep breathing and medication with nurse. Enjoys quiet music and finds it relaxing. Accepted printed information on aromatherapy. Made a goal to attempt simple guided imagery tomorrow. Accepts verbal praise and emotional support given. |
| | (g) Assess problem-solving ability and work with patient regarding improvement in this area. | (g) The ability to problem-solve increases the quality of decisions made and obtains better results for the individual in all areas of life. This will also help him gain more control over his life. | (g) Agrees that his ability to problem-solve has been compromised lately by his emotional state. |

*(continues)*

| Assessment Data: O = Objective, S = Subjective | Evidence-Based Interventions: | Rationales: | Patient Responses: |
|---|---|---|---|
| | 2(a) Teach patient importance of using relaxation and problem-solving techniques on a daily basis to increase success rate. | 2(a) The patient may not realize that these are valuable coping skills and strategies to use throughout life rather than only when experiencing problems. Over time the body and mind will be able to respond more quickly and provide a higher quality of relaxation that would not be achieved if only practiced inconsistently. | 2(a) Verbalizes understanding of need to continue with skills learned on a regular basis. |
| | (b) Encourage to return to previous hobbies and try new ones. | (b) Hobbies can provide healthy distraction and opportunities for social interaction and support. | (b) Agrees to try to play tennis when discharged and to learn to golf. |

**Evaluation:** 1. Has attempted using deep breathing, music, and simple meditation. Accepts information. Has a goal to try simple guided imagery while hospitalized.
2. Agrees to try to use deep breathing, music, and simple meditation as well as to resume playing tennis and to learn to play golf. Continue care plan and evaluate plan in 48 hours.

**Nursing Care Plan:** Major depression, single episode, severe, without psychotic features.
**Nursing Diagnosis:** Altered Nutrition: Less Than Body Requirements r/t decreased appetite s/t depressed mood AEB weight loss of 10 pounds.
**Outcomes** (include time frames): 1. Will eat at least 75% of all meals and snacks by the 3rd day of admission. 2. Will gain 1–2 pounds within 1 week of hospitalization.

| Assessment Data: O = Objective, S = Subjective | Evidence-Based Interventions: | Rationales: | Patient Responses: |
|---|---|---|---|
| 10-pound weight loss (O) Decreased appetite (S) Fatigue (S) | 1(a) Assess eating pattern for at least the past 3 days by having patient record what foods and the amounts he has eaten. | 1(a) This will help the nurse indentify patterns in food choices, food groups, and amount of each ingested. | 1(a) Needed some assistance from his roommate due to difficulty with memory. |
| | (b) Record food preferences and attempt to provide these or healthy versions of these. | (b) Providing food preferences increases chances the patient will eat and reinforces that the nurse cares about the patient. | (b) Expressed appreciation. |
| | (c) Teach importance of daily intake of essential nutrients to provide physical energy, regulate blood glucose levels; provide materials for cell growth and repair, and production of neurotransmitters needed for mental health. | (c) Providing information can improve understanding and increase chance of adherence to treatment. | (c) Stated he did not realize that not eating would affect his mental health. |
| | (d) Provide information on a balanced, low fat, low sodium diet and appropriate calorie intake while assisting with healthy menu choices. Introduce the food pyramid as a guide. | (d) Basic nutrition information is included in the scope of nursing. The patient does not show a need for a dietician referral at this time. If laboratory tests indicate deficits or if he fails to gain weight when eating an appropriate amount, a dietician referral should be requested. The food pyramid is an easy to use guide to healthy eating practices. | (d) Accepted information and verbalized understanding. Ate 75% of all meals and snacks during 2nd day of hospitalization. |
| | (e) Weigh daily before breakfast in a hospital gown and slippers on same scale. | (e) These methods help achieve more accurate results. | (e) Maintaining admission weight at this time. |

**Evaluation:** 1. Eating 75% of all meals and snacks by 2nd day of admission.
2. Maintaining admission weight. Continue care plan and evaluate in 48 hours.

# Question 9

a. Lexapro/escitalopram is an antidepressant, specifically a selective serotonin reuptake inhibitor (SSRI) that has less serious side effects than other types of antidepressants.

b. Medication must be taken exactly as prescribed to ensure maximum effectiveness and therapeutic blood level. It may take up to 4 or 5 weeks to experience a maximum therapeutic effect. The patient should not stop any medication without psychiatrist or psychiatric nurse practitioner's knowledge to help avoid a discontinuation syndrome. Many side effects can be treated if patients report them rather than just stopping the medication on their own.

c. Common side effects include nausea, vomiting, weight loss or gain, sexual side effects, restlessness, insomnia or drowsiness, vivid dreams or nightmares, fine tremor, dizziness, headache, paresthesias, feelings of electric shock sensations, myoclonus during sleep, bradycardia, or rash. *Caution:* Some patients, especially those under 18 years of age, have reported increased aggression, suicidal ideation or thoughts of harming others leading to mandatory "black box" warnings. These symptoms should be reported immediately. Precautions taken include informing patients and their families as well as more frequent assessment by the psychiatrist after discharge from the hospital (i.e., every week for the first 4 weeks).

d. The patient should avoid alcohol, illegal drugs, herbal preparations, OTC medications, or misuse of prescription medications. These will interfere with how well a medication works or may cause dangerous interactions. Combining Lexapro and Saint-John's-wort, a common herbal remedy for depression, may result in a potentially life-threatening reaction known as serotonin syndrome. This may also occur if a person uses illegal substances such as cocaine or ecstasy and if concurrently taking other types of antidepressants (such as tricyclics and MAOIs).

e. Signs and symptoms of serotonin syndrome include restlessness, excitement, agitation, mental confusion, delirium, fever, elevated blood pressure, muscle twitching, hyperreflexia, chills, nausea, and diarrhea. Some patients' symptoms may be prolonged or even fatal. Prevention, early recognition, and intervention are important.

f. If interested in trying complementary alternative treatment such as Saint-John's-wort he should discuss this with his psychiatrist before doing so on his own. Saint-John's-wort has been used as a monotherapy to treat mild depression, but can become dangerous if combined with traditionally prescribed antidepressants.

# Question 10

Most patients, and their families, benefit from some form of psychotherapy. Although medications help bring neurotransmitters back into balance, which in turn helps alleviate symptoms of mental illnesses, combining psychotherapy with medication has produced even greater success. Difficulty with coping, problem-solving, decision-making, anger management, difficult situations or people still remain and take much more time than is available during a brief hospitalization period. Medications help patients think more clearly, which increases their ability to learn new information and ways of dealing with life in general. Psychotherapy also provides much needed emotional support and a place to practice new ways of dealing with situations and people. During psychotherapy, the psychotherapist or counselor (i.e., psychologist, social worker, or APRN) accepts patients as they are without preconceived notions and uses a nonjudgmental attitude as part of the healing process. In addition, cognitive behavioral therapy (CBT), interpersonal psychotherapy (IPT), and supportive therapy are short-term psychotherapies that occur for a specified number of weeks and help patients learn ways of helping themselves after the psychotherapy sessions have been completed.

There are many types of psychotherapy depending on the theory used as the basis for development of a specific type. The methods used vary according to the specific type of psychotherapy (see the appendix to this book). Two specific types of psychotherapy have been offered to this patient: CBT and IPT.

The psychotherapist using CBT will encourage the patient to look at his own beliefs or perceptions that may be having an impact on his mood state. Beliefs and perceptions affect emotions and behavior or actions. However, such beliefs and perceptions may not be accurate or realistic and may sometimes lead a person to engage in unhealthy behaviors or miss opportunities in life. For example, a patient may believe that everyone must love him and if he is rejected his life will be a disaster. He may now perceive that his future is ruined and that there is no reason to go on living. Realistic examination of such a belief in light of factual information would show that this is not true. However, a person who clings to this belief would have certain emotions triggered, such as emotional devastation, worthlessness, anger, anxiety, powerlessness, helplessness, hopelessness, apathy, depression, and even suicidal thought. These emotions would in turn influence behavior or actions, such as failure to take care of basic needs or activities of daily living (ADLs), social withdrawal, problems in other relationships, decreased productivity at work or poor academic performance, refusal of help from others, decreased attempts to change the situation or reach out for help, or thinking of a ways to harm himself. The psychotherapist would explore other situations in the patient's life, pointing to examples when someone did not like or approve of the patient, yet he was able to go on with his life. The therapist would also teach the patient coping strategies and problem-solving skills in order to deal with unrealistic beliefs.

The psychotherapist would use interpersonal psychotherapy (IPT) to explore significant interpersonal relationships the patient is having difficulty with and their impact on the patient's symptoms. Potentially dysfunctional past relationships are explored to determine how the patient's current significant relationships are affected. Past relationships are not explored to the degree, intensity, or depth that they are in traditional psychoanalytic therapy because IPT and CBT are short-term psychotherapies. More emphasis is placed on current interpersonal relationships and the context they provide for the onset of the patient's mood disorder. For this patient, significant interpersonal relationships would include his parents, siblings, best friends, and former love relationships including the one he lost approximately 1 month ago. Social functioning including roles in the past and present would be explored. If a disagreement existed or exists between the patient and a significant person in his life, ways to deal with this situation are explored, including how to handle the situation, improving communication, or modifying expectations of how satisfactorily the situation will be resolved. The patient may need to learn new skills regarding communication, negotiating, and preserving self-esteem. He will experience relief of symptoms as a result of improved interpersonal relationships.

# Question 11

Anyone who is depressed is at risk for contemplating and committing suicide. Women attempt suicide more often than men, but more men are successful at committing suicide due to using more lethal methods. Unfortunately, even patients who have been hospitalized on a psychiatric unit where contraband is restricted have attempted to harm themselves, and even died, with whatever means have been available including putting small articles of clothing or latex gloves in their mouths causing suffocation, tying together shoe laces or bed sheets to hang themselves, and using common objects such as pencils or pens to stab themselves. Some patients do not trust healthcare professionals enough to confide in them regarding suicidal ideations or plans. It is imperative that nurses establish a therapeutic alliance with patients and be keen observers of patients' behavior that may be clues to this type of thinking. Patients with strong religious convictions, who at most times in their lives have been able to derive comfort and strength from their spirituality, in moments of severe emotional pain have impulsively harmed and even killed themselves just to stop the emotional pain. Therefore, patients who respond to questions about suicidal ideations and plans with statements that their religion would not allow them to think those thoughts or do such a thing still need to be closely monitored. As part of the verbal contract to not harm themselves, patients should also be asked if they would tell someone if they were to start having such thoughts.

These facts are sometimes difficult for students as well as experienced psychiatric/mental health nurses to deal with emotionally, making it necessary to draw on the support of fellow professionals and staff.

The patient has stated that he does not think he can refrain from acting upon feelings or impulses to harm himself. If even with the nurse's help he is unable to identify reasons for this and still cannot verbally contract to not harm himself, he will need to be placed on 1:1 observation, also referred to as constant observation (CO). This means that a staff member must be with the patient at all times within an arm's length away from the patient to maintain his safety, which is also explained to him. The staff member is also available to provide emotional support. This intervention is in the patient's best interest (i.e., beneficence) and is less restricting than placing him in a behavioral control room or giving him IM medication.

**Nursing Diagnosis:** Risk for Suicide r/t severe psychological loss AEB breakup of 2-year relationship with girlfriend approximately 1 month ago. Continue outcomes #1 and #2 from initial care plan.

| Assessment Data:<br>O = Objective,<br>S = Subjective | Evidence-Based<br>Interventions: | Rationales: | Patient<br>Responses: |
|---|---|---|---|
| (Refer to previous information.)<br>Date: _____<br>Agitated during visit with male friend (O)<br>Remained agitated and upset after male friend left (O)<br>Able to respond to nurse's offer to talk (O)<br>Unable to verbally contract to refrain from feelings or impulses to harm himself (S) | Date: _____<br>1(a) Assess if patient has a specific plan of how to hurt himself. | 1(a) The patient is unable to verbally contract to refrain from harming himself. He may be thinking of a specific plan and knowing this will help you provide for his safety. | 1(a) Denies specific plan to harm himself. Admits only to strong feelings and uncertainty about his ability to refrain from acting upon them. |
| | (b) Assist patient to verbalize feelings and what specifically triggered these feelings. | (b) Verbalizing feelings and identifying the actions leading up to these may help decrease their intensity and help identify more specific ways to deal with them. This in turn could help the patient gain more control over his feelings and decrease the possibility of acting upon them. | (b) States he feels hurt, angry, betrayed, and ashamed. Wonders why he did not realize what was happening between his previous girlfriend and another man. Blames himself for her behavior. |
| | (c) Place patient on 1:1 or COs; provide simple, concrete reasons for this action and criteria for discontinuing this level of safety precaution. | (c) This action provides even greater safety for the patient. Keeping explanations simple and concrete increases the patient's ability to understand the actions being taken on his behalf. The nurse has a legal and ethical responsibility to tell a patient why interventions are being implemented and the criteria for discontinuation (i.e., ability to refrain from harming self, ability to verbally contract not to harm self). | (c) Verbalizes understanding of reason for 1:1 or COs. Also states he feels safer with staff member continually present. |
| | (d) Continue to assess level of agitation and anxiety. | (d) Higher or increasing levels of agitation and anxiety increase the risk of the patient harming himself. | (d) Restless, increased muscle tension, suicidal ideations, and perceived inability to refrain from harming self indicate a +3 level of anxiety. No evidence of dissociation or psychosis noted. |

| Assessment Data:<br>O = Objective,<br>S = Subjective | Evidence-Based<br>Interventions: | Rationales: | Patient<br>Responses: |
|---|---|---|---|
| | (e) Offer prn medication if available and patient not responding to emotional support, therapeutic communication, or a calmer environment. | (e) Judicious use of prn medication can be useful in helping the patient regain control. It is used if other nonpharmacological methods are not effective or in conjunction with other methods for a synergistic effect. An antianxiety agent would be beneficial for this patient. Other patients experiencing psychotic thought disturbances or extremely agitated to the point of actually hurting themselves or others benefit from antipsychotic prn medications. | (e) The patient did not have prn medication orders when admitted, but is now ordered Ativan/lorazepam 1 mg po every 6 hours prn anxiety or agitation. Responding to quieter environment and therapeutic communication at this time. Aware he may have medication if needed, but declines offer at this time. |
| | (f) Assess patient's ability to verbally contract to refrain from acting upon feelings or impulses to harm himself. | (f) As the patient becomes calmer and less distraught he will be more able to verbally contract to refrain from acting upon feelings or impulses to harm himself. | (f) Remains unable to verbally contract to refrain from acting upon feelings or impulses to harm himself. |

**Evaluation:** 1. Calmer and remains free from self-harm.
2. Unable to verbally contract to refrain from strong feelings or impulses to harm himself. Prepare to place patient temporarily on 1:1 or COs until evaluated by psychiatrist. Continue care plan and evaluate every shift and prn.

**Nursing Diagnosis:** Ineffective Individual Coping r/t situational crisis perceived as overwhelming AEB suicidal ideations without a plan, poor academic performance, social withdrawal, decreased interest in hobbies, insomnia, and disheveled appearance following loss of long-term relationship approximately 1 month ago. Continue outcome #1 from initial care plan.

| Assessment Data:<br>O = Objective,<br>S = Subjective | Evidence-Based Interventions: | Rationales: | Patient Responses: |
|---|---|---|---|
| (Refer to previous information.)<br>Date: _____<br>Agitated during visit with male friend (O)<br>Remained agitated and upset after male friend left (O)<br>Girlfriend of 2 years had been seeing another man during part of the time they were together (S)<br>Recent girlfriend is now dating the man she was previously seeing while involved with patient (S)<br>Able to respond to nurse's offer to talk (O) | Date: _____<br>1(a) Take patient to a quieter area and attempt to engage in relaxation techniques he was practicing previously.<br><br>(b) Remind patient of earlier statements of feeling better after practicing newly learned techniques.<br><br>(c) Attempt to distract patient by engaging in conversation, watching TV, or playing cards with a small group of other patients.<br><br>(d) When patient is calmer, explore the validity of the information he received from his male friend. | 1(a) A calmer environment is less stimulating and can help the patient think more clearly. He is more likely to overreact to too many stimuli at this time that would increase his agitation, anxiety, and suicidal impulses.<br>(b) Helps the patient remember earlier successes and increases possibility of believing he can be successful again using these techniques.<br>(c) Offers other ways of coping and temporarily focusing on something else other than his own thoughts. Also provides social support from other patients.<br>(d) This helps the patient evaluate whether or not the information is accurate and if his thought processes are clear. Assists the patient with problem-solving skills. | 1(a) Responding to calmer environment. Less muscle tension noted and affect calmer.<br><br><br>(b) Admits he remembers feeling better and agrees to try deep breathing with soft music in the background.<br><br>(c) Talks with two other patients about the results of the football game last night on TV.<br><br>(d) Admits there is a slight chance the information is not true, but states he trusts his male friend. |

| Assessment Data:<br>O = Objective,<br>S = Subjective | Evidence-Based<br>Interventions: | Rationales: | Patient<br>Responses: |
|---|---|---|---|
| | (e) Help patient identify what he can and cannot control about the situation and reinforce what he can control. | (e) Much time and energy may be spent worrying about behaviors or situations we cannot control. This decreases how much time and energy is available for productive action and problem-solving. A person may remain emotionally and psychologically "stuck," focusing on what is unable to be controlled. This can add to their frustration, fatigue, powerlessness, and depressed mood. Focusing on what can be controlled—for example, choices you can make or how you respond to the situation or another person's behavior—gives an increased sense of control and a clearer view of reality. This increases a person's ability to more effectively make decisions, problem-solve, and feel more empowered to deal with the situation. | (e) States he does focus more on the negative aspects of the situation, which leads him to feel powerless and depressed. Agreed to work with the nurse to develop a list of what he can control in his life at this time. |

**Evaluation:** 1. Responding to calmer environment, therapeutic communication, presence of nurse, and social support of other patients. Using new coping techniques and starting to look at what he can control in his situation versus what he cannot control. Continue interventions from initial care plan and additional interventions. Evaluate every shift and prn. Continue this plan and evaluate in 48 hours.

# References

American Psychiatric Association. (2000). *Diagnostic and statistical manual of mental disorders* (4th ed.). Text Revision. Washington, DC: Author.

Antai-Otong, D. (2007, June). Psychopharmacology of bipolar disorders. Psychiatric Nursing Conference, New Orleans, LA.

Bezchlibnyk-Butler, K. Z., & Jeffries, J. J. (2005). *Clinical handbook of psychotropic drugs* (15th ed.). Ashland, OH: Hogrefe & Huber.

Boyd, M. A. (2008). *Psychiatric nursing: Contemporary practice* (4th ed.). Philadelphia, PA: Wolters-Kluwer/Lippincott Williams & Wilkins.

Carpenito-Moyat, L. J. (2008). *Nursing diagnosis: Application to clinical practice* (12th ed.). Philadelphia, PA: WoltersKluwer/Lippincott Williams & Wilkins.

Fischbach, F. (2004). *A manual of laboratory and diagnositic tests* (7th ed.). Philadelphia, PA: Lippincott Williams & Wilkins.

Fontaine, K. L., & Fletcher, J. S. (2003). *Mental health nursing* (5th ed.). Upper Saddle River, NJ: Pearson.

Fortinash, K. M., & Holoday Worret, P. A. (2007). *Psychiatric nursing care plans* (5th ed.). St. Louis, MO: Mosby, Elsevier.

Fox, R. (2007). Early, aggressive treatment of depression may prevent recurrence. *NeuroPsychiatry Reviews 8*(11), 9.

George-Gay, B., & Chernecky, C. C. (2002). *Clinical medical-surgical nursing: A decision making reference.* Philadelphia, PA: Saunders.

Grunebaum, M. F., & Mann, J. J. (2007). Safe use of SSRIs in young adults: How strong is evidence for new suicide warning? *Current Psychiatry 6*(11), 27–43.

Kelly, J. (2007). Genetic variation may impact response to antidepressants. *NeuroPsychiatry Reviews, 8*(1), 1–26.

Keltner, N. L. (2005). *Psychotropic drugs* (4th ed.). St. Louis, MO: Elsevier, Mosby.

Keltner, N. L., Schwecke, L. H., & Bostrom, C. E. (2007). *Psychiatric nursing* (5th ed.). St. Louis, MO: Elsevier, Mosby.

Kidd, P. S., & Wagner, K. D. (2001). *High acuity nursing* (3rd ed.). Upper Saddle River, NJ: Pearson.

La Torre, M. A. (2002). Integrated perspectives: Enhancing therapeutic presence. *Perspectives in Psychiatric Care, 38* (1), 34–36.

Lewis, S. M., Heitkemper, M. M., & Dirksen, S. R. (2004). *Medical-surgical nursing: Assessment strategies and management of clinical problems* (6th ed.). St. Louis, MO: Mosby.

Macneil, J. S. (2005). Psychotherapy can reduce mood disorder relapse. *Clinical Psychiatry News, 33*(8), 23.

Marcus, P. (2007, June). Suicidal ideation: Assessment and prevention. Psychiatric Nursing Conference, New Orleans, LA.

McKenry, L., Tessier E., & Hogan, M. (2006). *Mosby's pharmacology in nursing* (22nd ed.). St. Louis, MO: Mosby.

*Mosby's medical, nursing, and allied health dictionary,* (6th ed.). (2002). St. Louis, MO: Mosby.

Mullen, J., Endicott, J., Hirschfeld, R. M.,Yonkers, K., Tarcum, S., & Bullinger, A. L. (Eds.). (2004). *Manual of rating scales: For the assessment of mood disorders.* Wilmington, DE: Astrazeneca Pharmaceuticals.

O'Brien, P. G., Kennedy, W. Z., & Ballard, K. A. (2008). *Psychiatric mental health nursing: An introduction to theory and practice.* Sudbury, MA: Jones and Bartlett.

Sadock, B. J., & Sadock, V. A. (2003). *Kaplan and Sadock's synopsis of psychiatry: Behavioral sciences/clinical psychiatry* (9th ed.). Philadelphia, PA: Lippincott Williams & Wilkins.

Schultz, J. M., & Videbeck, S. L. (2005). *Lippincott's manual of psychiatric nursing care plans* (7th ed.). Philadelphia, PA: Lippincott Williams & Wilkins.

Shelton, R. C. (2006). Treatment-resistant depression: Are atypical antipsychotics effective and safe enough? *Current Psychiatry, 5*(10), 31–44.

Skarsater, I., Agren, H., & Dencker, K. (2001). Subjective lack of social support and presence of dependent stressful life events characterize patients suffering from major depression compared to healthy volunteers. *Journal of Psychiatric and Mental Health Nursing, 8,* 107–114.

Stein, J. (2007). Genes linked to suicidal thoughts during antidepressant therapy. *NeuroPsychiatry Reviews, 8*(11), 1–17.

Stevenson, M. (2007). Combination therapy effectively treats depressed adolescents. *Neuropsychiatry Reviews, 8*(1), 11.

Stong, C. (2006). Assessing suicide risk—separating attempts from ideation. *NeuroPsychiatry Reviews, 7*(8), 1–19.

Stuart, G. W., & Laraia, M. T. (2005). *Principles and practice of psychiatric nursing* (8th ed.). St. Louis, MO: Mosby, Elsevier.

Townsend, M. C. (2008). *Nursing diagnoses in psychiatric nursing* (7th ed.). Philadelphia, PA: F. A. Davis.

Varcarolis, E. M. (2006). *Manual of psychiatric nursing care plans* (3rd ed.). St. Louis, MO: Saunders, Elsevier.

Varcarolis, E. M., Carson, V. B., & Shoemaker, N. C. (2006). *Foundations of psychiatric mental health nursing: A clinical approach* (6th ed.). St. Louis, MO: Saunders, Elsevier.

Yigletu, H., Tucker, S., Harris, M., & Hatlevig, J. (2004). Assessing suicidal ideation: Comparing self-report versus clinician report. *American Psychiatric Nurses Association, 10*(1), 9–15.

# Web Sites

American Foundation for Suicide Prevention: www.afsp.org

American Psychiatric Association Continuing Medical Education (CME): www.psych.org/cme

American Psychiatric Association Databases PsycINFO: www.apa.org/psycinfo

Clinicaltrials.gov: www.clinicaltrials.gov

Psychiatry.com: www.psychiatry.com/index.php

U.S. National Institutes of Health Clinical Trials: www.clinicaltrials.gov

Your Total Health NBC and iVillage: yourtotalhealth.ivillage.com

# Telephone Hotlines

American Association of Suicidology: 1-202-237-2280; 1-800-SUICIDE; 1-800-273-TALK (8255); www.suicidology.org

National Alliance on Mentally Illness (NAMI): 1-800-950-NAMI; www.nami.org

National Suicide Emergency Hotline: 1-800-SUICIDE (1-800-784-2433)

Yellow Ribbon Suicide Prevention Campaign: (303) 429-3530; Ask4help@yellowribbon.org

# *Bipolar Disorder, Hyperthyroidism, and Marijuana Abuse*

## ANSWER KEY

## Questions 1 and 2

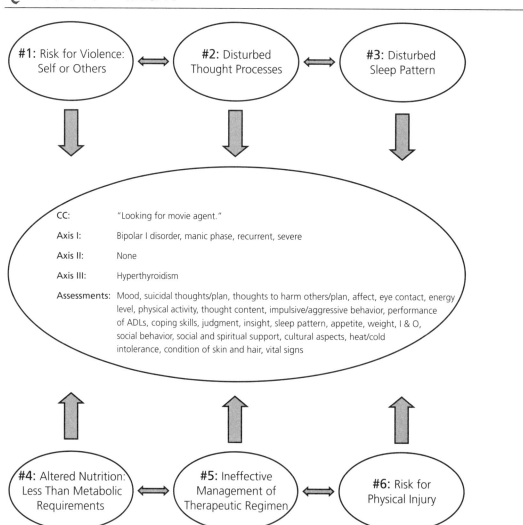

**#1:** Risk for Violence: Self or Others

**#2:** Disturbed Thought Processes

**#3:** Disturbed Sleep Pattern

| | |
|---|---|
| CC: | "Looking for movie agent." |
| Axis I: | Bipolar I disorder, manic phase, recurrent, severe |
| Axis II: | None |
| Axis III: | Hyperthyroidism |
| Assessments: | Mood, suicidal thoughts/plan, thoughts to harm others/plan, affect, eye contact, energy level, physical activity, thought content, impulsive/aggressive behavior, performance of ADLs, coping skills, judgment, insight, sleep pattern, appetite, weight, I & O, social behavior, social and spiritual support, cultural aspects, heat/cold intolerance, condition of skin and hair, vital signs |

**#4:** Altered Nutrition: Less Than Metabolic Requirements

**#5:** Ineffective Management of Therapeutic Regimen

**#6:** Risk for Physical Injury

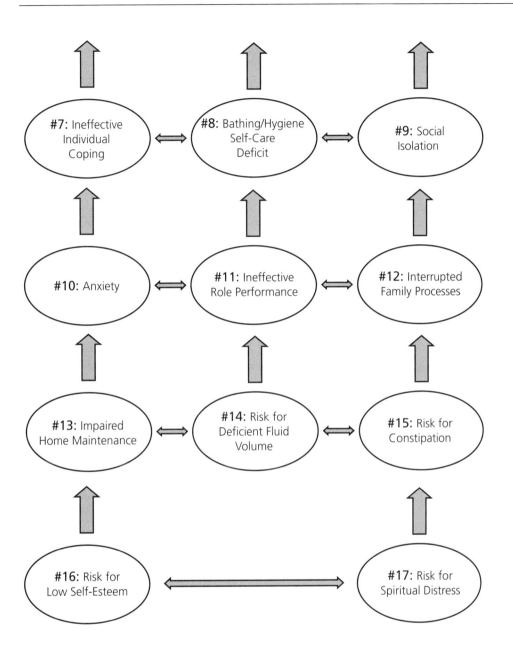

# Question 3

**Nursing Care Plan:** Bipolar I disorder, manic phase, recurrent, severe.
**Nursing Diagnosis:** Risk for Violence Toward Self or Others r/t decreased ability to control impulses and aggressive behavior s/t bipolar I disorder, manic phase AEB poor judgment, limited insight, minimizes danger to self, and nonadherence with treatment prescribed regimen.
**Outcomes** (include time frames): 1. Will remain free from self-harm and refrain from harming others during the intake assessment process and throughout hospitalization. 2. Will verbally contract with staff not to harm self or others every shift throughout hospitalization.

| Assessment Data: O = Objective, S = Subjective | Evidence-Based Interventions: | Rationales: | Patient Responses: |
|---|---|---|---|
| Grandiose (delusional) thinking (O) Severe, manic phase of bipolar I disorder (O) Psychomotor agitation during intake assessment—difficulty sitting still and singing at times (O) Labile mood (S) Very bright affect (O) Racing thoughts and FOI as evidenced by incomplete sentences and moving rapidly from one topic to another (O) Reports stopped taking Lithium because she did not like taking it and refuses to discuss other possible reasons (S) Denies need for treatment (S) | 1(a) Begin to develop a rapport and a therapeutic nurse/patient alliance that is the beginning of the therapeutic nurse/patient relationship.<br><br><br><br><br><br><br><br>(b) Perform a suicide risk assessment and obtain a verbal no harm to self or others contract with patient during the initial intake assessment process, every shift, and prn throughout hospitalization. | 1(a) Developing a rapport with the patient will assist in gaining the patient's trust and cooperation in the future. According to Peplau, the therapeutic nurse/patient relationship is the foundation that must be established to initiate future work in the healing process (Keltner, Schwecke, & Bostrom, 2008; O'Brien, Kennedy, & Ballard, 2008).<br><br>(b) Patients with Bipolar diagnoses are high risk for committing suicide due to extreme impulsivity during the manic phase or the severity of depression during the depressed phase. A behavior contract actively engages the patient in their treatment and encourages personal responsibility for their behavior. It also demonstrates staff involvement. The patient's condition may change, making it necessary to obtain another contract earlier than the next scheduled shift. | 1(a) Initially labile, intrusive, restless, irritable, and easily agitated. Tolerated nurse's presence as long as interactions were short and language simple and direct. Did accept the nurse's offer of help and reassurance of safety. Agreed to allow the nurse to work with her during hospitalization.<br><br><br>(b) Denies suicidal ideation and agreed to refrain from harming self and others. However, there is danger r/t labile mood, easily agitated and impulsivity inherent in bipolar disorder that requires she be monitored closely and the contract renewed prn as well as every shift. Least restrictive treatment must always be used, but if her condition worsens and her assessment information shows imminent danger—for example, inability to contract or engaging in impulsive aggressive behavior—she may require more intense measures for her safety as well as the safety of others (i.e., 1:1 or CO, prn medication, seclusion/behavioral control room, 4 or 5 point restraints). The ethical, legal |

| Assessment Data: O = Objective, S = Subjective | Evidence-Based Interventions: | Rationales: | Patient Responses: |
|---|---|---|---|
| | | | principle of beneficence is used as well as the law of least restrictive treatment to guide your interventions. |
| | (c) Maintain an environment free from potentially harmful objects. | (c) This decreases opportunities for the patient to harm herself or others. | (c) Has not engaged in any harmful behavior to self or others. |
| | (d) Initiate and maintain safety rounds or checks every 15 minutes. | (d) This measure ensures the patient's location and safety as well as the safety of other patients on the unit. | (d) More able to tolerate safety checks every 15 minutes as long as you do not engage her in conversation. |
| | (e) Decrease environmental stimuli (i.e., number of people in area, noise, light). | (e) A calm environment is less distracting or irritating and assists the patient to maintain control over impulsive or aggressive urges. | (e) Less psychomotor agitation and irritability noted. |
| | (f) Inform patient of unit rules regarding acceptable behavior and set limits when necessary. | (f) This lets the patient know what is or is not acceptable and assists her to act in accordance with unit rules. | (f) Listened to short, basic explanation. More accepting of verbal redirection for intrusiveness. |
| | (g) Use a calm, matter-of-fact tone of voice when interacting with this patient. Refrain from arguing or engaging in power struggles with her. | (g) Because of labile mood, irritability, and increased energy level, it is not unusual for patients diagnosed with bipolar I or II disorder, manic phase, to argue with staff and engage in power struggles related to unit rules. | (g) Fewer attempts to engage in power struggles. More accepting of verbal directives. |
| | (h) Administer scheduled and prn medication as ordered. Reinforce need to take medication consistently no matter how she feels. | (h) The patient has stopped taking her medication and it will take time for a therapeutic blood level to be reached in order to manage her symptoms. Most patients do not like to take medication due to the side effects or they do not believe they are ill and need medication. Failure to take medication or stopping medication on their own is a major cause of relapse and readmission. | (h) Initially refused medications, stating she did not need them and she did not like to take them. Now more cooperative about taking medication. |

*(continues)*

| Assessment Data:<br>O = Objective,<br>S = Subjective | Evidence-Based<br>Interventions: | Rationales: | Patient<br>Responses: |
|---|---|---|---|
| | (i) When scheduling this patient for group activities or therapies keep the group size small and limit the amount of time that the group meets. | (i) This will provide the patient with needed therapy and assist her to focus, but it will decrease the risk of becoming overwhelmed and agitated as a result of too many environmental stimuli. | (i) Able to tolerate groups lasting no longer than 20 minutes each, with three other patients attending. |
| | (j) Plan psychoeducation groups on topics of diagnosis, medication, coping skills, problem solving, anger management, relapse prevention, signs and symptoms of relapse, and healthy lifestyle behaviors. | (j) Psychoeducation is an important part of both inpatient and outpatient treatment. Nurses provide psychoeducation in one-on-one and group settings as well as for families. | (j) Initially denied needing information, but as mood becomes more even, expresses interest and participates in groups. Ambivalent about family being provided information. |
| | 2(a) Obtain a verbal no harm to self or others during the initial intake assessment process, every shift, and prn throughout hospitalization. | 2(a) See rationale for 1(b). | 2(a) Verbally contracted to refrain from harming self or others. |
| | (b) Continue therapeutic use of self to strengthen therapeutic nurse/patient alliance. | (b) This promotes and strengthens trust between the patient and nurse and also helps promote the healing process. | (b) Tolerates shorter, more frequent interaction with nurse and other staff. |

**Evaluation:** 1. Remains free from harm to self and has not attempted to harm others.
2. Verbally contracted to not harm self or others. Agreed to tell a staff member if she feels the urge to hurt herself or others. Continue care plan and evaluate every shift and prn if condition changes.

**Nursing Care Plan:** Bipolar I disorder, manic phase, recurrent, severe.
**Nursing Diagnosis:** Disturbed Thought Processes r/t biochemical alterations s/t bipolar I disorder, manic phase, AEB grandiose delusions of having a "movie agent," FOI, inappropriate dress, poor hygiene, and walking down a highway at 4 a.m. against traffic.
**Outcomes** (include time frames): 1. Will experience at least a 50% decrease, or cessation of, delusional thinking by the end of the 1st week. 2. Will dress in a more socially acceptable manner by the end of the 1st week. 3. Will bathe with assistance of staff on 1st day of admission.

| Assessment Data: O = Objective, S = Subjective | Evidence-Based Interventions: | Rationales: | Patient Responses: |
|---|---|---|---|
| Looking for "movie agent" (O) Racing thoughts and FOI as evidenced by incomplete sentences and moving rapidly from one topic to another (O) Singing at times during the intake interview (O) Wearing zebra striped coat, red negligee, and dirty high-top sneakers (O) Strong body odor, matted hair, smeared lipstick, and chipped fingernails (O) Walking down a highway against traffic at 4 a.m. (O) Rapid, pressured speech (O) Children in father's custody (O) Evicted from apartment 2 weeks ago (O) Denies need for treatment (S) States, "I'm too busy to bother eating." (S) | 1(a) Continue to assess for changes and themes in thought processes and thought content. | 1(a) This allows you to monitor if the patient's condition is improving, worsening, or remaining the same. It also helps determine if there was a specific trigger that preceded the deterioration of her condition other than stopping her medication. Themes in delusional thinking help you identify not only triggers that initiate this type of thinking but also problematic issues the client is dealing with. | 1(a) Decreased frequency of verbalizations r/t movie agent. States she felt ignored by her family, but unable to make a connection between these feelings and grandiose thoughts. |
| | (b) Remind the patient of her surroundings and of who you are. | (b) This helps orient/reorient the patient to place and staff. It also helps reinforce that she is in a safe place with people who want to help her. | (b) Correctly states her location and the names of staff members. Admits to feeling safe in the hospital. |
| | (c) Assist the patient to differentiate between delusional thinking and reality-based thinking. | (c) Initially the patient will have difficulty determining which thoughts are real and which are delusional. This may be frightening and frustrating to the patient. The nurse can help the patient with this process while providing understanding and emotional support. | (c) Admits to having difficulty distinguishing between reality and her thoughts. States there are times when she realizes there is no movie agent. |
| | (d) Avoid arguing with the patient while reinforcing reality by providing factual information in a calm, nonjudgmental manner. (i.e., "In your record the | (d) This approach avoids upsetting or provoking the patient to become agitated while assisting to reorient her to reality. | (d) Initially became angry and upset when told it was documented that she was an unemployed homemaker. She more often reluctantly accepts this as reality. |

*(continues)*

| Assessment Data: O = Objective, S = Subjective | Evidence-Based Interventions: | Rationales: | Patient Responses: |
|---|---|---|---|
| | case manager documented that you are an unemployed homemaker.") (e) Decrease environmental stimulation (such as, noise, light, number of people in area). | (e) A calm environment decreases physical activity and anxiety that may be triggering delusional thinking. The patient may be using delusional thinking to cope with increased anxiety. | (e) Calm outward appearance, but becomes irritable quickly when the noise level on the unit increases or the lights are brighter or when additional people (such as visitors) are present on unit. |
| | (f) Perform a mental status exam every shift. | (f) The mental status exam includes areas such as thought processes, thought content including suicidal/homicidal ideations, speech, psychomotor activity, appearance, cognition, judgment, and insight. It can provide valuable information about whether the patient is improving. | (f) Decreased frequency of verbalizations r/t movie agent; admits to "sometimes" still thinking she has a movie agent and at other times realizes she does not; reports difficulty differentiating reality from delusions; oriented × 5; speech less rapid and pressured, more goal-directed, and sentences are more complete; less psychomotor agitation and intrusiveness in quiet, calm environment; remains easily distracted and reports difficulty concentrating, but thoughts have "slowed down"; continues to have difficulty participating in groups lasting longer than 20 minutes; judgment and insight fair; hygiene is improving and clothing is more appropriate. |
| | (g) Administer mood stabilizer and antipsychotic medications as ordered. | (g) There are many mood stabilizers available for the treatment of labile mood in bipolar disorders. Atypical SGAs and novel antipsychotics have been approved for monotherapy (without mood stabilizers) to treat both delusional thinking as well as labile mood. Older antipsychotics may also be | (g) Initially refused medications, stating she did not need them and she did not like to take them. Now more cooperative about taking medication. |

| Assessment Data: O = Objective, S = Subjective | Evidence-Based Interventions: | Rationales: | Patient Responses: |
|---|---|---|---|
| | | used with mood stabilizers for delusional thinking if other medications are not effective. | |
| | (h) Spend time 1:1 with patient in diversional activities such as listening to quiet music, participating in a relaxation exercise, or playing cards. | (h) This will help distract the patient, keep her focused in reality, and provide role modeling of social skills. | (h) Initially too restless, distracted, and irritable to concentrate for any length of time on an activity, but has improved to the point of being able to play cards with a staff member and attempt to learn deep breathing. At first insisted on listening to rock music but then did try listening to classical music. She found it "soothing," but she complained that she couldn't dance to it. |
| | (i) Teach patient to go to a quiet place and use diversional activities to cope when beginning to feel irritable, agitated, or anxious. | (i) Teaching patients ways to help themselves cope in appropriate activities helps engage them in their treatment and promotes independence. | (i) Has been going to her room or a quieter area of the dayroom when reminded to do so. |
| | (j) Engage patient in smaller group activities with two or three other clients for 20 to 30 minutes at a time until less distractible and attention span has increased. | (j) A patient in a manic phase is very distractible, irritable, labile, and has a limited attention span. Smaller groups for shorter periods of time are more beneficial than insisting she attend larger groups for longer periods that may cause her to become agitated. Groups assist the client to remain focused on reality, provide valuable education, and improve ability to function. | (j) Able to tolerate groups lasting no longer than 20 minutes each with three other patients attending. |
| | 2(a) Request additional clothing through social worker/case manager if no suitable clothing was brought to hospital. | 2(a) The social worker/case manager may be able to persuade her to give permission to contact patient's family, and be able to arrange for clothing and toiletries to be provided. There may also be funds available to provide certain items for indigent clients. | 2(a) Initially refused request to contact family members, but has given permission. Appropriate clothing obtained. |

*(continues)*

| Assessment Data:<br>O = Objective,<br>S = Subjective | Evidence-Based<br>Interventions: | Rationales: | Patient<br>Responses: |
|---|---|---|---|
| | (b) Assist patient to choose more socially appropriate clothing. | (b) Since the patient's thought patterns are altered, she will have difficulty making good choices or judgments. | (b) More accepting of assistance with choosing clothing that matches and is suitable for wearing out on unit. |
| | (c) Verbally praise patient for appropriate choices. | (c) This provides positive reinforcement for behavior you want her to repeat. | (c) Accepts and enjoys verbal praise. |
| | 3(a) Gather supplies and have bath/shower area ready before taking the client to the area. | 3(a) Being organized avoids any delay that can provide an opportunity for the client to become distracted and make it more difficult to refocus her back to the task of bathing. Patients in a manic phase are also easily irritated and any delays or disorganization could increase the client's irritation and possibly cause her to become agitated. | 3(a) Initially "too busy" to shower, but now accepts assistance with showering and requires limit setting as to the frequency and amount of time spent in the shower. |
| | (b) Tell the patient, "it's time to take a shower." | (b) Using simple, direct language makes it easier for her to understand what is expected of her. If you ask her if she is ready to bathe, she is more likely to say no as if it were a choice, making it that much more difficult to persuade her to take care of her hygiene. | (b) Now accepts verbal direction to take a shower and more willingly attends to personal hygiene. |

**Evaluation:** 1. By the end of the 1st week of hospitalization the patient demonstrates a reduction in delusional thinking, and she has mentioned feeling ignored by her family. Admits to having difficulty at times distinguishing between reality and delusions, but does realize at times that her thoughts are not based in reality. Speech is less rapid and pressured; using more complete sentences; flows more smoothly from one topic to another and is more goal directed. Able to tolerate 20-minute group sessions attended by three other patients by the end of the 1st week.
2. More appropriately dressed.
3. Free from body odor and appearance is clean. It may take longer for her appearance to be neat and well-groomed. Continue care plan and evaluate in 48 hours.

**Nursing Care Plan:** Bipolar I disorder, manic phase, recurrent, severe.
**Nursing Diagnosis:** Disturbed Sleep Pattern r/t increased energy level s/t manic phase of bipolar I disorder AEB walking down a highway against traffic at 4 a.m. and psychomotor agitation/difficulty sitting still and singing at times during intake assessment.
**Outcomes** (include time frames): 1. Will sleep at least 5 to 6 hours per night without awakening by the end of the 1st week.

| Assessment Data: O = Objective, S = Subjective | Evidence-Based Interventions: | Rationales: | Patient Responses: |
|---|---|---|---|
| Walking down a highway against traffic at 4 a.m. (O) Racing thoughts and FOI demonstrated by incomplete sentences and moving rapidly from one topic to another (O) Psychomotor agitation during intake assessment—difficulty sitting still, singing at times (O) | 1(a) Assess client's sleep pattern, including whether she takes naps during the day. | 1(a) Establishes baseline information. Daytime napping may have a negative effect on nighttime sleep pattern. | 1(a) Admitted that sleep pattern has been a problem at times and that she requires only 2 hours of sleep and occasionally stays awake for "a few days." When depressed may sleep as long as 10 hours without awakening. |
| | (b) Schedule a balance of activity and rest periods when client is in a manic phase. | (b) During manic episodes, the body expends a great amount of energy and clients risk becoming extremely fatigued physically without being able to stop activity on their own and will need assistance with balance. | (b) Initially laughed when nurse mentioned having a balance of activity and rest but agreed to "try" this. When informed of milieu therapy and schedule of group therapy, activities, meal, and shower times as well as rest periods and bedtime, she stated that she would "try" to follow a schedule. |
| | (c) Assist client in establishing a regular bedtime routine including a specific time to go to bed and awaken. | (c) A regular bedtime routine promotes sleep by signaling the body and mind that it is time to prepare for sleep. | (c) Admitted that she does not follow a regular schedule of activities, including specific times to go to bed and wake up. |
| | (d) Eliminate distracting noise. | (d) A client in a manic phase is easily distracted and experiences racing thoughts. Noise will increase this tendency, making it even more difficult to fall asleep. | (d) Admitted that loud noises keep her from falling asleep but is starting to fall asleep within 30 minutes after going to bed. |
| | (e) Work with typical side effects of medications as a therapeutic effect for insomnia. | (e) Mood stabilizers and antipsychotics cause drowsiness as an expected side effect. As client's body adjusts to the medication, this side effect will decrease, but by that time her sleep pattern should be more normal. Sleeping agents may not be ordered unless necessary and then | (e) Reported drowsiness during first few days of hospitalization that is starting to decrease. |

*(continues)*

| Assessment Data: O = Objective, S = Subjective | Evidence-Based Interventions: | Rationales: | Patient Responses: |
|---|---|---|---|
| | (f) Teach client the importance of getting enough sleep and avoiding triggering another manic episode.<br><br>(g) When the client's mood is more stable and she is experiencing fewer delusional and racing thoughts, teach various ways to promote sleep after discharge: reducing noise or using "white noise" (low speed fan); eliminating light in bedroom and caffeinated beverages from diet; getting regular exercise (avoid 2 hours before bedtime); eating a light snack but avoiding a heavy meal before bedtime; using relaxation exercises (such as deep breathing and progressive relaxation exercises) on a daily basis before bedtime; taking a warm bath; avoiding the use of sleep agents, including herbals, unless prescribed by psychiatrist; establishing and continuing a regular bedtime routine; going to bed and awakening around the same time on a consistent basis; and using the bedroom for sleep only rather than for watching TV. | it should be for a short amount of time or only prn to avoid disrupting REM stage sleep. Also, many sleep agents may be habit-forming.<br>(f) Sleep is restorative for body, mind, and spirit. Also, too little or inconsistent sleep may trigger a manic episode for many clients with bipolar disorders.<br>(g) The client should be as involved as possible in her care to promote collaboration to give her more control over her condition and to increase independence. | (f) Stated that she did not know this and was somewhat skeptical at first, but agreed to try getting at least 5 to 6 hours of sleep on a regular basis.<br><br>(g) Admitted to drinking at least 4 cups of regular coffee daily. Agreed to at least try to decrease this amount by half and gradually to eliminate caffeine altogether. Agreed to try to go to bed around the same time every night and awaken around the same time every morning. Stated she would like to try using a fan at night. Agreed that a warm bath would be relaxing. Agreed to refrain from taking any medications or herbal remedies without discussing them with her psychiatrist. Denies having had a TV in her bedroom before being evicted, but reports that she frequently fell asleep in front of the TV in her living room. Beginning to learn progressive relaxation exercises. |

| Assessment Data: O = Objective, S = Subjective | Evidence-Based Interventions: | Rationales: | Patient Responses: |
|---|---|---|---|
| | (h) Explore complementary therapies such as aromatherapy and meditation with client when mood is more stable. Caution to use only calming scents such as lavender, chamomile, or bergamot rather than rosemary or sage that can be more stimulating. | (h) Simple meditation techniques are easy to learn, and they promote relaxation of body, mind, and spirit as well as calming aromatherapy substances. Research shows that people who practice transcendental meditation have been able to lower their levels of catecholamines such as epinephrine and norepinephrine, which are catecholamines that are released by the adrenal medulla during sympathetic nervous system stimulation that occurs during hyperactive states including manic episodes. Because catecholamines also act as neurotransmitters, an excess would contribute to the symptoms of a manic phase. | (h) Stated that she used to like to use lavender bath salts and that she might like to try to learn to mediate when her thoughts are clearer. |

**Evaluation:** 1. Sleeping 4 hours per night without awakening by the end of the 1st week. Continue care plan and evaluate in 72 hours.

# Question 5

a. This medication must be taken exactly as prescribed to ensure maximum effectiveness and to maintain a therapeutic blood level. No medication should be stopped without psychiatrist or psychiatric nurse practitioner's knowledge to help avoid a discontinuation syndrome. Many side effects can be treated if patients report them rather than just stopping the medication on their own.

b. When starting this medication, patients may experience fine hand tremors, nausea, mild diarrhea, polydipsia and polyuria, and some diaphoresis. These symptoms usually are transient.

c. Because weight gain may occur, it is important to exercise regularly and follow a low-fat, high-fiber diet.

d. Symptoms of lithium/Eskalith toxicity including diarrhea, vomiting, mental confusion, slurred speech, course hand tremors, muscle weakness and incoordination, difficulty walking, dizziness, sedation, and bradycardia.

e. Becoming dehydrated during hot weather will increase risk of toxicity.

f. Patients who become ill or have an illness accompanied by a fever or excessive diaphoresis should not make major changes in their water and salt intake *without* informing their psychiatrist. Any of these conditions will directly affect their lithium/Eskalith level, either increasing the risk of toxicity or causing the level to be too low and not effective for symptom control.

g. Some clients report a metallic taste in their mouth.

h. Avoidance of NSAIDS (i.e., Aspirin, Motrin/ibuprofen, Advil/naprosyn) while taking lithium/Eskalith due to risk for toxicity. Tylenol is acceptable as long as patient does not have history of liver problems.

i. Patient should avoid alcohol, illegal drugs, herbal preparations, and OTC medications or misuse of prescription medications. These will interfere with the therapeutic effect or may cause dangerous interactions.

j. Female patients should discuss the use of a reliable birth control method and discuss possibility of becoming pregnant with psychiatrist/physician. Lithium/Eskalith is teratogenic during the first trimester (causing possible cardiac birth defects).

k. Lithium/Eskalith blood levels will need to be monitored on a regular basis (therapeutic level $= 0.6–1.2$ mEq). There should be 8 to 12 hours between the last dose taken and the blood test. Patients who are routinely taking an evening dose of lithium/Eskalith will need to be sure to take the dose 8 to 12 hours before they are scheduled to have their blood test. They should not take the morning dose until their blood test is completed.

# Question 6

Depakote/valproic acid is an anticonvulsant medication frequently used as a mood stabilizer in the treatment of bipolar disorders. It may be prescribed in conjunction with another mood stabilizer such as lithium/Eskalith or as a monotherapy.

a. This medication must be taken exactly as prescribed to ensure maximum effectiveness and to maintain a therapeutic blood level. No medication should be stopped without psychiatrist or psychiatric nurse practitioner's knowledge to help avoid a discontinuation syndrome. Many side effects can be treated if patients report them rather than just stopping the medication on their own.

b. Side effects of Depakote/valproic acid include drowsiness, sedation, nausea, vomiting, weight gain, hair loss, and irregular menses in females.

c. Adverse effects include hepatotoxicity, blood dyscrasias such as decreased platelet activity and CBC with differential, and pancreatitis. It is important to report a tendency to bruise or bleed easily because this may be a sign of blood dyscrasias or hepatotoxicity. Symptoms of hepatoxicity include tendencies to bruise or bleed easily, anorexia, nausea, vomiting, abdominal pain/discomfort, jaundice, dark colored urine, and elevated LFTs. Symptoms of pancreatitis include abdominal pain/discomfort, anorexia, nausea, vomiting, elevated serum glucose, amylase and lipase, and decreased serum calcium.

d. Female patients should discuss use of a reliable birth control method and possibility of becoming pregnant with psychiatrist/physician. Depakote/valproic acid is teratogenic during the first trimester (causing possible neural tube birth defects, neurologic dysfunction/deficits, musculoskeletal, and cardiac defects).

e. Patients who experience GI upset should take medication with food.

f. Patients should avoid alcohol, illegal drugs, herbal preparations, and OTC medications, and misuse of prescription medications. These will interfere with how well their medication works or may cause dangerous interactions.

g. Depakote/valproic acid blood levels will need to be monitored on a regular basis (therapeutic level = 50–100 mcg; some texts may show 50–115 mcg, but currently the FDA recommended safe therapeutic level is 50–100 mcg). There should be 8 to 12 hours between the last dose taken and their blood test. If patients are routinely taking an evening dose of Depakote/valproic acid, they will need to be sure to take the dose 8 to 12 hours before they are scheduled to have their blood test. They should not take the morning dose of Depakote/valproic acid until their blood test is completed.

# Question 7

Pulse rate = 100, respirations = 24, and BP = 140/90 (many patients also experience elevated temperature), increased energy, labile mood/mood swings, disturbed sleep pattern, restlessness, easily distracted, undetermined amount of weight loss, and manic behavior.

a. Additional nursing diagnoses:

- Risk for Fatigue r/t increased metabolism and disrupted sleep pattern s/t hyperthyroidism AEB pulse rate = 100, respirations = 24, BP = 140/90, restlessness, psychomotor agitation, easy distractibility, and sleeping less than 5 to 6 hours per night.

- Imbalanced Nutrition: Less Than Body Requirements r/t increased metabolism and inconsistent eating pattern s/t bipolar I disorder, manic phase, and hyperthryroidism AEB self-report of being too busy to eat and undetermined amount of weight loss.

- Disturbed Sleep Pattern r/t increased metabolism and increased energy level s/t hyperthyroidism and manic phase of bipolar I disorder AEB restlessness, psychomotor agitation, and sleeping less than 5 to 6 hours per night.

# Question 8

Symptoms of hyperthryoidism include mood swings or labile mood, irritability, restlessness, psychomotor agitation, insomnia, fatigue, weight loss, and elevation in vital signs. These symptoms are similar to those seem in the manic phase of bipolar I disorder and, therefore, would intensify them.

# Question 9

Medication such as Propylthiouracil (PTU) or Tapazole/methimazole. Inderol/propranolol may be prescribed temporarily until the patient starts responding to PTU or Tapazole/methimazole. Continued monitoring of thyroid laboratory testing with a thyroid panel consisting of TSH, T3 uptake, total T3, total T4, free T4, and a total thyroxine index (FTI or T7). (Medication such as mood stabilizers, antipsychotics if needed, psychotherapy, and psychoeducation would be ordered to treat bipolar disorders.)

# Question 10

    a. What a diagnosis of hyperthyroidism means.

    b. Role of thyroid hormone in regulation of metabolism.

    c. Importance of normal levels of thyroid hormone.

    d. Problems caused by an excess of thyroid hormone.

    e. Signs and symptoms of hyperthyroidism.

    f. Effect of hyperthyroidism on bipolar I disorder during the manic phase.

    g. Dietary considerations, including eliminating caffeine, restricting seafood, increasing dietary complex carbohydrates and protein to provide additional calories for increased energy level while maintaining a low-fat diet; eating six smaller meals per day to provide a consistent source of energy.

    h. Scheduling rest periods alternating with periods of activity to prevent excess fatigue, and the need for routine blood tests to check thyroid functioning.

Medication teaching for propylthiouracil (PTU) or Tapazole/methimazole should include the following:

    a. Importance of taking medication exactly as prescribed and around the same time every day to ensure maximum effectiveness and therapeutic blood level. No medication should be stopped without prescribing physician's knowledge to help avoid a discontinuation syndrome. Many side effects can be treated if patients report them rather than just stopping the medication on their own.

    b. Patients who experience GI irritation may take medication with food even though it will affect the absorption rate of the medication. Patients need to inform prescribing physician if they need to take medication with food so that an appropriate dose may be prescribed to properly treat their condition.

    c. Patients should inform all healthcare providers of all medication they are taking.

    d. OTC medications should be avoided because many contain iodine or sympathomimetics such as pseudoephedrine, which can aggravate hyperthyroidism. Patients should also avoid Aspirin, which has an anticoagulant effect (may cause increased bruising and bleeding), alcohol, illegal drugs, and herbal preparations, or misuse of prescription medications. These will interfere with how well their medication works or may cause dangerous interactions.

    e. Adverse effects include nausea, vomiting, decreased taste, dizziness, skin rash, fever, agranulocytosis, leukopenia, thrombocytopenia, and bone marrow depression. Signs of agranulocytosis include sudden or quickly developing sore throat, fever, chills, or sores in the mouth. Signs of leukopenia include increased susceptibility to infection or more frequent infections and decreased WBC. Signs of thrombocytopenia include easy bruising or bleeding, decreased platelet count or increased PT and INR. Signs of bone marrow depression include bleeding from gums, delayed healing, and leukopenia.

# Question 11

Fatigue, lethargy, decreased rate and force of cardiac contractions, anemia, somnolence, impaired memory, slow speech, decreased motivation, decreased affect, muscle weakness, weight gain, constipation, decreased appetite, cold intolerance, loss of hair, coarse skin, and decreased deep tendon reflexes on physical examination. These symptoms are similar to those seen in the depressed phase of bipolar I disorder and, therefore, would intensify them.

   a. Synthroid/levothyroxine is commonly used. Monitoring of thyroid function with blood tests specifically the TSH which is abnormally high in untreated or insufficiently treated hypothyroidism and the FT3 evaluate the effectiveness of medication therapy. A low-calorie, high-fiber diet will be ordered to assist with weight loss and constipation, yet still provide for patient's metabolic needs. Frequent rest periods to help with fatigue should be scheduled between group therapy, activities, and appropriate exercise times. Memory aids may be helpful for impaired memory.

The results of laboratory/diagnostic tests obtained in the ER are available:

CBC: RBCs = 4.5 (women = 3.6–5, men 4.2–5.4), Hgb = 12 (women = 12–16, men = 14–18), Hct = 37% (women = 36–48%, men = 42–52%)

Electrolytes: Na = 138 (135–145), K = 4.0 (3.5–5.3), Ca (total) = 9 (8.8–10.4), Mg = 2 (1.8–2.6)

Glucose = 80 (70–110)

WBCs = 6 (4.5–10.5)

BUN = 12 (6–20)

Creatinine = 1.0 (0.8–1.2)

GFR = 125 (125 ml per hour; normal range adjusted by individual laboratories to account for the aging process)

Albumin = 2.8 (3.5–4.8)

Total protein = 5 (6–8)

TSH = 0.1 (0.4–4.2)

Total T3 = 225 (80–200)

T3 Uptake = 10 (0.9–1.10)

Total T4 = 60 (5.4–11.5)

Free T4 = 5 (0.7–2)

Free thyroxine index (FTI or T7) = 6 (1.5–4.5)

Lithium level = 0 (0.6–1.2)

BAL/BAC = 0 (0)

B-HCG = negative (negative)

RPR = pending (negative)

VDRL = pending (negative)

UA = pending (negative)

UDS/urine toxicology = pending (negative)

CXR = bilateral views normal (normal/absence of pathology)

EKG/ECG = normal sinus rhythm (normal sinus rhythm or NSR)

# Question 12

The lithium level of "0" provides objective evidence that corroborates the patient statement of not taking her medication. The creatinine, BUN, and GFR measure kidney function. Normal kidney function must be established for the patient to be safely restarted on lithium therapy to avoid toxicity. Also, there have been cases where patients on long-term lithium therapy have developed kidney damage. If kidney function is already compromised, the psychiatrist would not order lithium therapy.

# Question 13

To determine if the patient has been drinking, taking illegal drugs, abusing someone else's prescribed pain medications, or is adherent with certain types of prescribed medications (such as tricyclic antidepressants). Many patients deny unhealthy behavior when questioned, yet their laboratory test results show the opposite.

# Question 14

The B-HCG is a pregnancy test obtained by taking a blood sample. Because many psychotropic medications can be teratogenic, especially during the first trimester of pregnancy, it is very important to know if a female is pregnant. The RPR and VDRL are blood tests for syphilis and should be negative. Many patients in a manic phase experience hypersexuality. When this is combined with impulsivity and poor judgment, there may be increased involvement in sexual activities and risk for not only pregnancy but STDs as well. If other STDs are suspected (such as chlamydia, gonorrhea, and trichomonas/trichomoniasis), you should request a gynecological consult or testing by the primary care provider.

# Question 15

The abnormal results are most likely related to her report of being too busy to eat along with her increased activity level and metabolism. This patient will require increased dietary sources of protein and you would ask the psychiatrist to order a diet high in protein for her. Her albumin level is not low enough to require IV supplementation. The UA results showed no signs of infection, but the urine toxicology/urine drug screen (UDS) was positive for tetrahydrocannabinol (THC) indicating marijuana use.

# Question 16

There is no specific detoxification regimen to treat marijuana use or abuse because there are no medically life-threatening withdrawal signs and symptoms from this substance. However, using marijuana is an unhealthy coping strategy. Many patients diagnosed with bipolar disorders use, abuse, or become dependent on illegal substances, alcohol, or prescription medications because of impulsivity, poor judgment, poor insight, or attempting to self-medicate psychotic symptoms. When the patient's mood is more stable, her thoughts less delusional, and her ability to concentrate is improved, she will benefit from psychotherapy with a professional addictions counselor. Support groups for addiction behavior led by laypeople are also extremely helpful not only to help with refraining from using a substance but also to provide much needed emotional support and a sense of family for those with disrupted family systems.

    a. Ineffective Individual Coping r/t impulsivity, poor judgment, and poor insight; and increased stress s/t manic phase of bipolar I disorder AEB walking on highway at 4 a.m., indifferent to danger or risk for injury, and eviction from apartment 2 weeks ago.

# Question 17

Discharge planning should include a follow-up appointment with a psychiatrist to monitor her progress, manage her psychotropic medications, and monitor lithium and valproic acid blood levels as well as other pertinent abnormal laboratory and diagnostics results. A referral for a follow-up appointment should be scheduled with a primary care physician (if patient's hyperthyroidism is difficult to control, an endocrinology consult should also be planned) to monitor the hyperthyroidism, manage medications, and monitor thyroid function laboratory studies. Social work/case management referral prior to discharge for financial, healthcare insurance, payment for medication, and housing needs.

a. At this time the patient needs more supervision than she has had, especially since her family is not directly involved in her life or care. A group home may be an appropriate option until her condition improves to the point of trying to live independently again. The possibility of increased family involvement in the future, even living with a relative, should also be explored with the patient and social worker/case manager.

b. Follow up appointments with a psychiatrist, primary care physician, and possibly an endocrinologist as previously mentioned; referral for psychotherapy including individual, group, and family counseling by a psychologist, social worker, or APRN; partial hospitalization/day treatment program 5 days/week for at least 6 weeks; refer to answer to question 16 related to marijuana use. Referral for ongoing intensive outpatient case management to be continued when partial hospitalization has been completed and vocational rehabilitation evaluation for potential future education and employment.

c. Refer to community agencies for clothing, food, transportation, and any additional housing assistance needs.

d. Support groups such as National Alliance on Mental Illness (NAMI) for continued education and support for both the patient and family, Emotions Anonymous, and religious organizations. Alcoholics Anonymous (AA), Narcotics Anonymous (NA), and Al-Anon may be suggested as needed.

# References

American Psychiatric Association. (2000). *Diagnostic and statistical manual of mental disorders* (4th ed.). Text Revision. Washington, DC: Author.

Antai-Otong, D. (2007, June). Psychopharmacology of bipolar disorders. Psychiatric Nursing Conference, New Orleans, LA.

Aubry, J., Ragama-Pardos, E., Favre, S., Menzinger, M., Muscionico, M., Sanchez, S., Gex-Fabry, M., Ferrero, F., & Bertschy, G. (2003). Efficacy and safety of olanzapine plus valproate in the treatment of acute mania: An open study. *International Journal of Psychiatry in Clinical Practice*, 7, 131–134.

Bezchlibnyk-Butler, K. Z., & Jeffries, J. J. (2005). *Clinical handbook of psychotropic drugs* (15th ed.). Ashland, OH: Hogrefe & Huber.

Boyd, M. A. (2008). *Psychiatric nursing: Contemporary practice* (4th ed.). Philadelphia, PA: Wolters-Kluwer/Lippincott Williams & Wilkins.

Carpenito-Moyat, L. J. (2008). *Nursing diagnosis: Application to clinical practice* (12th ed.). Philadelphia, PA: WoltersKluwer/Lippincott Williams & Wilkins.

Chung, H., Culpepper, L., De Wester, J. N., Grieco, R. L., Kaye, N. S., Lipkin, M., Rosen, S. J., & Ross, R. (2007, Nov). Part 3: Clinical management of bipolar disorder: Achieving best outcomes through a collaborative care model. *Supplement to Current Psychiatry*, S11–18.

Chung, H., Culpepper, L., De Wester, J. N., Grieco, R. L., Kaye, N. S., Lipkin, M., Rosen, S. J., & Ross, R. (2007). Part 4: Treatment by phase: Pharmacologic management of bipolar disorder. *Supplement to Current Psychiatry*, S19-32.

Dunn, K., Elsom, S., & Cross, W. (2007). Self-efficacy and locus of control affect management of aggression by mental health nurses. *Issues in Mental Health Nursing, 28*(2), 201–217.

Fischbach, F. (2004). *A manual of laboratory and diagnositic tests* (7th ed.). Philadelphia, PA: Lippincott Williams & Wilkins.

Fontaine, K. L., & Fletcher, J. S. (2003). *Mental health nursing* (5th ed.). Upper Saddle River, NJ: Pearson.

Fortinash, K. M., & Holoday Worret, P. A. (2007). *Psychiatric nursing care plans* (5th ed.). St. Louis, MO: Mosby, Elsevier.

George-Gay, B., & Chernecky, C. C. (2002). *Clinical medical-surgical nursing: A decision making reference*. Philadelphia, PA: Saunders.

Geracioti, T. D., Jr. (2006). Identifying hyperthyroidism's psychiatric presentations. *Current Psychiatry, 5*(12), 84–92.

Keltner, N. L., Schwecke, L. H., & Bostrom, C. E. (2007). *Psychiatric nursing* (5th ed.). St. Louis, MO: Mosby, Elsevier.

Kidd, P. S., & Wagner, K. D. (2001). *High acuity nursing* (3rd ed.). Upper Saddle River, NJ: Pearson.

Krakowski, M. (2007). Violent behavior: Choosing antipsychotics and other agents. *Current Psychiatry 6*(4), 63–70.

Kupfer, D. J. (2004, June). Bipolar depression: The clinician's reference guide (BD-CRG). *Current Psychiatry*.

La Torre, M. A. (2002). Integrated perspectives: Enhancing therapeutic presence. *Perspectives in Psychiatric Care, 38*(1), 34–36.

Lewis, S. M., Heitkemper, M. M., & Dirksen, S. R. (2004). *Medical-Surgical nursing: Assessment strategies and management of clinical problems* (6th ed.). St. Louis, MO: Mosby.

Macneil, J. S. (2005). Psychotherapy can reduce mood disorder relapse. *Clinical Psychiatry News, 33*(8), 23.

Marcus, P. (2007, June). Suicidal ideation: Assessment and prevention. Psychiatric Nursing Conference, New Orleans, LA.

McKenrey, L., Tessier, E., & Hogan, M. (2006). *Mosby's pharmacology in nursing* (22nd ed.). St. Louis, MO: Mosby.

Merriman, J. (2007). Clock gene disruption may produce mania symptoms in patients with bipolar disorder. *NeuroPsychiatry Reviews, 8*(6), 18.

*Mosby's medical, nursing, and allied health dictionary* (6th ed.). (2002). St. Louis, MO: Mosby.

Mullen, J., Endicott, J., Hirschfeld, R. M., Yonkers, K., Tarcum, S., & Bullinger, A. L. (Eds.). (2004). *Manual of rating scales: For the assessment of mood disorders*. Wilmington, DE: Astrazeneca Pharmaceuticals.

O'Brien, P. G., Kennedy, W. Z., & Ballard, K. A. (2008). *Psychiatric mental health nursing: An introduction to theory and practice*. Sudbury, MA: Jones and Bartlett.

Sadock, B. J., & Sadock, V. A. (2003). *Kaplan and Sadock's synopsis of psychiatry: Behavioral sciences/clinical psychiatry* (9th ed.). Philadelphia, PA: Lippincott Williams & Wilkins.

Schultz, J. M., & Videbeck, S. L. (2005). *Lippincott's manual of psychiatric nursing care plans* (7th ed.). Philadelphia, PA: Lippincott Williams & Wilkins.

Sirven, J. I. (2007). Dangerous duo: Anti-epileptics plus herbals. *Current Psychiatry, 6*(7), 116.

Stein, J. (2007). Genes linked to suicidal thoughts during antidepressant therapy. *NeuroPsychiatry Reviews, 8*(11), 1, 16–17.

Stong, C. (2006). Assessing suicide risk-separating attempts from ideation. *NeuroPschiatry Reviews, 7*(8), 1, 19.

Stong, C. (2007). Bipolar disorder underrecognized, poorly treated. *NeuroPschiatry Reviews, 8*(6), 1, 18.

Stuart, G. W., & Laraia, M. T. (2005). *Principles and practice of psychiatric nursing* (8th ed.). St. Louis, MO: Mosby, Elsevier.

Thompson, J., McFarland, G. K., Hirsch, J. E., & Tucker, S. M. (2002). *Mosby's clinical nursing,* (5th ed.). St. Louis, MO: Mosby.

Townsend, M. C. (2008). *Nursing diagnoses in psychiatric nursing* (7th ed.). Philadelphia, PA: F. A. Davis.

Tugrul, K. (2003). The nurse's role in the assessment and treatment of bipolar disorder. *Journal of the American Psychiatric Nurses Association, 9*(6), 180–186.

U.S. Department of Health and Human Services, National Institutes of Health. (2006, September). Bipolar disorder exacts twice depression's toll in workplace: Productivity lags even after mood lifts. Retrieved September 1, 2006, from http://www.nih.gov/news/pr/sep2006/nimh-01.htm

U.S. Department of Health and Human Services, National Institutes of Health. (2006, March). Study sheds light on medication treatment options for bipolar disorder. Retrieved March 29, 2006, from http://www.nih.gov/news/pr/mar2007/nimh-28.htm

Varcarolis, E. M. (2006). *Manual of psychiatric nursing care plans* (3rd ed.). St. Louis, MO: Saunders, Elsevier.

Varcarolis, E. M., Carson, V. B., & Shoemaker, N. C. (2006). *Foundations of psychiatric mental health nursing: A clinical approach* (6th ed.). St. Louis, MO: Saunders, Elsevier.

Yigletu, H., Tucker, S., Harris, M., & Hatlevig, J. (2004). Assessing suicidal ideation: Comparing self-report versus clinician report. *American Psychiatric Nurses Association, 10*(1), 9–15.

# Web Sites

American Foundation for Suicide Prevention: www.afsp.org

American Psychiatric Association Continuing Medical Education (CME): www.psych.org/cme

American Psychiatric Association Databases PsycINFO: www.apa.org/psycinfo

Clinicaltrials.gov: www.clinicaltrials.gov

Psychiatry.com: www.psychiatry.com/index.php

U.S. National Institutes of Health Clinical Trials: www.clinicaltrials.gov

Your Total Health NBC and iVillage: yourtotalhealth.ivillage.com

# Telephone Hotlines

American Association of Suicidology: 1-202-237-2280; 1-800-SUICIDE; 1-800-273-TALK (8255); www.suicidology.org

National Alliance on Mentally Illness (NAMI): 1-800-950-NAMI; www.nami.org

National Suicide Emergency Hotline: 1-800-SUICIDE (1-800-784-2433)

Yellow Ribbon Suicide Prevention Campaign: (303) 429-3530; Ask4help @yellowribbon.org

# CHAPTER 3

# Psychotic and Medical Disorders: Schizophrenia and Hypertension

## ANSWER KEY

## Question 1

Not at this time. The patient is cooperative, and although frightened and paranoid, not physically aggressive or verbally threatening to harm anyone or himself. The medication administered and brief time of physical restraint in the emergency room was effective. However, he experiences paranoid delusions and his behavior is unpredictable making him a high risk for violence that he perceives as acting to protect himself. It is necessary to monitor him closely (i.e., with 15-minute safety checks/rounds). If he becomes agitated and aggressive and lesser restrictive methods are not effective, he may at that time need to be placed in a seclusion or behavioral control room with physical restraints.

## Question 2

The patient has been ill for several years, making his condition chronic. Positive symptoms include paranoid and bizarre delusions of a midget with sharp, pointed teeth from another planet in a spaceship trying to kill him; looking over his shoulder to see if someone is sneaking up behind him, recurring visual hallucinations involving a midget, and interpreting the attempts of staff members to assist him as threatening; he responds with physically aggressive behavior to protect himself.

Negative symptoms include flat affect, poor eye contact, needing more reminders to bathe and change clothing, and difficulty adjusting to changes in his social environment such as a new resident being admitted to the same assisted living facility.

## Questions 3, 4, and 5

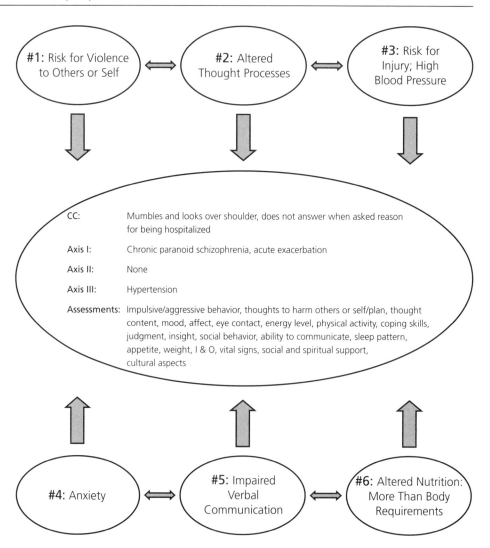

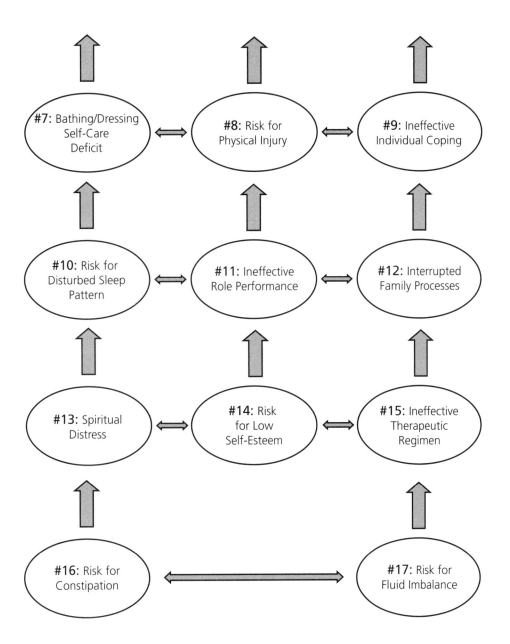

**Nursing Care Plan:** Chronic paranoid schizophrenia, acute exacerbation.
**Nursing Diagnosis:** Altered Thought Processes r/t biochemical alterations affecting sensory perception and recent stressor s/t chronic paranoid schizophrenia AEB thoughts of midget with sharp, pointed teeth from another planet traveling in a spaceship and trying to kill him; looking over shoulder and mumbling to himself during intake assessment; around the anniversary date of being evacuated during a hurricane, and running away from assisted living facility within a few days of the admission of a new resident.
**Outcomes** (include time frames): 1. Will experience at least a 50% decrease in paranoid delusions and visual hallucinations by the end of the 1st week.

| Assessment Data: O = Objective, S = Subjective | Evidence-Based Interventions: | Rationales: | Patient Responses:* |
|---|---|---|---|
| Paranoid delusions of midget from another planet trying to kill him (S) Visual hallucinations of midget with sharp, pointed teeth (S) Frightened during intake assessment (O) Looking over shoulder and mumbling to himself during intake assessment (O) Needing additional reminders to bathe and change clothes (O) Flattened affect (O) Poor eye contact (O) New resident admitted to same assisted living facility 2 days ago (O) Around the anniversary date of being evacuated during a hurricane (O) | 1(a) Perform mental status exam at admission and every shift including thought processes, thought content, and speech for indications of paranoid delusions and visual or command auditory hallucinations.

(b) Continue therapeutic use of self to strengthen therapeutic nurse/patient alliance.

(c) Tell the patient you want to help him and keep him safe. | 1(a) This will establish a baseline of information, help you evaluate if his psychosis is improving, worsening, or remaining the same. Treatment and nursing interventions will be adjusted depending on many factors including the results of the mental status exam.
(b) This promotes and strengthens trust between the patient and nurse. Paranoid patients have great difficulty trusting anyone, which makes it difficult for them to obtain treatment, accept any help offered, and make significant progress toward healing.
(c) If you can convince the patient that you sincerely want to help him, it will help increase his ability to trust you and possibly be more open with his thoughts and feelings. This helps you not only to assess him more accurately but also to anticipate potential problems and to intervene early to prevent escalation of paranoia or agitation. | 1(a) Continues to have paranoid delusions and visual hallucinations. Denies auditory or command hallucinations.

(b) Initially tolerated the presence of a nurse and one other staff member. By 3rd day able to tolerate the additional presence of two more staff members.

(c) Nodded his head when asked if he believes the nurse wants to help him. |

*Patient responses are examples of what students would look for to decide whether their planned interventions were successful, needed more time, or needed to be changed. Responses will vary depending on the patient.

| Assessment Data:<br>O = Objective,<br>S = Subjective | Evidence-Based<br>Interventions: | Rationales: | Patient<br>Responses: |
|---|---|---|---|
| | (d) Use simple words and direction when communicating with patient. | (d) Simple words and directions increase a patients' abilities to understand and follow especially when they are experiencing competing internal stimuli such as delusional thinking, hallucinations, cognitive deficits, or problems with correct perception. Patients diagnosed with schizophrenia have "concrete" versus "abstract" thinking and interpret what is said literally, which also makes it necessary to communicate with them in simple, direct language. | (d) Follows directions and is cooperative at this time. |
| | (e) Use a calm, matter-of-fact tone of voice, consistent manner, and open, relaxed body posture when interacting with this patient. Refrain from arguing with patient about delusions and hallucinations. | (e) Strong feelings—whether positive or negative—are transmitted as energy. Patients with any type of psychiatric illness are very sensitive to specific and general environmental changes, including how they are approached, voice tone, and nonverbal communication such as the body language of healthcare professionals. If a patient feels threatened or intimidated, use a calm, matter-of-fact tone of voice and an open, relaxed body posture to transmit a therapeutic feeling of calmness and safety to the patient. This helps decrease the risk of escalating his behavior or triggering agitation. Also, because the patient truly believes his delusions and hallucinations are real, | (e) Responds well to calm, matter-of-fact tone of voice, and open, relaxed body posture. Less muscle tension and improved eye contact noted during interaction. |

*(continues)*

| Assessment Data: O = Objective, S = Subjective | Evidence-Based Interventions: | Rationales: | Patient Responses: |
|---|---|---|---|
| | | arguing with him to the contrary is not therapeutic and will only increase the risk of escalating his behavior or triggering agitation and even physical aggression. It may also erode his trust in you. | |
| | (f) Present simple facts and use therapeutic communication techniques when assisting patient to focus on reality-based topics; refrain from arguing with patient about delusions and hallucinations. | (f) Simple facts support reality and make it easier to lead the patient gently to examine his thoughts and perceptions. As medication blood levels increase, he will be increasingly more able to at least try to do this. Some patients will have complete relief of psychotic symptoms while others will have a decrease in psychotic symptoms to the point that they no longer interfere with their ability to perform daily tasks. Some patients report the psychotic symptoms are still present, but they realize they are not real and are able to function in spite of the symptoms. | (f) Having difficulty accepting another possible explanation for his delusions and visual hallucinations. |
| | (g) Explore the meaning of the paranoid delusions and visual hallucinations to the extent the patient is able to tolerate this. | (g) Psychological theories explain that psychotic symptoms may be the brain's way of coping with intense feelings or severe stressors—from feelings of inferiority, fear, and anxiety to threats to integrity or sense of self, and significant losses. Themes in the delusions or hallucinations are clues to what they mean or the purpose they serve for the patient. | (g) Nodded head when asked if he was afraid of being hurt and feeling less safe lately. Does not elaborate when answering questions. |

| Assessment Data: O = Objective, S = Subjective | Evidence-Based Interventions: | Rationales: | Patient Responses: |
|---|---|---|---|
| | (h) If patient is disoriented or confused, orient to day, date, time, and place every shift and prn unless this increases his agitation. | (h) Someone who is psychotic may or may not also be disoriented or confused. Many patients with bizarre thoughts and behavior amazingly are oriented in all spheres. However, if they are not, they need to be reoriented. | (h) Oriented × 5 even though still not aware of why he has been hospitalized. |
| | (i) When in dayroom, dining room, or hallways, refrain from laughing, documenting, or speaking so that the patient cannot hear you. | (i) Paranoid patients frequently misinterpret environmental stimuli and cues. They will assume you are laughing at them, talking negatively about them, purposely talking about them so that they cannot hear you, or documenting negative information about them. This may undermine their trust in you and risk triggering agitation or even physical aggression. | (i) Remains paranoid and sensitive to the behavior of all staff members. |
| | (j) Decrease environmental stimuli (e.g., number of people in an area, noise, light). | (j) Many patients experience increased frequency of psychotic symptoms in noisy, chaotic environments. This intervention helps decrease the risk of triggering the patient's psychotic symptoms as well as agitation or aggressive behavior. | (j) Easily startled; starts to pace or retreats to his own room when more than two other patients are in the dayroom; withdraws to his room during visiting hours. |
| | (k) Perform necessary frequent observation in a less obvious manner from a safe distance. | (k) Paranoid patients are very sensitive to even normal eye contact and are convinced they are being watched for some negative or harmful reasons. However, they need to be observed frequently due to safety concerns for everyone on the unit including | (k) Becomes hypervigilant and more paranoid if he perceives staff members are "following" him. |

*(continues)*

| Assessment Data:<br>O = Objective,<br>S = Subjective | Evidence-Based<br>Interventions: | Rationales: | Patient<br>Responses: |
|---|---|---|---|
| | (l) Administer scheduled and prn medication as ordered. Reinforce need to take medication consistently no matter how he feels. | themselves. This can be done from a suitable distance that permits both visualization of the patient and physical closeness to be able to intervene when necessary. (l) Even though he has been receiving medication from the assisted living facility staff, he is experiencing an increase in symptoms and needs to achieve an increased steady blood level to help decrease his delusional and abnormal thinking. Most patients do not like to take medication because of the side effects or because they do not believe they are ill and need medication. Failure to take medication or stopping medication on their own is a major cause of relapse and readmission. | (l) After much persuasion, takes medication after examining it and the packaging. |
| | (m) Encourage and remind patient to attend groups with a small number of participants and a time frame of approximately 20 minutes. | (m) In the past, mental healthcare professionals did not believe patients diagnosed with schizophrenia would derive much benefit from attending group psychotherapy or psychoeducation. More current thinking and recommendations do include group psychotherapy and psychoeducation not only for the families of these patients but also for the patients as well. Supportive group therapy, social skills, coping skills, relaxation techniques, | (m) More comfortable attending groups toward end of 1st week. Initially able to tolerate sitting in group for only 5 minutes but now is able to stay for 20 minutes with four other patients. Asks an appropriate question about the topic being discussed. |

| Assessment Data: O = Objective, S = Subjective | Evidence-Based Interventions: | Rationales: | Patient Responses: |
|---|---|---|---|
| | | enhanced problem-solving skills, planning simple goals, and information related to medications and diagnosis provided in smaller groups, over a shorter time span, and in a consistent environment are more helpful than previously thought. More research is needed in this area. | |
| | (n) When patient is more comfortable on the unit, help him to differentiate reality from delusions and hallucinations. | (n) The nurse's presence helps reinforce reality, but over time patients will need to be able to learn how to distinguish between thoughts and experiences that they are having that are based in reality and those that are not even if they never totally stop having psychotic symptoms. This will help them to be able to function more normally on a day-to-day basis. Learning how to focus and how to ask others if they are having similar experiences may be initiated during hospitalization and continued during outpatient psychotherapy and psychoeducation sessions. | (n) Beginning to work with primary nurse, psychologist, and OT. Will need to continue practicing techniques learned in outpatient therapy. |

**Evaluation:** Has started to make progress, but remains very paranoid. Less frequent verbalizations related to delusions and hallucinations but content remains the same. Able to tolerate the presence of two other patients in the dayroom, but starts to pace or withdraw to his own room if more patients are present or during visiting hours. Although initially suspicious, he is taking medication and tolerating mouth checks. Able to attend two groups per day by the end of the 1st week of hospitalization and now able to tolerate 20 minutes of group time with four other patients. Continue care plan and evaluate in 72 hours.

**Nursing Care Plan:** Chronic paranoid schizophrenia, acute exacerbation.

**Nursing Diagnosis:** Risk for Injury r/t increased blood pressure and history of smoking over the past 22 years s/t history of hypertension AEB blood pressure of 168/90 even when taking Coreg/carvedilol 25 mg po bid, potential side effect of orthostic hypotension from Risperdal/risperidone 2 mg po bid, and received Ativan/lorazepam 2 mg IM in emergency room prior to being brought to the psychiatric/mental health unit.

**Outcomes** (include time frames): 1. Will have SBP of less than 140 and DBP less than 90 within 24 hours of admission. 2. Will remain free from serious medical consequences of elevated blood pressure.

| Assessment Data: O = Objective, S = Subjective | Evidence-Based Interventions: | Rationales: | Patient Responses: |
|---|---|---|---|
| Admission BP = 168/90 (O) Admission pulse = 96 (O) History of hypertension (O) Prescribed and receiving Coreg/carvedilol 25 mg po bid (O) Prescribed and receiving Risperdal/risperidone 2 mg po bid (O) Received Ativan/lorazepam 2 mg IM in emergency room (O) Briefly restrained physically in emergency room (O) History of chronic paranoid schizophrenia (O) Experiencing an increase in psychotic symptoms (O) Agitated and physically aggressive with assisted living facility staff (O) Weighs 250 pounds and is 6 ft. tall (O) Has smoked 1½ packs of cigarettes per day over past 22 years (O) | 1(a) Recheck BP and pulse 2 hours after admission while continuing to obtain vital signs every shift as ordered. | 1(a) Even though the patient's orders include vital signs every shift, the nurse may and is responsible to obtain information and evaluate the patient's condition more frequently if indicated. The pulse rate may be abnormally low, and the elevated blood pressure shows the body's attempt to compensate. Frequently patients' mental and emotional states affect their physical state (including vital signs). The patient should still be closely monitored due to a history of hypertension, current medication to treat hypertension, and past problems with medical signs and symptoms being ignored in psychiatric/mental health settings to the detriment of the patient's physical condition. The number of patients with both psychiatric and medical illness is increasing. The nurse in any setting working within the RN scope of practice defined by the state of licensure must be aware of and provide care for all the | 1(a) BP 140/90 when rechecked 2 hours after admission. Continue to obtain vital signs every shift as ordered and prn if indicated. |

| Assessment Data:<br>O = Objective,<br>S = Subjective | Evidence-Based<br>Interventions: | Rationales: | Patient<br>Responses: |
|---|---|---|---|
| | | patient's diagnoses and needs. If unable to do so, the nurse is responsible to notify nursing management as well as the psychiatrist and other healthcare providers involved in the patient's treatment to avoid actual or potential harm. | |
| | (b) Administer scheduled doses of Coreg as ordered. | (b) The patient has a history of hypertension and needs to maintain a consistent blood level of medication to help control his blood pressure. | (b) Taking scheduled doses of Coreg when offered. |
| | (c) Administer prn Catepres, notify physician as ordered, and recheck BP and pulse 60 minutes after administering. | (c) The onset of action for Catepres is 30 to 60 minutes. It is important to bring the blood pressure into more normal limits to avoid serious medical consequences including CVA, MI, and kidney or eye damage. | (c) BP 140/90, prn Catepres not needed at this time. Continue to obtain vital signs every shift as ordered and prn if indicated. |
| | (d) Use a calm, matter-of-fact tone of voice, consistent manner, and open, relaxed body posture when interacting with this patient. | (d) This will help increase the patient's emotional comfort level, which will have a relaxing effect on his body. | (d) Responds well to calm, matter-of-fact tone of voice, and open, relaxed body posture. Exhibits less muscle tension and improved eye contact during interaction. |
| | (e) Suggest refraining from smoking until BP has decreased, using a nicotine patch while hospitalized, and pursuing a smoking cessation plan after discharge. Explain that smoking privileges may be withheld if BP becomes dangerously high to prevent serious life-threatening complications. | (e) Unfortunately many patients diagnosed with psychiatric illnesses smoke. Asking them to stop smoking when experiencing psychiatric crises is frequently too much to expect. It may be better to discuss smoking cessation or reduction as a possible outpatient goal. Some patients agree to try using a nicotine patch as a step toward smoking cessation. However, | (e) Does not want to stop smoking, but agrees to wait to smoke until his BP and pulse are rechecked. |

*(continues)*

| Assessment Data:<br>O = Objective,<br>S = Subjective | Evidence-Based<br>Interventions: | Rationales: | Patient<br>Responses: |
|---|---|---|---|
| | | there may be times when patients' physical conditions (such as chest pain, elevated BP, or signs of impending CVA or MI) take precedence over their emotional states and rights and smoking privileges are withheld to prevent life-threatening situations. In such cases, when patients have not had an opportunity to smoke for several hours, their anxiety will increase since they are used to smoking frequently. | |
| | (f) Teach relaxation techniques, including deep breathing and even simple meditation or yoga. | (f) Relaxation techniques decrease mental and emotional stress and trigger a physical relaxation response. | (f) Focuses only on learning deep breathing at this time. |
| | (g) Assist patient with meal and snack choices that are within the low-sodium, low-fat diet ordered. | (g) Decreasing sodium intake leads to decreased water retention. Decreased fat intake can help decrease weight. Both strategies can result in decreased blood pressure. Unfortunately, many psychotropic medications cause weight gain as a side effect. Some of the newer, atypical antipsychotics can also cause increased blood glucose and cholesterol levels leading to weight gain. Some sources show Risperdal as having mixed results related to causing increased blood glucose or cholesterol. Other sources show Risperdal does increase glucose levels. | (g) Accepts assistance with choosing meal and snack options within personal preferences. |

| Assessment Data: O = Objective, S = Subjective | Evidence-Based Interventions: | Rationales: | Patient Responses: |
|---|---|---|---|
| | (h) Monitor I & O every shift. | (h) Excessive water intake can lead to increased weight and blood pressure. Some patients diagnosed with schizophrenia also have problems with "water intoxication"—pathologically drinking such large quantities of water that it affects their physical health by decreasing electrolyte levels and increasing blood pressure. | (h) Accepts monitoring of I & O; within normal limits. |
| | (i) Weigh every 3 days as ordered or daily if gaining 2 pounds or more. | (i) Weight gain of 2 pounds or more may indicate water retention and have an effect on blood pressure. | (i) Maintains weight at 250 pounds. |

**Evaluation:** Blood pressure is elevated, but it is not at an immediately dangerous level. Patient is a smoker. Stress and anxiety levels may still be contributing to elevation. Continue to monitor vital signs q shift and prn as indicated. Continue care plan and evaluate q shift and prn.

# Question 6

a. The patient is experiencing EPS, more specifically tardive dyskinesia (TD). Some forms of EPS such as dystonia or akasthesia occur much sooner in treatment. Other forms of EPS such as TD can occur weeks or even a year later. Risperdal/risperidone is the most likely choice. Although it is true that Zyprexa/olanzapine in any form can also cause EPS, even if given as a prn dose, it is less likely to than Risperdal/risperidone. There is no information in the scenario as to whether or not he was given Zyprexa/olanzapine. The patient has been taking Risperdal/risperidone, and the dose was increased upon admission. He also has a history of receiving Haldol/haloperidol and Thorazine/chlorpromazine. Either of these medications would be even more likely to cause EPS. The patient may also be experiencing a cumulative effect of antipsychotic medication over time.

b. The term EPS refers to various types of abnormal, involuntary movements that are a result of adverse antipsychotic medication effects related to blocking the neurotransmitter dopamine or unmasking of abnormal movement already present when antipsychotic medication is administered. General categories of EPS include dystonic reactions or dystonia, akasthesia, akinesia, tardive dyskinesia, and pseudoparkinsonism.

Dystonic reactions or dystonia are muscle spasms or uncoordinated spastic muscle movements that can involve the face, tongue, extraocular muscles (e.g., during oculogyric crisis), trachea/larynx (e.g., laryngospasm), esophagus, neck (e.g., torticollis), thorax/respiratory muscles (e.g., respiratory problems), trunk (e.g., opisthotonus or arching of the back), or pelvis (e.g., swaying or difficulty walking). These reactions can be very frightening for patients, but they are easily treated.

Akasthesia is described as motor restlessness. Patients have difficulty sitting still or staying in one position for any length of time, and they may pace, fidget, shift their weight frequently from one foot to another, tap their foot, or be unable to sit still in a chair. They may also say that they feel as if they are going to "jump out of" their "skin." These reactions can cause extreme distress for the patient to the point of preferring to be ill rather than experience this side effect or even contemplating suicide. Early identification of akasthesia as well as any EPS is extremely important for the patient's well-being and increased adherence to prescribed treatment.

Akinesia refers to a decrease in motor movement or muscle weakness. The patient may complain of fatigue or tiring easily with physical activity.

Tardive dyskinesia (TD) refers to abnormal or purposeless muscle movements including the extremeties, trunk, face, jaw, and oral-buccal muscles, causing rocking or twisting motions, pelvic thrusting or gyrations, tremors, tongue darting or writhing, spastic facial movements, frowning, blinking, blowing, teeth grinding, lip smacking, or chewing movements when there is no food or gum in the mouth. This type of EPS may be irreversible, and it may also be extremely distressing for the patient. Medication may be given to counteract the adverse effects, and the dose of the prescribed antipsychotic may be decreased or totally discontinued. Unfortunately, regardless of these efforts the TD symptoms may be permanent.

Pseudoparkinsonism refers to signs and symptoms similar to those seen in Parkinson's disease, including slow motor movements, tremors, muscle rigidity, cogwheel rigidity, stooped posture, shuffling gait, facial masking or flattened affect, and pill rolling finger movements. Medication may be given to counteract the adverse effects, and the dose of the prescribed antipsychotic may be decreased or totally discontinued.

    c. An AIMS test is used to identify abnormal movements prior to a patient beginning antipsychotic medication therapy, and periodically (e.g., at 6-month intervals) to promote early identification of EPS or identify worsening of EPS already present due to medication adverse effects or prior disease states. An AIMS test should also be performed on a patient who has had an increase in the dose of an antipsychotic medication and is experiencing symptoms.

    d. Oral medications used as standard practice to treat or prevent the development of EPS are usually anticholinergics including Cogentin/benztropine, Symmetrel/amantadine, Parlodel/bromocriptine, Artane/trihexiphenidyl, Kemedrin/procyclidine, or Akineton/biperiden. In an emergency situation where the patient is experiencing life-threatening respiratory symptoms, laryngospasm, pain, or extreme emotional distress, Cogentin/benztropine or the antihistamine Benadryl/diphenhydramine are given IM.

In the past patients who were receiving antipsychotic medications, but were not experiencing EPS were frequently also ordered anticholinergic medications as a way to prevent the development of EPS. Unfortunately, such medications also had side effects, including blurred vision, dry mouth, urinary retention, constipation, mental confusion, psychosis, disorientation, and delirium. Currently the wisdom of using anticholinergics at all for EPS is being questioned, and these medications are ordered only when the patient starts to experience early EPS and they are withdrawn as soon as possible.

# Question 7

    a. Blurred vision, dry mouth, urinary retention, constipation, mental confusion, psychosis, delirium, or disorientation. The patient's I & O, bowel pattern, and mental status should be assessed every shift by the nurse. The patient should be taught to increase water intake, but not to the point of increasing weight or blood pressure. In such cases, patients may suck on ice chips or sugar-free hard candy to relieve dry mouth.

# Question 8

CBC: RBCs = 5 (women = 3.6–5, men 4.2–5.4), Hgb = 16 (women = 12–16, men = 14–18), Hct = 46% (women = 36–48%, men = 42–52%)

Electrolytes: Na = 140 (135–145), K = 4.2 (3.5–5.3), Ca (total) = 9.6 (8.8–10.4), Mg = 2.2 (1.8–2.6)

Glucose = 108 (70–110)

WBCs = 8 (4.5–10.5)

BUN = 16 (6–20)

Creatinine = 0.9 (0.8–1.2)

GFR = 125 (125 ml per hour; normal range adjusted by individual laboratories to account for the aging process)

ALT/SGPT = 10 (4–36)

AST/SGOT = 20 (0–35)

Total cholesterol = 200 (140–199)

HDL/HDL-C = 35 (women = 35–80, men = 35–65)

LDL = 130 (below 130)

Triglycerides = 150 (below 150)

Total cholesterol/HDL ratio = 4.2 (Men age 40–69 years equal to or below 4.2 means they have excellent protection against risk for cardiovascular disease; women age 40–69 years equal to or below 3.0 means they have excellent protection against risk for cardiovascular disease.)

RPR = negative (negative)

VDRL = negative (negative)

The patient has borderline high total cholesterol, LDL, triglycerides, and a total cholesterol/HDL ratio. He has a low normal HDL/HDL-C level. These levels will need continued monitoring because many psychiatric patients are at risk for developing metabolic syndrome due to side effects of psychotropic medications as well as the signs and symptoms of psychiatric illness that may interfere with healthy lifestyle behaviors.

# Question 9

a. Autonomic nervous system reactivity (sympathetic) including high fever, tachycardia, and elevated blood pressure as well as muscle rigidity described as "lead pipe rigidity," respiratory difficulty, diaphoresis, confusion, delirium, elevated CPK levels, WBCs, hyperkalemia, and hyponatremia. Cases of NMS in patients receiving atypical antipsychotic medications have been missed in early stages because of relying on the fact that NMS occurs less often in patients prescribed atypical antipsychotics versus traditional ones. It is still important for the nurse to be aware of this possibility and assess these patients for signs and symptoms of NMS. NMS is treated by withdrawing antipsychotic medication, providing supportive physical care including intravenous therapy and mechanical ventilation if needed, and Dantrium/dantrolene as well as Parlodel/bromocriptine. Fatalities have occurred.

b. Blood dyscrasias are pathological conditions that occur where any part of the blood components are caused to become abnormal in structure, quality, or function. Such conditions may be caused by hemolytic destruction (hemolytic anemia low RBCs), bone marrow suppression and aplastic anemia (decreased production/low RBCs or maturation of RBCs); destruction or suppression of WBC/neutrophil production/function (leukopenia or agranulocytosis most often seen with Clozaril/clozapine) or inhibition of platelet aggregation (decreased ability to clot) and decreased platelet count (thrombocytopenia). Signs and symptoms may include easy bruising, bleeding into soft tissues or prolonged bleeding after trauma, or greatly increased susceptibility to infection, possibly life threatening.

c. Patients who have at least three of the following conditions may be diagnosed with metabolic syndrome: a BMI score of at least 25, elevated blood glucose, elevated triglycerides, hypertension, and increased insulin levels. Previously termed "central obesity" and "syndrome X," metabolic syndrome increases a patient's risk of developing Type II DM or cardiovascular disease later in life, and there is an increased risk with some atypical antipsychotics. Patients prescribed these atypical antipsychotics are not only experiencing weight gain, but also increased blood glucose and cholesterol levels. Abdominal adipose cells are more metabolically active than those in other regions of the body, which leads to weight gain.

d. Clozaril/clozapine, Zyprexa/olanzapine, and more recently Risperdal/risperidone.

e. Geodon/ziprasidone has been noted to cause abnormal EKG/ECG results specifically prolongation of the QT or QTc interval causing increased risk for cardiac arrhythmias. According to the literature, many other atypical and traditional antipsychotics may also cause cardiac arrhythmias, but currently with atypical antipsychotics this is occurring with Geodon/ziprasidone and has led psychiatrists to obtain an EKG/ECG before initiating this medication or if a patient becomes symptomatic while receiving this medication.

# Question 10

Yes, current thinking is that even patients diagnosed with schizophrenia can benefit from psychotherapy and psychoeducation both during hospitalization and after discharge on an outpatient basis. The therapy and education will need to be tailored for the individual patient's abilities and needs. The families of patients diagnosed with schizophrenia require support and education as well.

Individual, group, and family psychotherapy and psychoeducation should be planned for and provided. Modified CBT, IPT, and supportive group therapy; OT to enhance social skills and skills needed for obtaining or maintaining employment (e.g., completing a job application and interview; getting along with coworkers), and psychoeducation including information on medications, signs and symptoms of schizophrenia; relapse signs and symptoms as well as how to prevent relapse; coping skills, relaxation techniques, enhanced problem-solving skills, simple goal planning, learning how to focus on reality while ignoring delusions or hallucinations, and how to differentiate between reality and psychotic symptoms; finding referral information for support groups, medication, and financial assistance as well as any basic needs. Referrals for religious-based organizations would be appropriate if patients are not religiously preoccupied or have delusions with religious themes. Assertive Community Treatment (ACT) helps patients with chronic mental illness by bringing needed therapies and services directly to them so that they do not have to go to several locations for treatment and services.

a. Initially 5 days per week for at least 1 month would be appropriate, followed by evaluation for potentially decreasing services to 3 days per week.

Also the National Alliance on Mental Illness (NAMI) provides education, advocacy, and support for all types of mental illness. The organization, which has local and state chapters across the United States, is available for patients, family members, friends, and anyone interested in helping those with mental illness.

# References

American Psychiatric Association. (2000). *Diagnostic and statistical manual of mental disorders* (4th ed.). Washington, DC: Author.

American Psychiatric Association. (2004). *Practice guidelines for the treatment of patients with schizophrenia* (2nd ed.). Washington, DC: Author.

Antai-Otong, D. (2004). *Psychiatric emergencies: How to accurately assess and manage the patient in crisis.* Eau Claire, WI: PESI Heatlthcare.

Appel, S. J., Jones, E. D., & Kennedy-Malone, L. (2004). Central obesity and metabolic syndrome: Implications for primary care providers. *Journal of the American Academy of Nurse Practitioners, 16*(8), 335–342.

Beebe, L. H. (2003). Health promotion in persons with schizophrenia: Atypical medications. *Journal of the American Psychiatric Nurses Association, 9*(4),115–121.

Beebe, L. H. (2007). Beyond the prescription pad: Psychosocial treatments for individuals with schizophrenia. *Journal of Psychosocial Nursing, 45*(3), 35–43.

Bezchlibnyk-Butler, K. Z., & Jeffries, J. J. (2004). *Clinical handbook of psychotropic drugs* (14th ed.). Ashland, OH: Hogrefe & Huber.

Bezchlibnyk-Butler, K. Z., & Jeffries, J. J. (2005). *Clinical handbook of psychotropic drugs* (15th ed.). Ashland, OH: Hogrefe & Huber.

Bradshaw, T., Lovell, K., & Harris, N. (2005). Healthy living interventions and schizophrenia: A systematic review. *Journal of Advanced Nursing, 49*(6), 634–654.

Carpenito-Moyat, L. J. (2008). *Nursing diagnosis: Application to clinical practice* (12th ed.). Philadelphia, PA: WoltersKluwer/Lippincott Williams & Wilkins.

Courey, T. J. (2007, July/August). Detection, prevention, and management of extrapyramid symptoms. *Journal for Nurse Practitioners, JNP,* 464–469.

Fischbach, F. (2004). *A manual of laboratory and diagnositic tests* (7th ed.). Philadelphia, PA: Lippincott Williams & Wilkins.

Fontaine, K. L., & Fletcher, J. S. (2003). *Mental health nursing* (5th ed.). Upper Saddle River, NJ: Pearson.

George-Gay, B., & Chernecky, C. C. (2002). *Clinical medical-surgical nursing: A decision-making reference.* Philadelphia, PA: Saunders.

Keltner, N. (2005). Genomic influences on schizophrenia-related neurotransmitter systems. *Journal of Nursing Scholarship, 37*(4), 322–328.

Keltner, N. L., Schwecke, L. H., & Bostrom, C. E. (2007). *Psychiatric nursing* (5th ed.). St. Louis, MO: Mosby, Elsevier.

Kidd, P. S., & Wagner, K. D. (2001). *High acuity nursing* (3rd ed.). Upper Saddle River, NJ: Pearson.

Krakowski, M. (2007). Violent behavior: Choosing antipsychotics and other agents. *Current Psychiatry, 6*(4), 63–70.

La Torre, M. A. (January-March, 2002). Integrated perspectives: Enhancing therapeutic presence. *Perspectives in Psychiatric Care, 38*(1), 34–36.

Lewis, S. M., Heitkemper, M. M., & Dirkson, S. R. (2004). *Medical-Surgical Nursing: Assessment Strategies and Management of Clinical Problems* (6th ed.). St. Louis, MO: Mosby.

Marcus, P. (2007, June). Suicidal ideation: Assessment and prevention. Psychiatric Nursing Conference, New Orleans, LA.

McKenrey, L., Tessier, E., & Hogan, M. (2006). *Mosby's pharmacology in nursing* (22nd ed.). St. Louis, MO: Mosby.

Meyer, J. (2004). Managing metabolic risks of antipsychotic therapy. *A Supplement to Clinical Psychiatry News, Clinical Update Continuing Education, 3.*

Mullen, J., Endicott, J., Hirschfeld, R. M., Yonkers, K., Tarcum, S., & Bullinger, A. L. (Eds.). (2004). *Manual of rating scales: For the assessment of mood disorders.* Wilmington, DE: Astrazeneca Pharmaceuticals.

Nihart, M. A. (2007, June). Pyschopharmacology updat(e) Psychiatric Nursing Conference, New Orleans, LA.

Nihart, M. (2007). Update: Neurobiological advances in understanding schizophrenia. Psychiatric Nursing Conference, New Orleans, LA.

O'Brien, P. G., Kennedy, W. Z., & Ballard, K. A. (2008). *Psychiatric mental health nursing: An introduction to theory and practice.* Sudbury, MA: Jones and Bartlett.

Sadock, B. J., & Sadock, V. A., (2003). *Kaplan and Sadock's synopsis of psychiatry: Behavioral sciences/clinical psychiatry* (9th ed.). Philadelphia, PA: Lippincott Williams & Wilkins.

Stong, C. (2006). Assessing suicide risk-separating attempts from ideation. *NeuroPschiatry Reviews, 7*(8), 1, 19.

Stuart, G. W., & Laraia, M. T. (2005). *Principles and practice of psychiatric nursing* (8th ed.). St. Louis, MO: Mosby, Elsevier.

Townsend, M. C. (2008). *Nursing diagnoses in psychiatric nursing* (7th ed.). Philadelphia, PA: F. A. Davis.

Varcarolis, E. M. (2006). *Manual of psychiatric nursing care plans* (3rd ed.). St. Louis, MO: Saunders, Elsevier.

Varcarolis, E. M., Carson, V. B., & Shoemaker, N. C. (2006). *Foundations of psychiatric mental health nursing: A clinical approach* (6th ed.). St. Louis, MO: Saunders, Elsevier.

Wynd, C. (2005). Guided health imagery for smoking cessation and long-term abstinence. *Journal of Nursing Scholarship, 37*(3), 245–250.

Yigletu, H., Tucker, S., Harris, M., & Hatlevig, J. (2004). Assessing suicidal ideation: Comparing self-report versus clinician report. *American Psychiatric Nurses Association, 10*(1), 9–15.

# Web Sites

American Heart Association: www.americanheartassociation.org

American Psychiatric Association Continuing Medical Education (CME): www.psych.org/cme

American Psychiatric Databases: www.apa.org/psycinfo

American Psychological Association: www.apa.org

Clinicaltrials.gov: www.clinicaltrials.gov

National Alliance on Mental Illness: www.nami.org

Psychiatry.com: www.psychiatry.com

United States Department of Health and Human Services, Substance Abuse and Mental Health Services Administration: www.samhsa.gov

Your Total Health NBC and iVillage: yourtotalhealth.ivillage.com

# Personality Disorders and Substance Abuse: Borderline Personality Disorder and Methamphetamine Abuse

## ANSWER KEY

## Question 1

You would explain and reassure her that everyone cares about her and is willing to listen to her. You may also need to verbally reinforce the idea that there are appropriate times and areas on the unit to talk. The patient may have insisted that a nurse or staff member should have time to talk to her when it was not appropriate, including times when the nurse or staff member were with another patient, preparing a shift report, leaving at the end of their shift, admitting or discharging patients, or intervening in a potential emergency situation. The patient may not have been willing to wait until a nurse or staff member was available to spend time with her. She may also have misinterpreted what the nurse or staff member said to her during their time together as not caring about her.

## Question 2

You would gently explain the difference between therapeutic relationships and social relationships. Reinforce that your relationship with her is a therapeutic one and try to direct the conversation to what friends she is planning on seeing once she discharged.

# Question 3

The difference in behavior the patient displayed in responses toward the nurse and psychologist would best be explained by the cognitive distortion dichotomous thinking and the behavioral phenomenon "splitting." Dichotomous thinking has caused the patient to now view the nurse as "all bad" because of the nurse's response and her refusal to meet the patient socially after discharge. The patient views the psychologist as the "only true friend" she has on the unit and, therefore, is "all good." The patient's view of the psychologist may change if the psychologist says or does something the patient disagrees with.

# Question 4

Signs and symptoms of borderline personality disorder for this patient would include a history of self-mutilation and recently cutting herself after a fight with her boyfriend; intense anger in response to the nurse's reply that all the staff care about the patient and refusal to meet the patient socially after discharge; engaging in splitting behavior and dichotomous thinking, as evidenced by her very different responses to the nurse and the psychologist; manipulative behavior and making statements that she will kill herself if no one cares about her; financial problems; and methamphetamine abuse.

# Question 5

You will need to be empathetic and use therapeutic communication to find out exactly why she perceives that no one cares about her. You will again reinforce that all the nurses and staff members care about her even though she may not perceive this to be true. She should also be assessed for suicidal ideations and plans, even though she may be trying to manipulate the nurse, due to impulsivity that is a symptom of borderline personality disorder.

# Question 6

Signs and symptoms of methamphetamine intoxication or being "high" would include restlessness; euphoria; excess energy; psychosis; anxiety; mood swings; increased blood pressure, pulse, and respirations; possibly increased temperature; dental decay if methamphetamine is smoked rather than ingested orally or used intravenously; open areas on face and extremities if picking or scratching skill due to visual hallucinations of bugs crawling on skin or tactile hallucinations of crawling skin sensations; and needle tracks if IV drug use has been involved.

Signs and symptoms of methamphetamine withdrawal would include fatigue, low energy level, depressed mood, and insomnia.

# Question 7

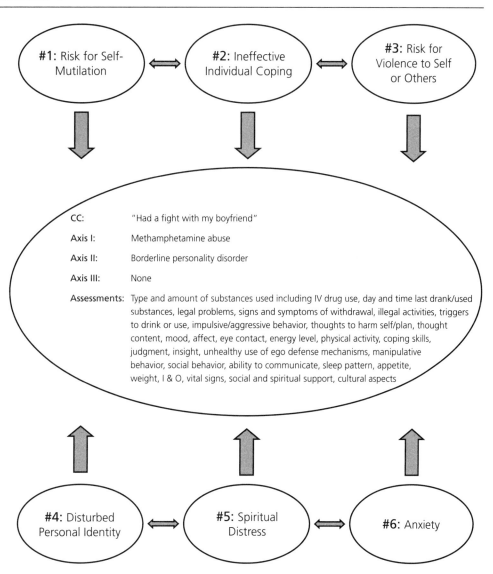

CC:            "Had a fight with my boyfriend"

Axis I:        Methamphetamine abuse

Axis II:       Borderline personality disorder

Axis III:      None

Assessments:  Type and amount of substances used including IV drug use, day and time last drank/used substances, legal problems, signs and symptoms of withdrawal, illegal activities, triggers to drink or use, impulsive/aggressive behavior, thoughts to harm self/plan, thought content, mood, affect, eye contact, energy level, physical activity, coping skills, judgment, insight, unhealthy use of ego defense mechanisms, manipulative behavior, social behavior, ability to communicate, sleep pattern, appetite, weight, I & O, vital signs, social and spiritual support, cultural aspects

#1: Risk for Self-Mutilation

#2: Ineffective Individual Coping

#3: Risk for Violence to Self or Others

#4: Disturbed Personal Identity

#5: Spiritual Distress

#6: Anxiety

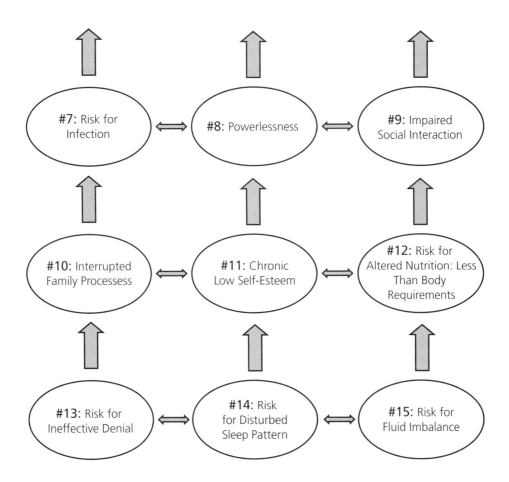

# Questions 8 and 9

|  | | | |
| --- | --- | --- | --- |
| **Nursing Care Plan:** Methamphetamine abuse, borderline personality disorder. **Nursing Diagnosis:** Risk for Self-Mutilation r/t impulsivity, anxiety, fear of abandonment, and disturbed personal identity s/t borderline personality disorder and methamphetamine abuse AEB cutting self after fight with boyfriend and history of self-mutilation. **Outcomes** (include time frames): 1. Will refrain from engaging in self-mutilation behaviors upon admission, every shift, and throughout hospitalization. | | | |
| **Assessment Data:** O = Objective, S = Subjective | **Evidence-Based Interventions:** | **Rationales:** | **Patient Responses:*** |
| Cut self after fight with boyfriend (O) History of self-mutilation (O) Engages in splitting behavior (O) History of sexual and physical abuse (O) | 1(a) Begin to develop a rapport and a therapeutic nurse/patient alliance that is the beginning of the therapeutic nurse/patient relationship. | 1(a) Developing a rapport with the patient will assist in gaining the patient's trust and cooperation in the future. Patients with borderline PD have trust issues that need to be dealt with in order for healing to occur. | 1(a) Somewhat distrustful but agrees to work with the assigned primary nurse during this hospitalization. |
| | (b) Initiate and maintain safety rounds or checks every 15 minutes. (c) Obtain a verbal contract with patient every shift and prn to seek out staff to talk rather than engage in self-mutilation. | (b) This measure ensures the patient's location and safety. (c) This patient is a high risk for self-mutilation. A behavior contract actively engages patients in their treatment and encourages personal responsibility for their behavior. It also demonstrates staff involvement. The patient's condition may change making it necessary to obtain another contract earlier than the next scheduled shift. | (b) States that she thinks having to have someone "watch" her "all the time" is "stupid." (c) Reluctantly contracts verbally to seek out staff rather than engage in self-mutilation. |
| | (d) Maintain an environment free from potentially harmful objects. | (d) This decreases opportunities for the patient to harm herself or others. | (d) Initally complained about not being able to have her own hair dryer with a long cord in her room, but later stated she understood the unit safety rules. |
| | (e) Assign the same nurses and other staff members to work with this patient throughout | (e) In addition to milieu therapy, this helps provide important consistency that the patient needs and | (e) Accepting of assigned nurses and staff members at this time. Attempted to obtain permission from a nurse *(continues)* |
| *Patient responses are examples of what students would look for to decide whether their planned interventions were successful, needed more time, or needed to be changed. Responses will vary depending on the patient. | | | |

| Assessment Data: O = Objective, S = Subjective | Evidence-Based Interventions: | Rationales: | Patient Responses: |
|---|---|---|---|
| | her hospitalization. When assigned primary nurses are not working, other nurses should defer any major decisions or requests from the patient to the primary assigned nurses. | helps reduce manipulative behavior. | temporarily assigned to the unit for one shift for personal possessions in locked area. |
| | (f) Observe patient both when she is aware and unaware of being observed. | (f) The patient's behavior may be different when she knows she is being observed versus when she does not know she is. This is true of patients who engage in manipulative behavior. | (f) Noted to be laughing and flirting with male patients on the unit, but when aware that staff is observing her behavior abruptly stops. |
| | (g) Explore reasons for engaging in self-mutilation. | (g) Patients engage in self-mutilation for various reasons including using it as a way to express intense emotions they cannot verbalize, attempting to manipulate someone else's behavior to fulfill patients' unmet needs or to not abandon/leave them; to decrease anxiety or to cause a physical release of endorphins that will in turn increase their mood. | (g) States that she "feels better" after she cuts herself and that her boyfriend usually feels sorry for her when she does this. |
| | (h) Understand that the patient may engage in manipulative or immature behavior when she feels personally or psychologically threatened. | (h) Patients with borderline PD freqently engage in immature behavior related to disturbed personal identify formation and regression to an earlier psychosocial developmental stage. | (h) Displays behavior seen in adolescent girls. Brought large stuffed animal collection along with her personal belongings at admission. Insists on having all 20 stuffed animals in her room. Remains on telephone longer than unit rules allow and complained to psychiatrist that she had been verbally redirected to allow someone else to use the telephone. |
| | (i) Perform a mental status exam every shift; ask the patient if she is aware that she has cut herself only after she has done so. | (i) The mental status exam includes areas such as thought processes and thought content, including suicidal/homicidal | (i) The patient shows poor judgment and poor insight regarding problem-solving and need for hospitalization. Denies any hallucinations or |

| Assessment Data: O = Objective, S = Subjective | Evidence-Based Interventions: | Rationales: | Patient Responses: |
|---|---|---|---|
| | | ideations, speech, psychomotor activity, appearance, cognition, and judgment and insight. Some patients engage in self-mutilation in response to auditory command hallucinations or during periods of dissociation. If hallucinations or dissociation is occurring, the patient will need treatment for these additional problems. | dissociative symptoms. Denies suicidal or homicidal ideations/plans. Dresses in seductive manner on unit and accepted verbal redirection for this. The remainder of the mental status exam is normal. |
| | (j) Assess anxiety level every shift and prn. | (j) As the patient's anxiety level increases, so does her risk of engaging in self-mutilation. | (j) Rates anxiety level an "8" on a scale of 0–10 where 0 = none and 10 = extremely severe. |
| | (k) Using a matter-of-fact tone of voice and nonjudgmental attitude, set limits on the patient's self-destructive behavior. | (k) The patient must not be allowed to engage in harmful or manipulative behavior. Using a matter-of-fact tone of voice and nonjudgmental attitude will help prevent the patient from perceiving the nurse as challenging, which could lead to a power struggle. | (k) Voiced her disagreement with the "rules," especially those related to telephone times and visiting hours. |
| | (l) Assist the patient to express feelings and fears of abandonment verbally and through the use of role-play, journaling, music, and drawing. | (l) These are healthy/adaptive ways of expressing feelings versus self-destructive/maladaptive means. | (l) Has difficulty expressing feelings, especially intense emotions including anger and love. Has difficulty talking about past sexual and physical abuse, but states that she does talk to her outpatient therapist about these issues "sometimes." Willing to try new ways of expressing her feelings. Stated that she fears being alone for the rest of her life. At times uncomfortable accepting emotional support from nurses and other staff members. |

*(continues)*

| Assessment Data:<br>O = Objective,<br>S = Subjective | Evidence-Based<br>Interventions: | Rationales: | Patient<br>Responses: |
|---|---|---|---|
| | (m) Explore the patient's concept of self and share how the staff sees her. | (m) Understanding how the patient views herself will help you begin to change her distorted perceptions by presenting reality. This process will take much time and will also be explored in psychotherapy. Even though patients engage in destructive ways of managing intense feelings or fears, they are also ashamed of their behavior and need to feel accepted as human beings deserving of care. | (m) Has a poor self-concept and difficulty identifying personal strengths. |
| | (n) Teach patient the difference between healthy and unhealthy boundaries. Guide patient in seeing where she has established unhealthy boundaries. | (n) Patients with borderline PD have established unhealthy boundaries and need education and assistance with understanding the difference between healthy and unhealthy. | (n) States that her outpatient therapist has mentioned these concepts, but still having some difficulty with how to establish healthy boundaries with people she had unhealthy ones with previously. |
| | (o) Teach patient anger management skills. | (o) Mismanagement of intense anger leads patients with borderline PD to act impulsively and destructively. | (o) Identifies own problem with anger management and willing to learn how to deal with this problem. |
| | (p) Remind patient to use techniques learned in DBT to decrease urges or engaging in self-mutilation. | (p) Dialectical behavioral therapy (DBT) is a type of long-term psychotherapy developed by M. Linehan specifically for the treatment of patients diagnosed with borderline PD. This therapy combines CBT with the concept of mindfulness. Patients are also taught techniques including impulse control, self-soothing, and how to appropriately ask for what they need. | (p) Admits that some of the DBT techniques she has learned are helpful if she is able to "remember to use them." |

**Evaluation:** 1. Has refrained from engaging in self-mutilation even though at times displaying immature and inappropriate behavior. Rates anxiety level an "8" on a scale of 0–10 where 0 = none and 10 = extremely severe. Contracted verbally to seek out staff rather than engage in self-mutilation, but did so reluctantly. Remains high risk for self-mutilation. Continue care plan and evaluate plan every shift and prn.

**Nursing Care Plan:** Methamphetamine abuse, borderline personality disorder.

**Nursing Diagnosis:** Ineffective Individual Coping r/t maladaptive coping strategies and poor problem-solving skills s/t borderline personality disorder and methamphetamine abuse AEB abusing methamphetamine, self-mutilation, and anxiety.

**Outcomes** (include time frames): 1. Will learn at least two positive coping strategies to continue using after discharge.

| Assessment Data: O = Objective, S = Subjective | Evidence-Based Interventions: | Rationales: | Patient Responses: |
|---|---|---|---|
| Methamphetamine abuse (O) UDS positive for amphetamines (O) Cuts self after fight with boyfriend (O) History of self-mutilation (O) Methamphetamine abuse (O) Difficulty expressing and dealing with intense emotions (O) History of sexual and physical abuse (O) | 1(a) Maintain an open, nonjudgmental attitude yet maintain appropriate professional boundaries when interacting and assessing patient. | 1(a) This is not only a therapeutic approach, but also a way to help the patient feel accepted and more willing to work with the nurse toward treatment goals and be more accepting of treatment in general. | 1(a) Positive response to nurse and other staff members' open, nonjudgmental attitude. |
| | (b) Assist to identify triggers to use methamphetamine and engage in other self-destructive behavior including self-mutilation. | (b) Once triggers are indentified, the nurse can work with the patient on ways to avoid these if possible or deal with them in ways that do not lead her to drink and abuse prescription pain medications. | (b) Identifies arguments with her boyfriend and feeling rejected by her family as triggers. At the suggestion of the nurse, agrees to a family meeting before being discharged with the approval of the psychiatrist. |
| | (c) Assess the patient's level of self-esteem. Assist with using personal strengths to obtain benefits of treatment. | (c) Some patients who abuse/depend on substances have very low self-esteem and use substances to cope. They need help believing they deserve help and can change. Many struggle with emotional dependency issues, dependent personality disorders, antisocial personality disorders, or anxiety. This patient also has to deal with issues related to childhood sexual and physical abuse that contribute to her poor self-concept and low self-esteem. | (c) Admits to having low self-esteem and difficulty identifying personal strengths. Agreed that she is intelligent and artistic when these strengths were identified by the nurse. Denies any physical attractiveness. Stated that she would think about attending a support group for survivors of sexual and physical abuse after discharge. |

*(continues)*

| Assessment Data:<br>O = Objective,<br>S = Subjective | Evidence-Based<br>Interventions: | Rationales: | Patient<br>Responses: |
|---|---|---|---|
| | (d) In psychoeducation, groups present topics that include self-esteem, taking personal responsibility for decisions and actions, empowerment, problem-solving methods, social skills, and anger and impulse management. | (d) These are important areas for patients with borderline PD and those with substance abuse problems to learn about and deal with. | (d) Attends psychoeducation group when reminded to do so. States that her outpatient therapist has been working with her regarding taking personal responsibility for her own decisions and actions. |
| | (e) Teach patient stress reduction and relaxation techniques including deep breathing, progressive relaxation exercises, meditation, yoga, guided imagery, appropriate exercise, aromatherapy, warm baths/showers, journaling, time management, financial budgeting, proper rest/sleep, attending to spiritual needs, and taking up new hobbies. | (e) These techniques provide healthier coping strategies for the patient. Also, some patients who abuse/depend on substances have problems with anxiety and these strategies will help decrease their anxiety. | (e) Already uses deep breathing, meditation, and journaling. Practicing progressive relaxation exercises and taking warm baths in the evening. Expresses interest in learning how to manage her time and money and taking a yoga class. |
| | (f) Assess social support network. | (f) Social support is important for emotional, mental, and physical healing. It also is important in preventing relapse and maintaining hope. Many patients with Borderline PD or Substance Abuse/Dependence have limited or no social support. | (f) Reports that her boyfriend is her strongest support. States that she has no close nonromantic friends to confide in and feels rejected by her family. |
| | (g) Discuss with patient healthy ways of maintaining relationships and coping with rejection. | (g) Patients with borderline PD alternately display clinging then pushing away behaviors in interpersonal relationships. One moment they are asking the person to stay and not leave and the next moment they are demanding that they leave them. This is confusing to others and increases the likelihood of the other person | (g) Admits to having difficulty maintaining relationships and engaging in both clinging and pushing away type behavior with her boyfriend and friends. Expresses interest in learning new behavior. |

| Assessment Data: O = Objective, S = Subjective | Evidence-Based Interventions: | Rationales: | Patient Responses: |
|---|---|---|---|
| | (h) Provide information on 12-step program support groups such as NA. Teach the importance of this type of support, including the role of a sponsor. | ending the relationship, which reinforces the patient's expectations of being rejected and abandoned. The patient needs to be clear and direct in her requests and actions with others. (h) Even though NA stands for Narcotics Anonymous, the addiction process is the same for any substances of abuse, and 12-step programs have provided successful methods to achieve and maintain abstinence along with a type of support that only those who also struggle with the same problems can give. | (h) States that she went to NA "a few times," but she "didn't get much out of it." Agreed to try going to a different group. |

**Evaluation:** 1. At this time practicing progressive relaxation exercises and taking warm baths in the evening. Expresses interest in learning how to manage her time and money and taking a yoga class. Continue care plan and evaluate in 48 hours.

**Nursing Care Plan:** Methamphetamine abuse, borderline personality disorder.
**Nursing Diagnosis:** Risk for Violence Toward Self or Others r/t difficulty regulating intense emotions and feelings of rejection and impulsivity s/t borderline personality disorder and methamphetamine abuse AEB cutting self after fight with boyfriend, intense reaction to the nurse's inability to have a social relationship with her, making statements such as, "If nobody here cares about me I might as well kill myself!," and a history of self-mutilation.
**Outcomes** (include time frames): 1. Will remain free from self-harm and refrain from harming others during the intake assessment process and throughout hospitalization.

| Assessment Data: O = Objective, S = Subjective | Evidence-Based Interventions: | Rationales: | Patient Responses: |
|---|---|---|---|
| Cuts self after fight with boyfriend (O) History of self-mutilation (O) Difficulty expressing intense emotions verbally or other healthy ways (O) Intense anger expressed toward nurse (O) Methamphetamine abuse—if intoxicated would potentially be violent (O) UDS positive for amphetamines (O) | 1(a) Continue to develop a rapport and a therapeutic nurse/patient alliance that is the beginning of a therapeutic relationship. (b) Perform a suicide risk assessment and obtain a verbal no harm to self or others contract with patient during the initial intake assessment process, every shift, and prn throughout hospitalization. | 1(a) This will help increase the patient's trust which can be used therapeutically to help her express herself or to cope in more adaptive ways rather than resorting to using violence. (b) Patients with borderline PD are at high risk for committing suicide or harming others due to extreme impulsivity, intense anger, and difficulty tolerating intense emotions. Also Substance abuse decreases inhibitions and increases the patient's risk of harming herself or others. A behavior contract actively engages patients in their treatment and encourages personal responsibility for their behavior. It also demonstrates staff involvement. The patient's condition may change making it necessary to obtain another contract earlier than the next scheduled shift. | 1(a) Upon admission was distrustful of nurses, but has agreed to work with them. Slowly becoming less distrustful and sharing more information about herself. (b) Verbally contracts to not harm self or others. Agrees to seek out staff to talk if she has suicidal thoughts, thoughts to harm others, or feels increased frustration or anger. |
| | (c) Maintain an environment free from potentially harmful objects. | (c) This decreases opportunities for the patient to harm herself or others. Even in a protective environment patients have managed to find some way to harm themselves or others making it important | (c) Unhappy that glass perfume bottles were locked in a secure area. |

| Assessment Data: O = Objective, S = Subjective | Evidence-Based Interventions: | Rationales: | Patient Responses: |
|---|---|---|---|
| | | to be vigilant in efforts to maintain a safe environment. Literally anything may be used if patients are truly intent on harming themselves. | |
| | (d) Initiate and maintain safety rounds or checks every 15 minutes. Assess for possibly needing to be placed on 1:1 or constant observation (COs). | (d) This measure ensures the patient's location and safety as well as the safety of other patients on the unit. While it may be true that some patients crave attention and try to manipulate nurses or other staff members, it is best to lower the risk of the patient attempting to harm herself or others. If the patient wants to be placed on 1:1 or COs for attention, she will soon grow tired of someone watching her that closely and being with her at all times at arm's length and will ask for this to be discontinued. | (d) Continues to say that needing someone to monitor her every 15 minutes is "stupid." No indication for 1:1 or COs at this time. |
| | (e) Decrease environmental stimuli (i.e., number of people in area, noise, light). | (e) A calm environment is less distracting or irritating and assists the patient to maintain control over impulsive or aggressive urges. | (e) Responds well to a calm environment. Less body tension noted. |
| | (f) Use a calm, matter-of-fact tone of voice when interacting with this patient and setting limits on her behavior. Refrain from arguing or engaging in power struggles with her. | (f) Because of difficulty tolerating intense emotions or limits on their actions, it is not unusual for patients with borderline PD to argue with staff and engage in power struggles related to unit rules. | (f) Less challenging behavior noted when nurse and other staff members use a calm, matter-of-fact tone of voice. |
| | (g) Encourage patient to use relaxation techniques, anger management, impulse control, and DBT techniques on a regular basis and when she feels | (g) The patient needs to use other methods to cope adaptively with stress, frustration, anger, or any intense emotion. Over time she will become more able | (g) Starting to use newly learned relaxation techniques and DBT techniques from out-patient therapy. |

*(continues)*

| Assessment Data:<br>O = Objective,<br>S = Subjective | Evidence-Based<br>Interventions: | Rationales: | Patient<br>Responses: |
|---|---|---|---|
| | stressed, frustrated, or angry or has other intense emotions.<br><br>(h) Administer scheduled and prn medication as ordered. Reinforce need to take medication consistently no matter how she feels. | to tolerate these feelings and react less often without thinking first about the consequences of her actions.<br>(h) A therapeutic, steady blood level must be achieved and maintained to help control her symptoms. There are also times when additional medication is needed if nonpharmacological methods are not effective in reducing anxiety. Increased anxiety can cause a patient to react impulsively without thinking, including actions that would harm themselves or others. | (h) Adheres to medication regimen. Accepts prn medication when offered, but does not ask for medication. |

**Evaluation:** 1. Remains free from harm to self or others. Continue care plan and evaluate in 24 hours.

# Question 10

There is a tendency for nurses to be judgmental of and disgusted by the behaviors of patients diagnosed with borderline personality disorder and to try avoid working with them. Another common reaction is to feel sorry for these patients and engage in rescuing behavior. Either extreme decreases the nurse's ability to be therapeutic. Transference and countertransference may also occur. It is very important to verbalize your feelings toward and thoughts about this patient to your fellow nurses, members of the treatment team, and other staff members. Verbalizing, discussing, and listening to each other will provide a more realistic appraisal of patients and your response to them.

These types of patients become very adept at manipulating and splitting staff, which may cause tension and disagreements among nurses and staff members. It is important not only to be aware of this but to guard against it, recognize it, and deal with it for the benefit of all of the staff and the patient. Maintaining a consistent approach, following the nursing care plans as well as the treatment team plan, and assisting each other to keep a realistic view of the patient will help decrease the effect and amount of patient manipulation. Protecting your own mental, physical, and spiritual health by engaging in various healthy lifestyle behaviors is important no matter what type of patient you work with and no matter what area of nursing you practice in. Because nurses vicariously witness and absorb negative energy or emotional trauma, it is necessary for them to release all this for their own mental, physical, and spiritual health. There are also times when nurses and staff members seek individual professional counseling on their own. This is perfectly acceptable and sometimes necessary to maintain mental integrity.

# References

Agency for Healthcare Research and Quality. (2006, June). *Mental health conditions and substance abuse. The guide to clinical preventive services 2006: Recommendations of the U.S. preventive services task force.* U.S. Dept. of Health and Human Services. Retrieved October 24, 2008, from http://www.ahrq.gov/clinic/uspstf/uspstopics.htm

American Psychiatric Association. (2000). *Diagnostic and statistical manual of mental disorders* (4th ed.). Washington, DC: Author.

Antai-Otong, D. (2004). *Psychiatric emergencies: How to accurately assess and manage the patient in crisis.* Eau Claire, WI: PESI Heatlthcare.

Clements, P. T. (2005, April). Working with individuals who have low impulse control. Psychiatric Nursing Conference, New Orleans.

Clements, P. T. (2007, June). Exploring and examining the development of personality disorders. Psychiatric Nursing Conference, New Orleans, LA.

Delaune, S. C. (2007, June). Setting effective professional boundaries: Walking the line and knowing where it is! Psychiatric Nursing Conference, New Orleans, LA.

Dunn, K., Elsom, S., & Cross, W. (2007). Self-efficacy and locus of control affect management of aggression by mental health nurses. *Issues in Mental Health Nursing, 28*(2), 201–217.

Fischbach, F. (2004). *A manual of laboratory and diagnositic tests* (7th ed.). Philadelphia, PA: Lippincott Williams & Wilkins.

Grunebaum, M. F., & Mann, J. J. (2007). Safe use of SSRIs in young adults: How strong is evidence for new suicide warning? *Current Psychiatry, 6*(11), 27–28, 35–37, 40–43.

Gupta, N. E. (2006, August). The crystal meth users in your practice. *The Clinical Advisor, 9*(8), 25–29.

Keltner, N. L., Schwecke, L. H., & Bostrom, C. E. (2007). *Psychiatric nursing* (5th ed.). St. Louis, MO: Mosby, Elsevier.

La Torre, M. A. (2002). Integrated perspectives: Enhancing therapeutic presence. *Perspectives in Psychiatric Care, 38*(1), 34–36.

Lewis, S. M., Heitkemper, M. M., & Dirksen, S. R. (2004). *Medical-surgical nursing: Assessment and management of clinical problems* (6th ed). St. Louis, MO: Mosby.

Marcus, P. (2007, June). Suicidal ideation: Assessment and prevention. Psychiatric Nursing Conference, New Orleans, LA.

*Miller-Keane encyclopedia of medicine, nursing and allied health* (7th ed.). (2003). Philadelphia: Elsevier Science, Saunders.

Myers, D. G. (2004). *Psychology* (7th ed.). New York: Worth Publishers.

Naegle, M. A., & Erickson D'Avanzo, C. (2001). *Addictions and substance abuse: Strategies for advanced practice nursing.* Upper Saddle River, NJ: Pearson Education.

O'Brien, P. G., Kennedy, W. Z., & Ballard, K. A. (2008). *Psychiatric mental health nursing: An introduction to theory and practice.* Sudbury, MA: Jones and Bartlett.

Sadock, B. J., & Sadock, V. A. (2003). *Kaplan and Sadock's synopsis of psychiatry: Behavioral sciences/clinical psychiatry* (9th ed.). Philadelphia, PA: Lippincott Williams & Wilkins.

Stong, C. (2006). Assessing suicide risk-separating attempts from ideation. *NeuroPschiatry Reviews, 7*(8), 1, 19.

Stuart, G. W., & Laraia, M. T. (2005). *Principles and practice of psychiatric nursing* (8th ed.). St. Louis, MO: Mosby, Elsevier.

Townsend, M. C. (2008). *Nursing diagnoses in psychiatric nursing* (7th ed.). Philadelphia, PA: F. A. Davis.

Varcarolis, E. M. (2006). *Manual of psychiatric nursing care plans* (3rd ed.). St. Louis, MO: Saunders, Elsevier.

Yigletu, H., Tucker, S., Harris, M., & Hatlevig, J. (2004). Assessing suicidal ideation: Comparing self-report versus clinician report. *American Psychiatric Nurses Association, 10*(1), 9–15.

# Web Sites

American Heart Association: www.americanheartassociation.org

American Psychiatric Association Continuing Medical Education (CME): www.psych.org/cme

American Psychiatric Databases: www.apa.org/psycinfo

American Psychological Association: www.apa.org

Centers for Disease Control and Prevention: www.cdc.gov

Clinicaltrials.gov: www.clinicaltrials.gov

Healthy People 2010: www.healthypeople.gov

National Institute on Alcohol Abuse and Alcoholism, National Institutes of Health: www.niaaa.nih.gov

National Institute on Drug Abuse, National Institutes of Health: www.nida.nih.gov

Psychiatry.com: www.psychiatry.com

United States Department of Health and Human Services, Substance Abuse and Mental Health Services Administration: www.samhsa.gov

Your Total Health NBC and iVillage: yourtotalhealth.ivillage.com

# CHAPTER 5

# Eating Disorders: Anorexia Nervosa

## Question 1

CBC: RBCs = 3.2 (women = 3.6–5, men 4.2–5.4), Hgb = 11 (women = 12–16, men = 14–18), Hct = 34% (women = 36–48%, men = 42–52%), MCV = 70 (82–100), MCH = 20 (26–34), and MCHC = 28 (32–36)

Electrolytes: Na = 148 (135–145), K = 2.8 (3.5–5.3), Ca (total) = 10.8 (8.8–10.4), Mg = 2.8 (1.8–2.6)

Glucose = 64 (70–110)

WBCs = 6 (4.5–10.5)

BUN = 4.5 (6–20)

Creatinine = 1.0 (0.8–1.2)

GFR = 125 (125 ml per hour; normal range adjusted by individual laboratories to account for the aging process)

Albumin = 2.4 (3.5–4.8)

Total protein = 4.8 (6–8)

TSH = 2.0 (0.4–4.2)

Total T3 = 125 (80–200)

T3 Uptake = 1.0 (0.9–1.10)

Total T4 = 60 (5.4–11.5)

Free T4 = 1.0 (0.7–2)

UDS/urine toxicology = + for amphetamines (negative)

EKG/ECG = abnormal, irregular rate, bradycardia, flattened T wave (normal, NSR)

# Question 2

A nutrition stabilization contract is a behavioral contract that is used in behavioral therapy. Included in the contract are items such as the behavior identified as needing to be changed, specific goals, ways to reach those goals, rewards and consequences for work toward goals, or sabotage behaviors. In this case it would be specific to nutritional needs including agreeing to eat a specific number of calories per day to be gradually increased to not only help the patient attain a normal body weight, but also repair damage to the body that has occured. The contract would also include refraining from engaging in compensatory behaviors and rewards for refraining. Rewards cannot be anything related to food. The nutrition stabilization contract would be formulated as a collaborative effort with the patient and encourages patient responsibility and accountability for their own behavior.

# Question 3

Patients with eating disorders obsess about their weight. They weigh themselves daily and possibly more often. Visualizing the number on the scale can negatively reinforce the cognitive distortion that they still weigh too much. If they are experiencing healthy weight gain, it may be too frightening for them to see the number and it may cause them to relapse into old, unhealthy behaviors.

Weighing the patient before breakfast will provide a more accurate weight. Patients wearing hospital gowns will be less able to hide objects in clothing pockets or shoes to add to their weight, giving a false impression that they are making progress.

# Question 4

Patients who have AN restrict food. They are adept at hiding food in the buccal pouch of their mouths or in napkins or pockets to dispose of later in any available receptacle, including trashcans, toilets, sinks, and even potted plants. Also, if patients have the AN subtype of binging/purging they will use the bathroom to dispose of food they have actually eaten through self-induced vomiting. (The same would be true of patients diagnosed with BN.)

# Question 5

Food diaries are used as assessment and teaching tools. Patients not only record what they actually eat, including calories and food groups, but also feelings and situations that accompany the feelings. Triggers that increase anxiety and provoke use of compensatory behaviors can be identified through these diaries. Diaries are reviewed with patients to help them verbalize strong emotions, explore sensitive issues, and look at healthier, more adaptive ways of coping rather than using the maladaptive coping of the eating disorder.

# Questions 6 and 7

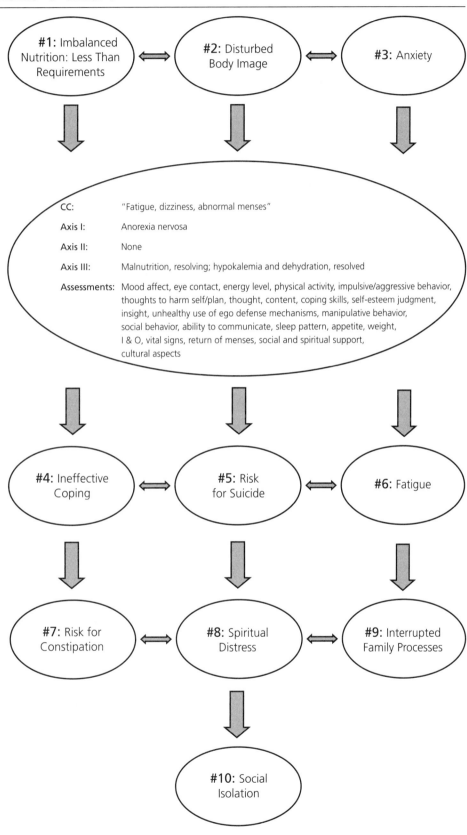

CC:        "Fatigue, dizziness, abnormal menses"

Axis I:    Anorexia nervosa

Axis II:   None

Axis III:  Malnutrition, resolving; hypokalemia and dehydration, resolved

Assessments: Mood affect, eye contact, energy level, physical activity, impulsive/aggressive behavior, thoughts to harm self/plan, thought, content, coping skills, self-esteem judgment, insight, unhealthy use of ego defense mechanisms, manipulative behavior, social behavior, ability to communicate, sleep pattern, appetite, weight, I & O, vital signs, return of menses, social and spiritual support, cultural aspects

#1: Imbalanced Nutrition: Less Than Requirements

#2: Disturbed Body Image

#3: Anxiety

#4: Ineffective Coping

#5: Risk for Suicide

#6: Fatigue

#7: Risk for Constipation

#8: Spiritual Distress

#9: Interrupted Family Processes

#10: Social Isolation

# Questions 8 and 9

**Nursing Care Plan:** Anorexia nervosa, malnutrition, resolving; hypokalemia and dehydration, resolved.
**Nursing Diagnosis:** Imbalanced Nutrition: Less Than Body Requirements r/t excessive fear of gaining weight s/t anorexia nervosa AEB compensatory behaviors of reported daily intake of 600 calories, overexercising, abusing OTC diet pills and diuretics, and remaining abnormal laboratory test results: RBCs = 3.2, Hgb = 11, Hct = 34%, MCV = 70, MCH = 20, MCHC = 28; albumin = 2.4, and total protein = 4.8.
**Outcomes** (include time frames): 1. Will eat at least 75% of all meals and snacks in 72 hours. 2. Will gain at least 2 lbs. during 1st week of hospitalization.

| Assessment Data: O = Objective, S = Subjective | Evidence-Based Interventions: | Rationales: | Patient Responses:* |
|---|---|---|---|
| Reported daily intake of 600 calories (S) Admits to overexercising at least 3 hours per day (S) Reported abuse of OTC diet pills and diuretics (S) Complains about fatigue (S) Complains about dizziness (S) Reports abnormal menses (S) Admission weight less than 85% of ideal body weight (O) Poor skin turgor (O) Remaining abnormal laboratory test results: RBCs = 3.2, Hgb = 11, Hct = 34%, MCV = 70, MCH = 20, MCHC = 28; albumin = 2.4, and total protein = 4.8 (O) Initial laboratory and diagnostics test results also showed electrolyte imbalance, UDS + for amphetamines, and abnormal ECG/EKG (O) | 1(a) Strict monitoring of intake and output every shift. (b) Maintain constant observation during all meal and snack times every shift. (c) Observe for behaviors such as taking a longer than normal time to finish meals and cutting food into very small pieces. (d) Encourage patient to continue eating even if she complains that she feels "full" after only a few bites of food. | 1(a) This helps provide a more accurate account of what the patient is eating, drinking, and eliminating. (b) Patients with eating disorders can be very manipulative because they believe they have to engage in this behavior and will take every opportunity to hide and later get rid of food. It only takes a few seconds to put food in a pocket or napkin to be disposed of later. (c) Patients with eating disorders try to take a very long time to eat to avoid having to finish a meal or snack. Frequently they cut food up into very small pieces making it look like they have eaten more than they actually have. This also takes up time during the meal. (d) Patients frequently complain of being full after eating only a small amount of food. They restrict their food intake and it makes sense that | 1(a) States "this is silly," but compliant with measuring and recording of all intake and output. (b) Unhappy about being on constant observation during all meal and snack times. (c) Observed cutting up food into very small pieces during meals. (d) Frequently states that she feels full during meals after eating only a few bites of food. Requires much encouragement to continue eating. |

*Patient responses are examples of what students would look for to decide whether their planned interventions were successful, needed more time, or needed to be changed. Responses will vary depending on the patient.

| Assessment Data: O = Objective, S = Subjective | Evidence-Based Interventions: | Rationales: | Patient Responses: |
|---|---|---|---|
| | | they would "feel" full, but they are misinterpreting the presence of food in their stomachs for being "full." | |
| | (e) Continue constant observation and restrict access to bathroom for at least 1 hour after all meal and snack times. | (e) Patients are adept at hiding food in the buccal pouch of their mouths, napkins, or pockets to dispose of later in any available receptacle including trashcans, toilets, sinks, and even potted plants. Also, if patients have the subtype of binging/purging, they will use the bathroom to dispose of food they have actually eaten through self-induced vomiting. (The same would be true of patients diagnosed with BN). | (e) Unhappy regarding continued constant observation and restriction of access to bathroom after all meals and snacks. States that her parents do not do that. |
| | (f) Encourage to keep up with food diary entries and if willing to explore contents of food diary. | (f) Food diaries are used as assessment and teaching tools. Patients not only record what they actually eat, including calories and food groups, but also feelings and situations that accompany the feelings. Triggers that increase anxiety and provoke use of compensatory behaviors can be identified through these diaries. Patients discuss the contents of food diaries with psychotherapists, psychiatrists, and nurses. Any discussion with patients should be followed up with careful documentation in patient records and notification of the treatment team. Although the food | (f) Has been making daily entries in her food diary. |

*(continues)*

| Assessment Data: O = Objective, S = Subjective | Evidence-Based Interventions: | Rationales: | Patient Responses: |
|---|---|---|---|
| | | diaries contain information related to food intake, the focus of discussion should be on the accompanying feelings and thoughts recorded. | |
| | (g) Assist with meal planning and healthy food choices while attempting to include patient preferences. | (g) Many patients do no know what healthy meal planning and choices consist of and need assistance with this. Including patient preferences when possible increases chances of patient cooperation and adherence. | (g) States that she did not know she needed to eat so much protein every day. States that she thought all protein was "high fat." |
| | (h) Administer Prozac 60 mg po daily as ordered. | (h) Prozac frequently is used in the treatment of eating disorders with doses at the higher end of the recommended dose range (e.g., 60–80 mg po daily). Prozac is protein-bound in the bloodstream. The patient needs to have enough protein intake for Prozac to be effective. | (h) Agreeable to taking Prozac at this time. |
| | (i) Administer nutritional supplements if ordered. | (i) Nutritional supplements such as Ensure or Boost may be needed initially to provide enough calories, vitamins, and minerals until patients are eating more normally and regularly. | (i) At this time the patient does not have an order for nutritional supplements other than a multivitamin with iron. |
| | (j) Offer emotional support when patient complains of abdominal pain when eating and drinking fluids. | (j) Patients frequently complain of abdominal pain when first starting to eat more normally again. They also frequently complain of constipation while waiting for their body to reestablish a normal bowel pattern again following laxative abuse. | (j) Frequently complains of abdominal pain after meals. |
| | (k) Ask about her family's attitudes toward food. | (k) In families of patients with eating disorders, | (k) States that her family frequently celebrates with food |

| Assessment Data:<br>O = Objective,<br>S = Subjective | Evidence-Based<br>Interventions: | Rationales: | Patient<br>Responses: |
|---|---|---|---|
| | | there may be too much emphasis on food, or there is too much concern about becoming overweight. Frequently another family member has an eating disorder or engages in eating disorder type behavior. | and that she has overweight relatives. |
| | 2(a) Weigh twice weekly before breakfast after emptying bladder on the same scale with her back to the scale. | 2(a) Patients with eating disorders obsess about their weight. They weigh themselves daily and possibly more often. Weighing the patient before breakfast using the same scale will provide a more accurate weight. Emptying the bladder decreases the effect of drinking large amounts of water prior to being weighed in order to give a false impression of working toward weight goals. Visualizing the number on the scale can negatively reinforce the cognitive distortion that they still weigh too much. Also, if they are experiencing healthy weight gain, it may be too frightening for them to see the number and cause them to relapse into old, unhealthy behaviors. | 2(a) Asks to be weighed every day and disagrees that twice a week is enough. Becomes anxious when told she has gained a half a pound. |
| | (b) Patient should be wearing hospital gown only, without shoes, before being weighed. | (b) Patients wearing hospital gowns will be less able to hide objects in clothing pockets or shoes to add to their weight, giving a false impression that they are making progress. | (b) Asks why she can't be weighed in her regular clothing because that is what she does at home. Disagrees with explanation given. |

*(continues)*

| Assessment Data: O = Objective, S = Subjective | Evidence-Based Interventions: | Rationales: | Patient Responses: |
|---|---|---|---|
| | (c) Maintain nutrition stabilization contract. | (c) The nutrition stabilization contract is a behavioral therapy method that increases the success of patients reaching collaboratively established goals. It also encourages patients to take responsibility and accountability for their own behavior. | (c) Participates in the establishment of a nutrition stabilization contract. At this time she is adhering to the contract. States that she entered into the contract only "to keep my mother happy." |
| | (d) Reinforce psychiatrist's discussion of abnormal laboratory test results and danger to physical health. | (d) Many patients do not realize the negative effect their compensatory behaviors have on their physical health. They focus only on what they see are the benefits (i.e., weight loss). | (d) At this time the patient is in denial, as evidenced by her refusal to believe that her compensatory behaviors caused her abnormal laboratory test results either currently or while in the ICU. |
| | (e) Teach age-appropriate norms for exercise amount and type. | (e) Many patients do not know what is appropriate or normal regarding exercise amounts or type. | (e) Continues to state that she believes exercising for at least 3 hours a day is normal. |
| | (f) Teach guidelines regarding normal weight for height and body structure. | (f) Many patients do not know what is considered to be normal weight for their height and body structure. They look at media images and assume that the images are correct no matter what their own height, body structure, and genetics are. | (f) Disagrees with what is a normal weight range for her height and body structure. States that she is "too fat." |
| | (g) Discuss relationship between normal body weight and regular menses. | (g) Many patients do not know that body weight and nutrition have a correlation with their menses. | (g) Quietly stated that she did not know her body weight or nutrition had anything to do with her menses. |

**Evaluation:** 1. Eating less than 75% of all meals and snacks. May need additional nutritional supplements. 2. Has gained a half pound accompanied by increased anxiety. Continue plan and evaluate in 24 hours.

**Nursing Care Plan:** Anorexia nervosa, malnutrition, resolving; hypokalemia and dehydration, resolved.
**Nursing Diagnosis:** Disturbed Body Image r/t cognitive distortions AEB fear of gaining weight, states she thinks she is too fat in spite of weighing 85% less of her ideal body weight, and use of compensatory behaviors.
**Outcomes** (include time frames): 1. Will begin to examine her own beliefs about what her body should look like by the end of the 1st week of hospitalization. 2. Will state at least two positive aspects of self by the end of the 1st week of hospitalization.

| Assessment Data: O = Objective, S = Subjective | Evidence-Based Interventions: | Rationales: | Patient Responses: |
|---|---|---|---|
| Reports she thinks she is too fat (S) Reported use of compensatory behaviors (S) Weighs less than 85% of her ideal body weight (O) | 1(a) Ask patient to describe verbally and then to draw what she thinks the ideal body should look like.

(b) Ask patient to verbally describe and then draw what she thinks she looks like.



(c) Ask patient to compare her verbal descriptions and drawings of the ideal body and her own body.

(d) Discuss the differences between what she believes is the ideal body and her own body, but avoid minimizing her thoughts and feelings. State that you realize she believes this to be the truth. | 1(a) Patients frequently have unrealistic views of what an ideal body should look like. Unfortunately, this is made worse by media images. (b) Frequently patients have inaccurate, usually negative, views of what they think they look like.

(c) Comparing the two gives the nurse and the treatment team a better understanding of how distorted her thinking is. (d) Discussing the differences helps clarify her erroneous beliefs and can be the start of helping her examine her unrealistic thoughts. By not minimizing the patient's thoughts and feelings, you establish trust and show that you recognize that she believes her thoughts and feelings to be the truth. It also shows that you understand what she is saying without agreeing that it is the truth. It will take time, cognitive-behavioral psychotherapy, and psychoeducation to begin changing her thoughts and feelings. Arguing with her would not be therapeutic. | 1(a) She verbally describes and draws an extremely thin, tall female. She writes the word "BEAUTIFUL" in large capital letters. She herself is thin, but short in stature. (b) She verbally describes and draws an overweight body form that is even shorter than her actual height. She writes the words "FAT" and "UGLY" in large, capital letters. (c) There are major differences in the patient's view of the ideal body and her own body.


(d) Sat quietly and listened while the nurse talked about the differences. |

*(continues)*

| Assessment Data: O = Objective, S = Subjective | Evidence-Based Interventions: | Rationales: | Patient Responses: |
|---|---|---|---|
| | (e) Encourage the patient to verbalize feelings related to what she believes to be the ideal body and her own body. | (e) Verbalization of feelings helps clarify for the nurse and the treatment team what the patient's personal feelings and issues are related to the ideal body and her own body. This will be a starting point to build on in therapy. | (e) States that she feels worthless and ugly because her body does not look like what she imagines to be the ideal body. |
| | (f) Introduce facts and reinforce reality by telling her how you actually see her. Begin to assist patient to differentiate between facts, thoughts, and feelings. | (f) Patients mistake their own thoughts and feelings as reality and facts. When this is directly pointed out to them, they can begin to change. Initially they may disagree, but in time they eventually begin to see the difference. | (f) States that she believes her own thoughts and feelings are the truth because they are so strong. |
| | (g) Ask about her family's ideas about weight and body shape and size. | (g) Family and cultural influences are very strong. Overemphasis on physical attractiveness to the exclusion of other positive attributes can have negative effects on body image and self-esteem of children and adolescents. | (g) States that her mother is "always worried about her weight" and that there are overweight relatives in the family. "I don't want to look like them." |
| | 2(a) Ask patient to list both positive and negative attributes of herself. | 2(a) This gives a clear picture of how the patient thinks and feels about herself. Someone with a disturbed body image and low self-esteem will have great difficulty listing or identifying anything positive about themselves. They will also have great difficulty listing or identifying nonphysical attributes. | 2(a) Hesitant at first because she has not been asked to do this before. |
| | (b) Ask patient to separate all the identified positive and negative physical attributes. | (b) Many times there are many physical attributes but few nonphysical attributes. | (b) Listed mostly negative physical attributes and only a few nonphysical attributes. |
| | (c) Assist patient to focus on positive nonphysical attributes. | (c) The patient may not be used to thinking about herself in nonphysical | (c) Had difficulty with this but finally said, "Oh, I see what you mean." |

| Assessment Data: O = Objective, S = Subjective | Evidence-Based Interventions: | Rationales: | Patient Responses: |
|---|---|---|---|
| | (d) Describe what positive nonphysical attributes you identify in her. (e) Add positive physical attributes you recognize in her. (f) Assist patient to choose two positive attributes—either nonphysical or physical—from all the ones identified by both you and the patient. (g) Instruct patient to keep a list of these positive attributes with her and to look at it every time she starts to think or feel negatively about herself. (h) Ask patient to add at least one more positive attribute to the list each week. | terms and will need help thinking about herself in more than physical terms. (d) This will provide reality, facts, and positive feedback. (e) See (d). (f) This is a collaborative intervention while reinforcing positive attributes. (g) This provides positive reinforcement and helps decrease negative thinking. It is something the patient can do on her own. (h) This will build upon the initial activity and continually reinforce that the patient has several positive attributes. | (d) Sat quietly and listened as positive nonphysical attributes were identified. (e) See (d). (f) With encouragement and assistance, was able to choose her intelligence and musical abilities as positive nonphysical attributes. Also identified her hair and eyes as positive physical attributes. (g) Stated that she would try to do this. (h) Agrees to add to the list on a weekly basis. |

**Evaluation:** 1. Only beginning to differentiate between her own thoughts and feelings regarding the ideal body image versus a more realistic body image.
2. Able to identify two positive nonphysical attributes and two positive physical attributes with encouragement and assistance. Continue care plan and evaluate in 72 hours.

**Nursing Care Plan:** Anorexia nervosa, malnutrition, resolving; hypokalemia and dehydration, resolved.
**Nursing Diagnosis:** Anxiety r/t ineffective coping AEB stating she feels in control of her life as long as she controls her weight and cognitive distortions regarding body image.
**Outcomes** (include time frames): 1. Will identify at least three triggers of increased anxiety within 72 hours of admission. 2. Will state at least three healthy ways she can manage anxiety and stress within 72 hours of admission.

| Assessment Data:<br>O = Objective,<br>S = Subjective | Evidence-Based<br>Interventions: | Rationales: | Patient<br>Responses: |
|---|---|---|---|
| States that she feels in control of her life as long as she controls her weight (S)<br>Reported use of compensatory behaviors (S)<br>Weighs less than 85% of her ideal body weight (O)<br>Admitted to ICU prior to being transferred to the psychiatric unit (O)<br>Agreed to nutrition stabilization contract to please her mother (S) | 1(a) Explore what situations, events, or people trigger anxiety for this patient.<br><br>(b) Assist patient to rank stressors in order from the most to the least anxiety producing.<br><br>(c) Assist patient to verbalize thoughts and feelings related to stressors rather than weight or food.<br><br>(d) Assess risk for suicide and obtain a verbal no self-harm contract with patient every shift and prn.<br><br>(e) Maintain safety checks every 15 minutes and safe environment as ordered. | 1(a) Exploring specific triggers that increase anxiety will help clarify what precipitates the patient's use of compensatory behaviors and perpetuates the eating disorder.<br><br>(b) Ranking stressors in order will help later on to decide which stressors to work with in psychotherapy.<br><br>(c) The stressors and the accompanying thoughts and feelings are the real underlying issues. Many patients attempt to engage nurses and staff members in talking about weight and food, but that is just a digression that enables them to avoid thinking about and dealing with deeper problems.<br><br>(d) The patient is at risk for committing suicide. Patients with eating disorders not only are anxious but also impulsive. In addition, the patient is an adolescent and adolescents frequently engage in impulsive behavior.<br><br>(e) Again, the patient is anxious and prone to impulsive behavior. Closely monitoring her location, activity, and environment helps ensure safety. | 1(a) Able to identify situations such as family conflict, parental arguments, father traveling frequently related to work obligations, school, and time pressure as significant situations that trigger increased anxiety.<br>(b) Able to rank stressors with assistance.<br><br>(c) Tries to avoid talking about stressors once identified. Would rather talk about weight, physical appearance, and food.<br><br>(d) No history of prior suicide attempts, plans, or ideations. Denies suicidal ideations at this time. Able to contract verbally not to harm self. Agrees to tell a staff member if she has suicidal thoughts.<br><br>(e) Curious about reason for safety checks, but cooperative. |

| Assessment Data: O = Objective, S = Subjective | Evidence-Based Interventions: | Rationales: | Patient Responses: |
|---|---|---|---|
| | 2(a) Assess coping strategies used and discourage compensatory eating disorder behaviors. | 2(a) Positive, healthy coping strategies should be reinforced and encouraged. Negative, unhealthy coping strategies should be identified and replaced with positive ones. | 2(a) States that she used to enjoy playing the violin but has not done so for some time due to needing to exercise at least 3 hours each day. |
| | (b) Encourage patient to begin practicing the violin again; explain that it is not necessary to exercise at least 3 hours per day to be healthy. | (b) The patient needs encouragement to let go of unhealthy behavior and return to using a formerly helpful coping strategy. | (b) States that it would be nice to play her violin again. Plans to ask the psychiatrist if her parents can bring her violin to her while she is still hospitalized. Verbalizes understanding that if her request is granted she will have to be observed while playing and have the violin stored in a locked area because the strings on the instrument and the bow present a potential means of harming herself. |
| | (c) Begin teaching stress management techniques such as deep breathing exercises, progressive muscle relaxation exercises, meditation, guided imagery time management, journaling feelings and thoughts, and assertive communication techniques. Allow the patient to choose three to start with. | (c) There are many stress management options available to help the patient cope more adaptively with stress, decrease anxiety, and experience more control over her own reactions, thus empowering her. By starting with only three you can avoid overwhelming the patient; allowing her choices about which to begin with fosters collaboration. | (c) Expresses interest in learning healthy ways to cope and manage stress. Chooses to start with deep breathing, meditation, and guided imagery. |

**Evaluation:** 1. Identified five situations that trigger an increase in her anxiety and ranked them from highest to lowest in significance with assistance. Once identified, tries to avoid talking about them.
2. Choosing to learn deep breathing, meditation, and guided imagery techniques. Continue plan and evaluate in 48 hours.

# Question 10

The best sources would be Eating Disorders and Emotions Anonymous support groups in their community. Also, the local chapter of the National Alliance on Mental Illness (NAMI) is helpful for education as well as support.

The following Web sites can provide helpful information:

Anorexia and Related Disorders, Inc. (ANRED): www.anred.com

Eating Disorders Referral and Information Center: www.edreferral.com

The National Association of Anorexia and Associated Eating Disorders (ANAD): www.anad.org

The National Eating Disorders Association (NEDA): www.nationaleating disorders.org

# Question 11

Individual and group psychotherapy for the patient including CBT and IPT. Family counseling and psychoeducation including the following areas:

a. Signs and symptoms of eating disorders

b. Signs of relapse and relapse prevention

c. Exploring general family values

d. Exploring family beliefs surrounding food

e. Teaching goals:

- Stop focusing on eating.

- Give compliments for talents, abilities, or accomplishments, *not* appearance.

- Improve communication skills.

- Use stress reduction techniques and healthy coping strategies.

- Learn the difference between overinvolvement (enmeshment) and normal care and concern.

# References

Abayomi, J., & Hackett, A. (2004). Assessment of malnutrition in mental health clients: Nurses' judgement vs. nutrition risk tool. *Journal of Advanced Nursing, 45*(4), 430–437.

American Psychiatric Association. (2000). *Diagnostic and statistical manual of mental disorders* (4th ed.). Washington, DC: Author.

Bezchlibnyk-Butler, K. Z., & Jeffries, J. J. (2005). *Clinical handbook of psychotropic drugs* (15th ed.). Ashland, OH: Hogrefe & Huber.

Boyd, M. A. (2002). *Psychiatric nursing: Contemporary practice* (2nd ed.). Philadephia: Lippincott Williams & Wilkins.

Delaune, S. C. (2007, June). Presentation: Setting effective professional boundaries: Walking the line and knowing where it is! Psychiatric Nursing Conference, New Orleans, LA.

Dichter, J. R., Cohen, J., & Connolly, P. M. (2002). Bulimia nervosa: Knowledge, awareness, and skill levels among advanced practice nurses. *Journal of the American Academy of Nurse Practitioners, 14*(6), 269–275.

Fischbach, F. (2004). *A manual of laboratory and diagnositic tests* (7th ed.). Philadelphia, PA: Lippincott Williams & Wilkins.

Fontaine, K. L., & Fletcher, J. S. (2003). *Mental health nursing* (5th ed.). Upper Saddle River, NJ: Pearson.

Hoerr, S. L., Bokram, R., Lugo, B., Bivins, T., & Keast, D. R. (2002). Risk for disordered eating relates to both gender and ethnicity for college students. *Journal of the American College of Nutrition, 21*(4), 307–314.

Keltner, N. L., Schwecke, L. H., & Bostrom, C. E. (2007). *Psychiatric nursing* (5th ed.). St. Louis, MO: Mosby, Elsevier.

Lewis, S. M., Heitkemper, M. M., & Dirkson, S. R. (2004). *Medical-Surgical nursing: Assessment strategies and management of clinical problems* (6th ed.). St. Louis, MO: Mosby.

McKenry, L., Tessier, E., & Hogan, M. (2006). *Mosby's pharmacology in nursing* (22nd ed.). St. Louis, MO: Mosby.

O'Brien, P. G., Kennedy, W. Z., & Ballard, K. A. (2008). *Psychiatric mental health nursing: An introduction to theory and practice.* Sudbury, MA: Jones and Bartlett.

Sadock, B. J., & Sadock, V. A. (2003). *Kaplan and Sadock's synopsis of psychiatry: Behavioral sciences/clinical psychiatry* (9th ed.). Philadelphia, PA: Lippincott Williams & Wilkins.

Sadock, B. J., & Sadock, V. A. (2005). *Kaplan and Sadock's comprehensive textbook of psychiatry* (8th ed.). Philadelphia, PA: Lippincott Williams & Wilkins.

*Saunders 2005 nursing drug handbook.* St. Louis, MO: Mosby.

Varcarolis, E. M. (2006). *Manual of psychiatric nursing care plans* (3rd ed.). St. Louis, MO: Saunders, Elsevier.

Varcarolis, E. M., Carson, V. B., & Shoemaker, N. C. (2006). *Foundations of psychiatric mental health nursing: A clinical approach* (6th ed.). St. Louis, MO: Saunders, Elsevier.

# CHAPTER 6

# Substance Abuse/Dependence: Alcohol Dependence and Opiate Abuse

## ANSWER KEY

## Question 1

The patient did not reveal any information about his drinking to the employee assistance program counselor until the 4th week of counseling sessions. He may have feared being fired if this information were known. He did not reveal any information regarding opiate abuse until the social worker at the outpatient program interviewed him. Frequently patients with substance abuse/ dependence problems do not divulge complete information at the beginning of assessment and initial treatment. They may minimize the amount or frequency of use. This behavior may be due to several reasons, including extreme denial of the seriousness of their problem, fear of negative consequences such being fired, being rejected by nurses and other healthcare professionals, or being rejected and abandoned by family members or friends who do not abuse/depend on substances.

It is important to know exactly how much and how often a patient uses substances to be able to safely treat and care for withdrawal signs, symptoms, and impending medical complications. If a nurse has a nonjudgmental, accepting attitude and explains these reasons to patients, they usually are more cooperative and willing to share necessary information. People who abuse/depend on substances usually prefer certain types of substances, but if they are not able to obtain them, they will use any available psychoactive substance in order to achieve a similar feeling or avoid withdrawal. The other available substances may not even be in the same category (e.g., opiate, amphetamine, hallucinogen) as their preferred substances, and this can cause additional unexpected physical complications that may need to be treated as well to prevent further harm. It is much safer to know this in the beginning rather than have to suddenly deal with unexpected changes in the patient's condition later in the detoxification process.

# Question 2

a. What day and time the patient last drank and used OxyContin/oxycodone?

b. How much did he drink and use at that time compared to how much he usually drinks and uses?

c. What triggers to drink and use can he identify?

d. Does he currently use any other substances? What did he use in the past?

e. Has he ever had DTs when abstaining from drinking?

f. Has he ever experienced blackouts?

g. Does he drink to the point of passing out?

h. How old was he when he started drinking? When he started abusing OxyContin/oxycodone?

i. If he was originally prescribed OxyContin/oxycodone for pain at least 2 years ago, how has he been obtaining more of this medication?

j. Is he currently engaged in illegal activities (e.g., theft, prostitution, dealing/selling drugs) to obtain substances? In the past?

k. Does he have any current or past legal charges or problems?

l. Has he ever been treated for substance abuse/dependence problems?

m. Has he ever tried a 12-step program?

n. What was the longest period of sobriety or abstinence from any substance that he ever experienced? When was that and for how long?

o. If he had a period of sobriety or abstinence, what does he think triggered his current use/dependence?

p. Has he ever been diagnosed or treated for any other mental health problems or medical problems?

q. Does he currently, or has he ever, experienced signs and symptoms of depression or mania (refer to chapter on mood disorders )?

r. Is he being prescribed any other medication or under a physician's care for any other problems?

s. Is there any current or past use of IV drugs, tobacco products, OTC medications, herbals, steroids, or supplements?

# Question 3

Librium/chlordiazepoxide is classified as a benzodiazepine and causes decreased anxiety and sedation by binding to gamma-butyric acid (GABA) receptors in the brain. It is one of the medications routinely used to treat or prevent signs and symptoms of alcohol withdrawal (including seizures) during detoxification treatment. Typically the dose is tapered by decreasing it by half every 2 days until it is discontinued to allow the CNS to adjust to decreasing alcohol and benzodiazepine levels and to avoid seizures.

a. Other medications frequently used include Ativan/lorazepam, Serax/oxazepam, Tranxene/clorazepate, or Valium/diazepam.

# Question 4

Signs and symptoms of alcohol withdrawal include nausea, vomiting, diarrhea, diaphoresis, tremulousness, elevated vital signs, irritability, subjective feelings of restlessness or observable psychomotor agitation, impulsive behavior, verbal or physical agitation, hyperreflexia, insomnia, and headache. As withdrawal progresses, patients may develop auditor or visual hallucinations.

Patients who develop DTs will experience grand mal seizures, increased auditory or visual hallucinations, tactile hallucinations (e.g., sensations of skin crawling or bugs crawling on the skin), increased agitation, possible physical aggressiveness, confusion, disorientation, and cardiac arrhythmias. Death may result from cardiovascular complications or respiratory complications secondary to status epilepticus. DTs occur in a patient who drinks heavily.

a. Early withdrawal usually begins approximately 6 to 8 hours after the last drink, and it will peak 24 to 48 hours after that.

b. DTs may begin typically 48 hours after the last drink, peaking in 48 to 72 hours from the beginning signs of DTs.

# Question 5

Signs and symptoms of opiate withdrawal include restlessness, irritability, rhinorrhea (runny nose), lacrimation (tearing of eyes), diaphoresis, elevated vital signs, nausea, vomiting, diarrhea, myalgia (muscle aching), arthralgia (joint aching), goose bumps/gooseflesh; visual, auditory, or tactile hallucinations, and insomnia.

    a. Catepres/clonidine is ordered to control blood pressure and prevent a sudden increase in blood pressure due to opiate withdrawal. Sudden development of hypertension is the most potentially serious medical complication of opiate withdrawal.

# Question 6

Any patient who abuses or depends on substances is at risk for malnutrition as well as dehydration. Typically the patient prefers to spend money on substances rather than nutritious food and prefers to drink or use drugs rather than eat. Deficiencies of most vitamins and minerals, especially thiamine/vitamin $B_1$, magnesium, folic acid, and cyanocobalamin/vitamin $B_{12}$ frequently occur and may cause additional physical or mental symptoms. Thiamine, a water soluble vitamin, is important for protection of the peripheral nervous system and carbohydrate metabolism. It is given to prevent the development or worsening of Wernike-Korsakoff syndrome (see Glossary). The brain needs glucose to function and thiamine is needed for the process of making glucose available to the brain. Folic acid is important for the development of RBCs. Deficiencies of folic acid or cyanocobalamin/vitamin $B_{12}$ can cause certain types of anemia. Cyanocobalamin/vitamin $B_{12}$ also helps protect the CNS. Magnesium affects CNS and cardiac function.

    CBC: RBCs = 4.0 (men = 4.5–6.0, women = 4.2–5.4)

    Hgb = 11.0 (men = 14–18, women = 12–16)

    Hct = 36% (men = 42–52%, women = 37–47%)

    MCV = 100 (80–95; elevated in liver disease, alcoholism, folic acid, or vitamin $B_{12}$ deficiency)

    MCH = 48 (27–30; elevated in anemia, folic acid, or vitamin $B_{12}$ deficiency)

    Electrolytes: Na+ = 140 (135–145)

    K+ = 4.0 (3.5–5.3)

    Ca+ = 9.0 (total calcium 7.6–10.4)

    Mg+ = 2.0 (1.8–2.6)

    Cl = 99 (98–106)

Glucose = 140 (70–110)

BUN = 12 (10–20)

Creatinine = 0.9 (0.6–1.2)

GFR = 125 (125 ml per hour; normal range adjusted by individual laboratories to account for the aging process)

Total protein = 5.0 (6–8)

Albumin = 2.0 (3.5–5)

Globulin = 1.8 (2.3–3.4; needed for immune system, immunoglobulin production)

ALT/SGPT = 200 (4–36; liver damage/disease)

AST/SGOT = 400 (0–35; liver damage/disease)

BAL = 180 (0)

UDS = positive for alcohol (negative)

TSH = 2.3 (0.4–4.2)

Total cholesterol = 220 (140–199)

Triglycerides = 300 (below 150)

HDL = 25 (women = 35-80, men = 35–65)

LDL = 180 (below 130 is desirable, greater than 160 is a high risk for cardiovascular disease)

Total cholesterol/HDL ratio = 6.4 (men age 20–39 yrs. = greater than 6.1 is a very high risk for cardiovascular disease, women 20–39 yrs greater than 4.2 is a very high risk for cardiovascular disease)

HBsAg = negative (negative)

IgM anti HBc = negative (negative)

Anti-HCV = negative (negative)

# Question 7

The results of the RBCs, Hgb, Hct, MCV, and MCH are abnormal and indicate that the patient is experiencing signs of anemia. This is not an uncommon finding in patients who abuse/depend on alcohol and other substances. Further nursing assessment should be done for signs and symptoms of anemia. These results should be reported to the psychiatrist. The patient should be tested again and evaluated further after his nutrition improves.

The results of the ALT/SGPT, AST/SGOT are abnormal and indicate liver problems. This is also not uncommon in patients who abuse/depend on alcohol and other substances. Further nursing assessment should be done for signs and symptoms of liver disease. These results should also be reported to the psychiatrist. The patient will be tested again to assess for results trending up or down and corresponding development or abatement of signs and symptoms of liver disease. The psychiatrist may decrease the dose of Librium/chlordiazepoxide and other medications ordered or discontinue Librium/chlordiazepoxide and order Ativan/lorazepam due to the shorter half-life than Librium, if the test results show an increase or if the patient becomes overly sedated indicating difficulty metabolizing the medications.

The results of the IgM anti-HBc, HBsAg, and anti-HCV indicate that the patient does not have acute or chronic hepatitis B or C, nor is he a carrier. Patients who abuse/depend on alcohol or substances frequently have hepatitis secondary to the chemically irritating effects on the liver or unhealthy lifestyle behaviors (e.g., sharing needles, unsafe sex practices). The globulin test results are slightly low and may indicate a decreased ability to fight infection related to one type of immunity, but the WBC is normal providing another type of immunity.

# Question 8

A psychoeducation group for this patient and others with similar problems and test results should include the following topics:

    a. Diet

    b. Exercise

    c. Adaquate amount of sleep

    d. Stress reduction and relaxation techniques

    e. Coping skills

    f. Personal responsibility and empowerment

    g. Safe sex practices

    h. Social support

    i. Spirituality

# Questions 9 and 10

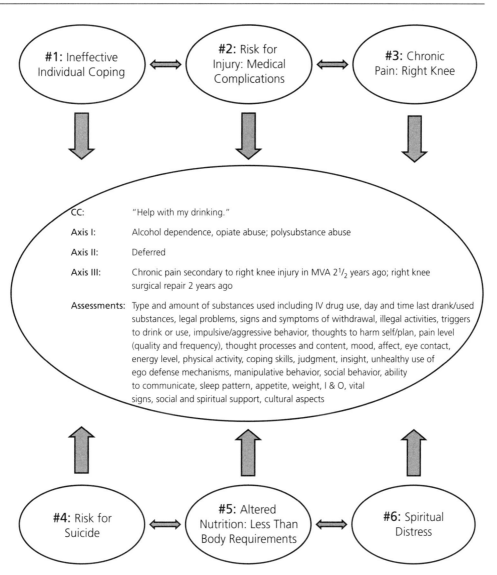

**#1:** Ineffective Individual Coping

**#2:** Risk for Injury: Medical Complications

**#3:** Chronic Pain: Right Knee

CC: "Help with my drinking."

Axis I: Alcohol dependence, opiate abuse; polysubstance abuse

Axis II: Deferred

Axis III: Chronic pain secondary to right knee injury in MVA 2½ years ago; right knee surgical repair 2 years ago

Assessments: Type and amount of substances used including IV drug use, day and time last drank/used substances, legal problems, signs and symptoms of withdrawal, illegal activities, triggers to drink or use, impulsive/aggressive behavior, thoughts to harm self/plan, pain level (quality and frequency), thought processes and content, mood, affect, eye contact, energy level, physical activity, coping skills, judgment, insight, unhealthy use of ego defense mechanisms, manipulative behavior, social behavior, ability to communicate, sleep pattern, appetite, weight, I & O, vital signs, social and spiritual support, cultural aspects

**#4:** Risk for Suicide

**#5:** Altered Nutrition: Less Than Body Requirements

**#6:** Spiritual Distress

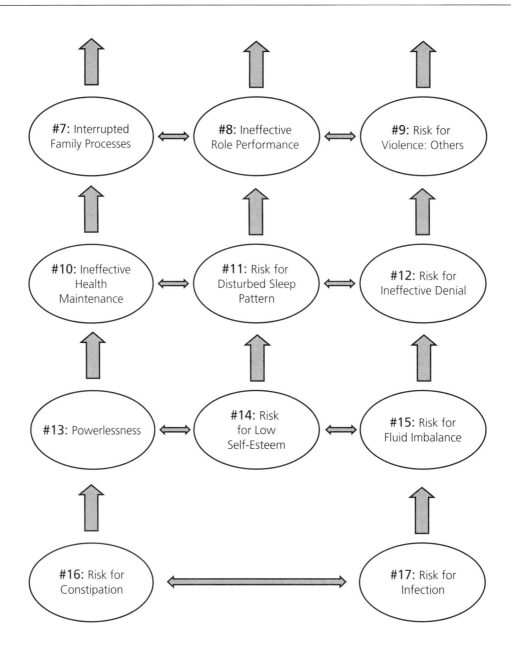

# Question 11

**Nursing Care Plan:** Alcohol dependence, opiate abuse; polysubstance abuse.
**Nursing Diagnosis:** Ineffective Individual Coping r/t poor judgment and problem-solving s/t divorce 6 months ago, and chronic knee pain following MVA 2½ years ago and surgery 2 years ago AEB drinking a fifth of vodka daily and taking eight 10 mg tablets of OxyContin/oxycodone; buying OxyContin/oxycodone on the streets.
**Outcomes** (include time frames): 1. Will verbalize understanding of the importance of taking personal responsibility for his own decision and actions r/t using alcohol and prescription pain pills to cope with problems by discharge. 2. Will attempt to learn at least two positive coping strategies to continue using after discharge.

| Assessment Data: O = Objective, S = Subjective | Evidence-Based Interventions: | Rationales: | Patient Responses:* |
|---|---|---|---|
| Drinks a fifth of vodka daily (O) Takes eight 10 mg tablets of Oxycontin daily (O) BAL/BAC = 180 (O) UDS positive for alcohol and opiates (O) Divorced 6 months ago (O) Chronic right knee pain following MVA 2½ years ago and surgery 2 years ago (O) | 1(a) Examine your own personal feelings and attitudes about substance abuse/dependence. Maintain an open, nonjudgmental attitude yet maintain appropriate professional boundaries when interacting with and assessing patient. | 1(a) Negative personal attitudes and stereotypes may cause nurses to engage in countertransference and interfere with their ability to be therapeutic and impede the patient's progress. This approach is therapeutic and will also help patients feel accepted and more willing to work with nurses toward treatment goals and be more accepting of treatment in general. | 1(a) Responds positively to open, nonjudgmental attitude by nurse and other staff members. States, "I feel like people here really want to help me." Verbalizes understanding of the differences between social and therapeutic relationships. |
| | (b) Begin to develop a rapport and a therapeutic nurse/patient alliance that is the beginning of the therapeutic nurse/patient relationship. | (b) Developing a rapport with the patient will assist in gaining the patient's trust and cooperation in the future. According to Peplau, the therapeutic nurse/patient relationship is the foundation that must be established to initiate future work in the healing process (Keltner, Schwecke, & Bostrom, 2007; O'Brien, Kennedy, & Ballard, 2008). | (b) Body posture more relaxed as interaction with admission nurse continues. Agrees to work with the nurse and adhere to the program rules. |
| | (c) Assist patient to identify triggers to drink and abuse prescription pain pills. | (c) Once triggers are identified, the nurse can work with the patient on ways to avoid these if possible | (c) Identified triggers to drink, including when his ex-wife picks up the children after his *(continues)* |

*Patient responses are examples of what students would look for to decide whether their planned interventions were successful, needed more time, or needed to be changed. Responses will vary depending on the patient.

| Assessment Data: O = Objective, S = Subjective | Evidence-Based Interventions: | Rationales: | Patient Responses: |
|---|---|---|---|
| | | or deal with them in ways that do not lead him to drink and abuse prescription pain medications. | visitation time with them and he is alone, spending too much time "thinking about what could have been." Identifies chronic knee pain as trigger to use OxyContin. Also admits that mixing alcohol and OxyContin "helps me forget my troubles." Insists this does not interfere with his performance at work. |
| | (d) Assess if experiencing cravings and suggest ways to deal with them, including distraction and relaxation techniques. Refer to the addictions counselor for further assistance. | (d) Cravings to drink or use drugs can be very strong and uncomfortable for the patient. It will be important for the patient to learn ways to deal with them while he is an inpatient so that he can continue to cope after discharge and decrease the risk of relapse. Addiction counselors have specialized education and experience, including confrontational techniques and 12-step programs, which help patients deal with problems directly related to their substance abuse/dependence including dealing with cravings, triggers, and relapse prevention strategies. Some addiction counselors are recovered alcoholics or addicts themselves. | (d) Admits to having cravings shortly after admission and feeling restless. |
| | (e) Assess the patient's level of self-esteem. Show him how to use personal strengths to obtain benefits of treatment. | (e) Some patients who abuse/depend on substances have very low self-esteem and use substances to cope. They need to realize that they deserve help and can change. Many struggle with emotional dependency issues, dependent | (e) Admits that the divorce "was a blow to my ego." After some thought, admits that he had some self-doubt when starting the current job he has, but since then is convinced that he is very capable of handling his responsibilities. |

| Assessment Data:<br>O = Objective,<br>S = Subjective | Evidence-Based<br>Interventions: | Rationales: | Patient<br>Responses: |
|---|---|---|---|
| | | personality disorders, anti-social personality disorders, or anxiety. | |
| | (f) Assess risk of suicide and maintain safety checks every 15 minutes. | (f) Many patients who abuse/depend on substances also have symptoms of undiagnosed depression. Substances decrease emotional inhibitions and can result in impulsive behavior. | (f) Denies having suicidal ideations or plans currently. Denies any past suicidal ideations or plans. Admits that he felt "pretty low" during his divorce, but never suicidal. Agrees to tell a staff member if he would start thinking about suicide. |
| | (g) Explore the patient's feelings and thoughts related to drinking and abusing prescription pain pills. | (g) Knowing how the patient feels and thinks can help with identifying reasons why the patient chooses this way to cope. | (g) States that alcohol and OxyContin are what has helped him the most so far, but admits it has "gotten out of hand." |
| | (h) Introduce the concept of personal responsibility or accepting responsibility for his own decisions and actions and overcoming the temptation to blame other people or circumstances for his substance abuse/dependence. | (h) Patients who abuse/depend on substances frequently attempt to explain their actions by blaming others or situations rather than taking responsibility themselves. | (h) States that he understands that it is important to take responsibility for himself and that he usually does so regarding work and child obligations, but had not thought about this in relationship to drinking and abusing OxyContin. |
| | (i) Assess social support network. | (i) Social support is very important for emotional, mental, and physical healing. It is also very important in preventing relapse and maintaining hope. | (i) States that during the divorce proceedings he went to stay with his younger brother and sister-in-law, but felt he was imposing on them after a few weeks. He also has a younger, unmarried sister in the area who he calls occasionally and his parents live 50 miles away. States that he usually sees his parents on holidays. All members of the family are "social drinkers," but he denies that that anyone is an alcoholic and that there are any family members who abuse drugs. States that his family is supportive of his seeking treatment. States he had close friends in college in |

*(continues)*

| Assessment Data: O = Objective, S = Subjective | Evidence-Based Interventions: | Rationales: | Patient Responses: |
|---|---|---|---|
| | | | another state, but since he moved back to his home area to work he has lost contact with them. "My wife was my best friend until the divorce." |
| | (j) Provide information about AA and NA as well as Al-Anon for the family. Teach patient the importance of this type of support, including the role of a sponsor. | (j) AA and NA are very successful 12-step programs led by laypersons who also have had substance abuse/dependence problems and are in recovery. They teach healthy coping, personal responsibility for actions, spirituality, and stress abstinence. Al-Anon and Alateen are very successful programs for supporting families and helping them cope. Sponsors are usually recovered alcoholics/addicts who will work one-on-one with a recovering person providing additional support and help dealing with cravings while expecting the person to take personal responsibility for their actions. | (j) States that he has heard of AA and NA but never thought he would need to go. Accepted information and said he would think about going. |
| | 2(a) Teach patient about alcohol-related diseases and dangers of mixing alcohol and opiates. | 2(a) Providing this information will help the patient understand that it is in his best interest to abstain from alcohol and to recognize the real danger of death from mixing alcohol and opiates. | 2(a) Stated that he had no idea how much damage alcohol could do to his body and mind. He did not realize that he could die from too much alcohol, especially when mixed with pain pills. |
| | (b) Explore better problem-solving strategies, including other possible ways the patient could have handled continued problems with pain control and the divorce. | (b) Patients who abuse/depend on substances have difficulty problem-solving and use substances to avoid dealing with their problems. They tend to repeat the same type of mistakes rather than learn better problem-solving skills unless they actively seek | (b) Agreed that he probably should have found another physician to treat his chronic knee pain when the surgeon stopped prescribing Oxycontin. Also agreed that he should have spent more time with his family of origin and made more of an effort to make new friends or spend less time alone. |

| Assessment Data:<br>O = Objective,<br>S = Subjective | Evidence-Based<br>Interventions: | Rationales: | Patient<br>Responses: |
|---|---|---|---|
| | | help to change their behavior. | |
| | (c) Teach stress reduction and relaxation techniques, including deep breathing, progressive relaxation exercises, meditation, yoga, guided imagery, appropriate exercise, aromatherapy, journaling, time management, financial budgeting, proper rest/sleep, attending to spiritual needs, and taking up new hobbies. | (c) These techniques provide patients with healthier coping strategies. Also, some patients who abuse/depend on substances have problems with anxiety and these strategies will help decrease this. | (c) Interested in learning new coping strategies. Learning deep breathing, progressive relaxation, and guided imagery. Requested information on yoga. States that he plans to go back to the gym that he used to work out in prior to the divorce. He will also seek help with time management as well as starting to budget his money. |
| | (d) Give positive feedback and verbal praise for attempts to learn and practice new stress reduction and relaxation techniques. | (d) This encourages the patient to keep trying to learn, reinforces learning, and improves his skills. | (d) Responds positively to verbal praise and feedback. Continues to practice new coping skills. |
| | (e) Teach patient the importance of using stress reduction and relaxation techniques on a regular basis after discharge to help prevent relapse and improve general health. | (e) The patient needs to have healthy coping strategies to replace unhealthy behavior or risk drifting back into previously used unhealthy habits. This also helps give him more control over his situation and empowers him. | (e) Verbalizes his understanding of the reason to use stress reduction and relaxation techniques on a regular basis after discharge. States that he understands how this can help him avoid starting drinking and abusing prescription pain pills again. |
| | (f) Teach patient the signs and symptoms of relapse to watch for. Include avoidance of triggers and establishing friendships with people who do not drink or use substances. | (f) Again, providing patient with this information helps give him more control over his situation and empowers him to avoid drifting back into using substances. | (f) Able to state several signs and symptoms to watch for. |

**Evaluation:** 1. Verbalizes understanding of the importance of taking personal responsibility for his own decision and actions. Was not aware of how significantly alcohol could affect his body and mind or the possibility of death due to excess alcohol or mixing alcohol with prescription pain pills. Accepted information on AA, NA, and Al-Anon but did not make a commitment to attend and obtain sponsors after discharge.
2. Has learned several positive coping strategies, including deep breathing, progressive relaxation, and guided imagery. Requested information on yoga. Planning to go back to the gym he used to work out in after discharge and to seek help with time and money management. Continue care plan and evaluate in 48 hours.

**Nursing Care Plan:** Alcohol dependence, opiate abuse; polysubstance abuse.
**Nursing Diagnosis:** Risk for Injury: Medical Complications r/t withdrawal from alcohol and opiates AEB admitting to drinking a fifth of vodka daily for the past year and taking eight 10 mg tablets of OxyContin/oxycodone daily for the past $1\frac{1}{2}$ years; reported last use of alcohol 4 hours prior to admission and last use of OxyContin/oxycodone 6 hours before admission.
**Outcomes** (include time frames): 1. Will remain free from serious medical complications including seizures, cardiovascular or respiratory complications during entire hospitalization.

| Assessment Data:<br>O = Objective,<br>S = Subjective | Evidence-Based<br>Interventions: | Rationales: | Patient<br>Responses: |
|---|---|---|---|
| Has drunk a fifth of vodka daily for the past year (O)<br>Takes eight 10 mg tablets of OxyContin daily for the past $1\frac{1}{2}$ years (O)<br>BAL/BAC = 180 (O)<br>UDS positive for alcohol and opiates (O)<br>Reported last use of alcohol 4 hours prior to admission (O)<br>Reported last use of OxyContin 6 hours before admission (O)<br>Denies history of DTs (S)<br>Denies history of blackouts (S)<br>Reports at least a 2-year history of drinking vodka (S)<br>Reports a $2\frac{1}{2}$ year history of using OxyContin initially prescribed after MVA and right knee surgery (S) | 1(a) Assess for signs and symptoms of withdrawal from alcohol and opiates upon admission, every shift and prn.<br>(b) Take vital signs every hour × 4 and prn if indicated; if stable, then every 2 hours × 4 and prn if indicated; if stable, then every 4 hours and prn if indicated × 72 hours.<br><br><br>(c) Place on seizure precautions and observe for tremulousness every shift and prn.<br><br><br><br>(d) Perform mental status exam every shift and prn if condition changes.<br><br><br><br><br><br><br>(e) Push fluids and maintain I & O every shift. | 1(a) This will enable the nurse to anticipate problems, prevent them, or intervene early to promote patient safety.<br>(b) Elevation in vital signs occurs during withdrawal from any substances. You may need to take them more often than at hourly intervals if they are abnormal to more closely monitor the patient's physical condition and intervene when needed.<br>(c) Seizures can occur during withdrawal from CNS depressants. Tremulousness is a sign of withdrawal from substances and can signal impending seizures or DTs.<br>(d) The mental status exam includes LOC, mood, psychomotor activity, and the presence or absence of hallucinations. During withdrawal from substances, the patient may become confused, disoriented, agitated, aggressive, and restless, and he may experience visual, auditory, or tactile hallucinations.<br>(e) These patients are frequently dehydrated which can cause electrolyte imbalances and increase mental confusion. If the | 1(a) Reports starting to feel restless. Slowly paces in day room. Denies other symptoms and none noted at this time.<br><br>(b) Vital signs T = 99, P = 90, R = 20, BP = 138/90.<br><br><br><br><br><br><br>(c) No tremulousness noted and patient denies tremors at this time.<br><br><br><br>(d) Normal results other than subjective report of patient starting to feel restless and objective sign that he is pacing slowly in day room.<br><br><br><br><br><br>(e) Has dry skin but normal turgor. Electrolytes WNL, RBCs, Hgb, and Hct decreased. Does not have overt signs of dehydration at this time. Oral |

| Assessment Data: O = Objective, S = Subjective | Evidence-Based Interventions: | Rationales: | Patient Responses: |
|---|---|---|---|
| | | patient cannot drink enough orally, IV therapy will be ordered by the psychiatrist or another physician if treated on a medical unit of a general hospital. | intake sufficient for metabolic needs. Denies constipation or diarrhea. |
| | (f) Ensure that ordered laboratory and diagnostic tests are performed and report abnormal results as soon as they are available. | (f) Delays in obtaining results directly affect the patient's care by potentially delaying treatment and leading to harmful circumstances for the patient. | (f) Laboratory/diagnostic tests performed and results obtained in standard amount of time. Has many abnormal results including elevated liver enzymes. Has normal physical assessment. |
| | (g) Decrease environmental stimuli. | (g) Environmental stimuli can help stimulate seizure activity. | (g) Adheres to unit policies related to providing a calm, low-stimulus environment. |
| | (h) Administer scheduled and prn medication as ordered and as indicated. | (h) This will help control withdrawal signs and symptoms, decreasing the risk of serious medical complications. | (h) Accepts scheduled medication. Prn medication not indicated at this time. Does not seek medication at this time. |
| | (i) Provide adequate nutrition for metabolic needs and weigh daily as ordered. | (i) Malnutrition and anemia will have a negative impact on patient's overall physical health, energy level, mood, and ability to concentrate and learn. | (i) The patient's laboratory results show signs of protein and vitamin deficiencies and decreased oxygen transport ability and anemia. Admission weight = 135 pounds; height = 5 feet, 9 inches. Admits to occasional fatigue and low energy levels. |
| | (j) Assess sleep pattern and promote improved sleep hygiene practices. | (j) Sleep is restorative, promotes physical and mental health, and increases energy and the ability to concentrate. Decreased amounts of sleep may trigger seizure activity. | (j) Complains of insomnia during 1st night after admission. Reports sleeping 5 hours, which coincides with night shift report. Agrees to avoid napping during the day and take a warm bath before going to bed tonight. |

**Evaluation:** 1. Remains free from serious medical complications of alcohol and opiate withdrawal, but has many abnormal laboratory and diagnostics tests results, which indicate potential for medical problems. Reports starting to feel restless; insomnia is validated by observation. Continue care plan and evaluate every shift and prn.

**Nursing Care Plan:** Alcohol dependence, opiate abuse; polysubstance abuse.
**Nursing Diagnosis:** Chronic Pain r/t injury s/t MVA $2^1/_2$ years ago regardless of surgical repair 2 years ago AEB slight limp when walking and unaware of being observed; admitting to drinking a fifth of vodka daily for the past year and taking eight 10 mg tablets of OxyContin/oxycodone daily for the past $1^1/_2$ years.
**Outcomes** (include time frames): 1. Will learn at least two new nonpharmacological ways to deal with chronic pain by discharge.

| Assessment Data: O = Objective, S = Subjective | Evidence-Based Interventions: | Rationales: | Patient Responses: |
|---|---|---|---|
| Reports MVA $2^1/_2$ years ago resulting in injury to right knee (S) Documentation of MVA in old records (O) Reports surgical repair of right knee 2 years ago (S) Faded surgical scar noted on right knee (O) Documentation of surgery in old records (O) Slight limp noted when walking and unaware of being observed (O) Has drunk a fifth of vodka daily for the past year (O) Has taken eight 10 mg tablets of OxyContin daily for the past $1^1/_2$ years (O) BAL/BAC = 180 (O) UDS positive for alcohol and opiates (O) Reports a $2^1/_2$ year history of using OxyContin initially prescribed after MVA and right knee surgery (S) Reports at least a 2-year history of drinking vodka (S) | 1(a) Assess quality, intensity, duration, and frequency of right knee pain every shift and prn. (b) Explore what methods the patient has used that have worked and not worked to relieve pain. (c) Using a nonjudgmental approach, teach patient about developing a tolerance to alcohol and opiates leading to increased use and the physical dangers this can lead to. | 1(a) The nurse needs to establish baseline information that will help with evaluation of the effectiveness of nursing care and treatment. (b) Patients use a variety of methods to relieve pain, including complementary and alternative methods. Some are healthy/adaptive while others are not. This patient already admits to abusing alcohol and Oxy-Contin to relieve pain. In desperation he may also be using other unhealthy/maladaptive ways to relieve his pain. (c) Some patients become desperate to relieve their pain and will use any means available. They do not think of the negative consequences or are not aware of them. Even though nurse and staff may not agree with their choices or would not engage in the same behaviors, being judgmental is not therapeutic and will negatively impact the nurse/patient relationship. Unfortunately many patients prescribed pain medication for legitimate reasons go on to abuse the medication if using it for the wrong reasons and not being truthful | 1(a) Reports intermittent, dull, aching pain. Rates pain a "6" on a scale of 0–10, with 0 = none and 10 = extremely severe. (b) States OxyContin and sometimes vodka "works the best." Admits that sometimes ice or OTC "Icy Hot" ointment works. (c) Admits to having increased the amount used in order to feel better. |

| Assessment Data:<br>O = Objective,<br>S = Subjective | Evidence-Based<br>Interventions: | Rationales: | Patient<br>Responses: |
|---|---|---|---|
| | | with the prescribing physician. | |
| | (d) Provide continued emotional support. | (d) The patient needs much emotional support not only to deal with chronic pain but also to try new ways of dealing with pain. | (d) Responds positively to emotional support. |
| | (e) Administer scheduled and prn medication as indicated. | (e) There are differing opinions among physicians as to the best way to treat patients with substance abuse/dependence problems and acute or chronic pain. This patient is prescribed Ultram, which will bind to mu receptors as OxyContin does but is not an opiate substance. There is some concern with the potential for abuse of Ultram and ordering a lower dose still within recommended range plus alternating the doses with ibuprofen will help control the patient's pain while controlling the amount of Ultram the patient is receiving. Additionally, since Ultram binds mu receptors, it may provide a secondary benefit in decreasing opiate withdrawal. | (e) States he receives "some relief" from Ultram, but not from ibuprofen. Rates his pain a "4." |
| | (f) Medicate patient 20 minutes before physical therapy sessions. | (f) Patients are understandably more cooperative and derive greater benefit from physical therapy if they are in less pain during sessions. | (f) Expresses appreciation for the nurse administering prn medication prior to physical therapy sessions. |
| | (g) Provide information and teach nonpharmacological methods of pain reduction and relief including deep breathing exercises, guided imagery, | (g) Providing information and teaching the patient about adapative versus maladaptive methods gives him more control over his pain relief. | (g) Is starting to use deep breathing and guided imagery in addition to prn medication. Learning exercises to use after discharge as well.<br><br>*(continues)* |

| Assessment Data:<br>O = Objective,<br>S = Subjective | Evidence-Based<br>Interventions: | Rationales: | Patient<br>Responses: |
|---|---|---|---|
| | medication, application of heat or cold if authorized by physician, and exercises recommended by physical therapist.<br>(h) Teach patient to avoid taking OTC medications including Tylenol/ acetominophen products.<br><br>(i) Observe for and teach patient to report easy bleeding, bruising, or abdominal pain. | (h) The patient has been drinking heavily for at least 2 years and now has elevated liver enzymes. Tylenol can be toxic to the liver and should be avoided.<br>(i) The patient is prone to developing gastritis, ulcers, or decreased amounts of clotting factors produced by the liver due to heavy alcohol consumption. He is currently ordered prn ibuprofen. You may need to hold the prn ibuprofen ordered and he may need to avoid NSAIDS. | (h) Stated that he was not aware that Tylenol could affect his liver. Agreed to avoid taking Tylenol and being more aware of OTC ingredients by reading the labels and asking questions.<br>(i) Agrees to report easy bleeding, bruising, or abdominal pain but denies any symptoms at this time. |
| | (j) Promote adequate rest and sleep. | (j) Fatigue and low energy decreases the patient's ability to deal with pain and increases the risk of using maladaptive coping methods and relapsing. | (j) Reported insomnia during 1st night after admission. Reports sleeping 5 hours, which coincides with night shift report. Agreed to avoid napping during the day and to take a warm bath before going to bed tonight. Asked about the possibility of the psychiatrist ordering a sleeping pill, but verbalized understanding when the nurse explained why this may not be a good idea at this time due to already receiving medication for withdrawal signs and symptoms. Verbalizes understanding that it will take time for his body to reestablish its own sleep pattern after being under the influence of substances for so long. |

**Evaluation:** 1. Reports some pain relief with Ultram, but not ibuprofen. Self-reported pain rating decreased from a 6 to a 4 on a scale of 0–10, with 0 = none and 10 = extremely severe. Going to physical therapy. Starting to use deep breathing and guided imagery in addition to prn medication. Learning exercises to use after discharge as well. Continue care plan and evaluate in 48 hours.

# Question 12

As stated above in the Rationales section of the Nursing Care Plan, AA and NA are very successful 12-step programs led by laypersons who also have had substance abuse/dependence problems and are in recovery. These programs require participants to admit they have no control over their alcohol or substance abuse/dependence and need help. Recovery is a lifelong process. Stressing abstinence, the programs teach healthy, adaptive ways of coping and personal responsibility for actions. They also provide much needed emotional support that is different from the confrontational style used by many addiction counselors. Both emotional support and confrontation are necessary. Sponsors are usually recovered alcoholics/addicts who will work one-on-one with a recovering person providing additional support and help dealing with cravings while expecting the person to take personal responsibility for their actions.

Al-Anon and Alateen are very successful programs for supporting the family and helping them cope. Codependency issues are also addressed in these groups. Many family members have taken on responsibilities and engage in behaviors that they believe will help the affected individual or keep the family together, but are actually not therapeutic and may even be harmful to the affected person and the family members. These support groups along with professional individual and family counseling are needed to deal with codependency.

The support of 12-step groups can help the patient maintain sobriety and also help his family deal with his substance abuse and dependence problems even though the divorce has already occurred. Strong emotions and situations that occurred during the marriage, and may still be occurring, need to be dealt with in order for everyone to heal and experience positive personal growth. The patient's ex-wife and children will also benefit from professional counseling to prevent possible future psychosocial developmental problems.

Maintaining sobriety and living drug-free can help decrease the number of substance-related accidents, injuries, and fatalities. The patient will be more likely to maintain employment, be more productive, and improve social relationships. Healthy individuals build healthy communities.

# Question 13

The patient is using the ego defense mechanism of denial. Denial is very strong in patients with substance abuse/dependence problems, but it is maladaptive and prevents them from either seeking or continuing in treatment. It is ineffective because it helps them delude themselves that they can stop abusing/depending on substances on their own without professional help, which increases their risk of relapse.

The patient is also displaying manipulative behavior by providing excuses to leave that seem to be valid and appealing to the healthcare staff, who understand and care about the well-being of his children.

# Question 14

The nurse and other healthcare staff will need to therapeutically convey their concern and empathy for him and his children. They must try to convince the patient that it truly is in his and his family's best interest to stay in treatment so that he can in the future be an even better person and father. This is difficult to do because the patient most likely is experiencing increased cravings to drink and use drugs. He may be becoming uncomfortable with the restrictions of the unit and the program. The nurse and other healthcare staff need to ask about cravings and the possibility of any other reasons for that patient asking to leave without insinuating that he wants to drink or use drugs. There may also be conditions from his employer—for example, that his employment will continue only if he receives and completes treatment for substance abuse/dependence. Sometimes asking the patients to at least wait to make a decision until talking to a psychiatrist is effective in causing them to delay an action or rethink their decisions.

If the patient continues to insist on leaving, the nurse needs to inform the patient of the dangers of not receiving full treatment, including medical risks to his physical health and increased risk of relapse. He should also be informed that many insurance companies refuse to pay for hospitalization and treatment if it is not completed because the chance of treatment success may be compromised if the patient refuses to participate. The nurse will also need to notify the psychiatrist that the patient is asking to leave treatment and document all the facts, including conversations with the patient, notification of the psychiatrist, and the psychiatrist's response.

# References

Alters, S., & Schiff, W. (2004). *Essential concepts for healthy living* (4th ed.). Sudbury, MA: Jones and Bartlett Publishers.

American Psychiatric Association. (2000). *Diagnostic and statistical manual of mental disorders* (4th ed.). Washington, DC: Author.

Antai-Otong, D. (2004). *Psychiatric emergencies: How to accurately assess and manage the patient in crisis.* Eau Claire, WI: PESI Heatlthcare.

Carpenito-Moyat, L. J. (2008). *Nursing diagnosis: Application to clinical practice* (12th ed.). Philadelphia, PA: Wolters Kluwer Lippincott Williams & Wilkins.

Delaune, S. C. (2007, June). Setting effective professional boundaries: Walking the line and knowing where it is! Psychiatric Nursing Conference, New Orleans, LA.

Dunn, K., Elsom, S., & Cross, W. (2007). Self-efficacy and locus of control affect management of aggression by mental health nurses. *Issues in Mental Health Nursing, 28*(2), 201–217.

Fischbach, F. (2004). *A manual of laboratory and diagnositic tests* (7th ed.). Philadelphia, PA: Lippincott Williams & Wilkins.

Fontaine, K. L., & Fletcher, J. S. (2003). *Mental health nursing* (5th ed.). Upper Saddle River, NJ: Pearson.

George-Gay, B., & Chernecky, C. C. (2002). *Clinical medical-surgical nursing: A decision-making reference.* Philadelphia, PA: Saunders.

Keltner, N. L., Schewecke, L. H., & Bostrom, C. E. (2007). *Psychiatric nursing* (5th ed.). St. Louis, MO: Mosby, Elsevier.

Kidd, P. S., & Wagner, K. D. (2001). *High acuity nursing* (3rd ed.). Upper Saddle River, NJ: Pearson.

Krakowski, M. (2007). Violent behavior: Choosing antipsychotics and other agents. *Current Psychiatry, 6*(4), 63–70.

La Torre, M. A. (2002). Integrated perspectives: Enhancing therapeutic presence. *Perspectives in Psychiatric Care, 38*(1), 34–36.

Marcus, P. (2007, June). Suicidal ideation: Assessment and prevention. Psychiatric Nursing Conference, New Orleans, LA.

McKenrey, L., Tessier, E., & Hogan, M. (2006). *Mosby's pharmacology in nursing* (22nd ed.). St. Louis, MO: Mosby.

National Institutes of Health (NIH). (2006, September 5). Early alcohol dependence linked to reduced treatment seeking and chronic relapse. (News release, pp. 1–2).

O'Brien, P. G., Kennedy, W. Z., & Ballard, K. A. (2008). *Psychiatric mental health nursing: An introduction to theory and practice.* Sudbury, MA: Jones and Bartlett.

Pender, N. J., Murdaugh, C. L., & Parsons, M. A. (2006). *Health promotion in nursing practice* (5th ed.). Upper Saddle River, NJ: Pearson.

*Saunders 2005 nursing drug handbook.* St. Louis, MO: Mosby.

Shaw, M. F., McGovern, M. P., Angres, D. H., & Rawal, P. (2004). Physicians and nurses with substance use disorders. *Journal of Advance Nursing, 47*(5), 561–571.

Stong, C. (2006). Assessing suicide risk—separating attempts from ideation. *NeuroPsychiatry Reviews, 7*(8), 1, 19.

Stuart, G. W., & Laraia, M. T. (2005). *Principles and practice of psychiatric nursing* (8th ed.). St. Louis, MO: Mosby, Elsevier.

Townsend, M. C. (2008). *Nursing diagnoses in psychiatric nursing* (7th ed.). Philadelphia, PA: F. A. Davis.

Varcarolis, E. M. (2006). *Manual of psychiatric nursing care plans* (3rd ed.). St. Louis, MO: Saunders, Elsevier.

Varcarolis, E. M., Carson, V. B., & Shoemaker, N. C. (2006). *Foundations of psychiatric mental health nursing: A clinical approach* (6th ed.). St. Louis, MO: Saunders, Elsevier.

Yigletu, H., Tucker, S., Harris, M., & Hatlevig, J. (2004). Assessing suicidal ideation: Comparing self-report versus clinician report. *American Psychiatric Nurses Association, 10*(1), 9–15.

# Web Sites

American Heart Association: www.americanheartassociation.org

American Psychiatric Association Continuing Medical Education (CME): www.psych.org/cme

American Psychiatric Databases: www.apa.org/psycinfo

American Psychological Association: www.apa.org

Centers for Disease Control and Prevention: www.cdc.gov

Clinicaltrials.gov: www.clinicaltrials.gov

National Institute on Alcohol Abuse and Alcoholism, National Institutes of Health: www.niaaa.nih.gov

National Institute on Drug Abuse, National Institutes of Health: www.nida.nih.gov

Psychiatry.com: www.psychiatry.com

United States Department of Health and Human Services, Substance Abuse and Mental Health Services Administration: www.samhsa.gov

Your Total Health NBC and iVillage: yourtotalhealth.ivillage.com

# Anxiety and Medical Disorders: Post-Traumatic Stress Disorder and Type II Diabetes Mellitus

## ANSWER KEY

## Question 1

At this time there is no treatment needed for the normal EKG/ECG and K+ results. Facility protocols typically initiate orders for CBG results greater than or equal to 400. These orders include obtaining a stat serum glucose and urine acetone. The physician should be notified of the results as soon as they are obtained, and documentation should include both the results and the notification. The patient already has a serum glucose level of 420. A serum acetone level would also be obtained to determine if the patient was experiencing DKA. Since the patient has a diagnosis of Type II DM, he would more likely have developed HHS. Typically CBGs may initially be performed every hour, depending on the patient's symptoms and the results of the CBGs. The frequency will be reduced to ac & hs when the results are closer to normal ranges. The patient is not unconscious and will be eating and receiving insulin.

After an initial dose of regular insulin is ordered and administered, an IV infusion of glucose may be ordered in addition to IVFs of l liter of 0.9% normal saline (NS) at 125 cc/hour additionally. A "sliding scale" of regular insulin will be used to help control glucose levels, with coverage starting at 201. When the patient's serum glucose is decreased to 250, the physician may change the IVFs to D5W to prevent hypoglycemia from too rapidly declining serum glucose levels. The patient's HgA1C level (glycosylated hemoglobin) will gradually become more normal when the patient's serum glucose is controlled. The HgA1C level shows the average serum glucose levels over the last 2 to 3 months giving a better clinical picture of serum glucose control. Normal values range from 4 to 6.7. Good diabetic control is considered to be in the range of 6.9 to 8.

# Question 2

The patient is an Iraq war veteran experiencing flashbacks, paranoia, nightmares, and difficulty sleeping, triggered by watching CNN coverage on television of the current situation in Iraq over the past 2 weeks. He is acting upon the flashbacks by patrolling his backyard at night, accusing his neighbor of helping enemy forces, and barricading himself in his home.

# Question 3

A voluntary admission is the least restrictive type of admission. At this time there is no indication that the patient is refusing treatment and he is no longer agitated or physically aggressive. Therefore, at this time it is both legal and safe. If the patient's condition would change, but he no longer wished to remain hospitalized, the psychiatrist has the option to initiate an involuntary commitment.

a. In most states patients who are voluntary admissions are legally able to sign a 72-hour notice indicating that they wish to leave at the end of that time. If patients elope, or leave without being formally discharged, their patient status is still a voluntary one. Every facility/organization has policies regarding elopement, but generally the nurse would notify the psychiatrist immediately as well as the unit nurse manager. The nurse would also notify the patient's next of kin or emergency contact person and try to determine where the patient would have gone. In addition, the nurse would contact the patient and try to talk him into coming back to the hospital. The medical physician should also be notified, especially if the patient has Axis III diagnoses. Documentation of the situation should include when the patient was last seen and his condition; how knowledge of the elopement was obtained; everyone who was notified; and whether or not the patient was able to be contacted. The psychiatrist will determine whether there are grounds to pursue an involuntary commitment, which may require that the patient be brought back to the hospital by the police, or to discharge the patient officially. (If the patient is on an involuntary commitment, the police will be notified to find the patient and bring him back to the hospital.)

For voluntary patients, facility policies vary as to whether or not the hospital administrator or CEO would be notified immediately. They would be made aware of the situation according to the facility policy time frame by the nurse manager or supervisor. If the patient has initially been involuntarily committed, the police and hospital administrator or CEO will be notified after notifying the psychiatrist.

# Questions 4 and 5

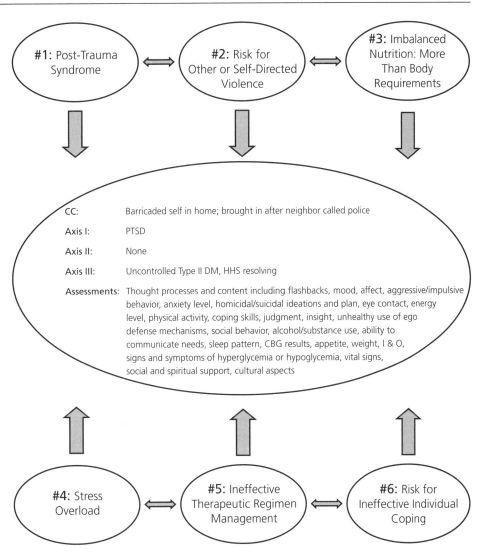

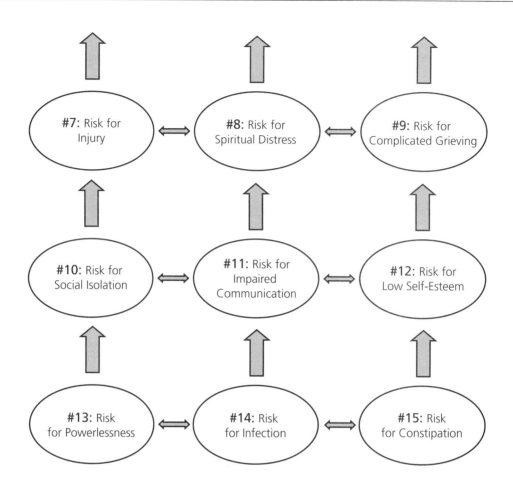

# Question 6

**Nursing Care Plan:** PTSD, uncontrolled Type II DM, HHS resolving.
**Nursing Diagnosis:** Post-Trauma Syndrome r/t intrusive memories of wartime s/t military deployment to Iraq AEB began prowling around the yard at night wearing camouflage attire, carrying a gun, looking for people who may be trying to harm him or others, accusing a neighbor of helping the enemy forces, and barricading self in own dwelling while threatening to shoot the police.
**Outcomes**: 1. Will tolerate the presence of and assistance from assigned nurses and other staff members on the unit within 48 hours of hospitalization. 2. Will report at least a 25% decrease in the frequency of flashbacks at the end of the 1st week of hospitalization.

| Assessment Data: O = Objective, S = Subjective | Evidence-Based Interventions: | Rationales: | Patient Responses:* |
|---|---|---|---|
| Prowling around the yard at night wearing camouflage attire (O) Carrying a gun (O) Paranoia (O) Accusing neighbor of helping enemy forces (S) Barricaded self in own dwelling and threatened to shoot police (O) Flashbacks (S) Nightmares (S) Signs and symptoms triggered by watching CNN television coverage of the current situation in Iraq (S) Diagnosis of PTSD (O) Stopped attending weekly support group (S) | 1(a) Begin to develop a rapport and trusting nurse/patient relationship by using yourself therapeutically. | 1(a) The therapeutic use of self, therapeutic listening (also referred to as active listening or attending skills) are the most important therapeutic tools the nurse can use when working with psychiatric/mental health patients. Using the self therapeutically can help the nurse begin to establish a rapport with the patient. Once rapport has been established, the nurse can build trust within the nurse/patient relationship. | 1(a) Tolerating the presence of the primary assigned nurse and other nursing staff. |
| | (b) Assign the same nurses and other staff to the patient when possible. | (b) This will help provide consistency of care for the patient and help reinforce the trusting relationship. | (b) Verbalizes understanding that the same nurses and other staff will be working with him. Agrees that it will be easier for him to know what to expect when working with the same people whenever possible. |
| | (c) Provide a calm, consistent milieu. | (c) This helps the patient feel calmer and helps decrease anxiety. It also helps him know what to expect, which in turn can help decrease episodes of escalating behavior or flashbacks. | (c) Hypervigilant and easily startled, but reacts favorably to calmer environment. *(continues)* |

*Patient responses are examples of what students would look for to decide whether their planned interventions were successful, needed more time, or needed to be changed. Responses will vary depending on the patient.

| Assessment Data: O = Objective, S = Subjective | Evidence-Based Interventions: | Rationales: | Patient Responses: |
|---|---|---|---|
| | (d) Use calm, nonthreatening approach; avoid sudden movements and keep your hands where the patient can see them during any interactions. | (d) These types of behaviors from nurses and staff members will help decrease the patient's anxiety, which in turn will help decrease episodes of escalation or flashbacks. | (d) Exhibits less muscle tension when approached in a calm, nonthreatening manner. |
| | (e) Reassure the patient that he is in a safe place and no harm will come to him here. | (e) Fear for his own safety will escalate his behavior and may lead to physical aggression. | (e) Appreciates being reminded of his safety. Shows relief and body posture is less tense. |
| | (f) Use clear, concise statements to explain all care and procedures before beginning. | (f) This approach will help ensure the patient's cooperation, decrease the chance of startling him or increasing his anxiety, and decrease the possibility of escalating behavior if he feels threatened. When patients are very anxious or feel threatened, their attention span becomes shorter and their focus becomes narrower, which makes it more difficult for them to understand what the nurse is saying or follow directions. | (f) Thanks nurse and other staff for explanations. Has been cooperative with assessments and care. |
| | (g) Assess readiness to talk about Iraq experiences. | (g) If the patient is not ready to talk about his experiences, forcing him will increase his anxiety, increase the risk of escalating aggressive behaviors and the occurrence of flashbacks, and undermine nurse/patient trust. | (g) Declines to talk about experiences in Iraq except to say that it is something he would like to "put behind me and move on." |
| | (h) If patient is unable to talk at this time, let him know you are available when he is ready. | (h) This type of response lets the patient know that you appreciate how difficult this must be for him and that you respect his wishes. It also lets him know that you care enough to be available in the future even though he is not ready at this time. This will | (h) Thanks nurse for being available, but still declines to talk about experiences. |

| Assessment Data: O = Objective, S = Subjective | Evidence-Based Interventions: | Rationales: | Patient Responses: |
|---|---|---|---|
| | | strengthen his trust and may make it easier for him to disclose his feelings when he is ready to talk. | |
| | (i) When patient indicates readiness to at least try to talk about experiences, use therapeutic communication to facilitate the patient's expression of feelings. | (i) Therapeutic communication will help the patient more easily express and explore feelings. It also helps the nurse be more accurate in gathering information and helping the patient problem-solve when needed. | (i) Declines to talk about experiences. |
| | (j) Avoid forcing the patient to talk about experiences. Be sensitive to emotional cues to stop the discussion and continue at another time. | (j) Forcing the patient to talk and being insensitive to his psychological and emotional pain is not therapeutic and is hurtful. It can be harmful to the patient and damage the trusting nurse/patient relationship. | (j) Changes the subject when anything related to Iraq is mentioned. Does not give a reason at this time about why he stopped attending the support group he previously was attending. |
| | (k) Offer emotional support when discussing psychologically and emotionally painful topics. Reassure the patient that he did what he had to do to survive in extreme circumstances. | (k) This approach shows that the nurse cares about the patient, has empathy for his painful feelings, and understands the sensitive nature of the topics being discussed. A long-range goal, using therapeutic communication and psychotherapy, is for the patient to begin to let go of some of the painful memories and replace them with positive experiences. | (k) Accepts some emotional support but attempts to maintain an outward appearance of emotional control. |
| | (l) Teach patient that the negative impact of the traumatic events can be decreased over time even though the past cannot be changed. | (l) This provides a realistic measure of hope that the future can be better without offering false reassurance. | (l) Admits that he does not believe that very much can be done to help him and therefore thinks it is best not to talk about it, but to focus instead on "getting on" with his life. Admits he is having problems with this approach. |
| | (m) Promote patient collaboration with treatment decisions. | (m) This will help continue to build trust between the patient, nurse, and all members of the treatment team. | (m) Appreciates being involved in treatment decisions. |

*(continues)*

| Assessment Data: O = Objective, S = Subjective | Evidence-Based Interventions: | Rationales: | Patient Responses: |
|---|---|---|---|
| | 2(a) Administer scheduled and prn doses of medication as ordered. | 2(a) Psychopharmacology is a major component of psychiatric/mental health treatment. Collaborative interventions using medication are of great benefit to patients. Because PTSD is difficult to treat, medications as well as other treatment must be tailored to the individual patient's needs and responses. The nurse must use good clinical judgment when assessing the patient's need for prn medication. | 2(a) Accepts medication ordered. Has received 1 prn dose of Zyprexa Zydis and 2 prn doses of Ativan since being transferred to this unit. |
| | (b) Temporarily eliminate viewing of all violence on television, including war and military news coverage. | (b) This removes a known trigger of the patient's symptoms. Over a period of time with the help of medications and psychotherapy, including desensitization therapy, certain types of television programming may be slowly introduced, depending upon how the patient responds. | (b) Verbalizes understanding of modifying television viewing and is cooperative. |
| | (c) Reassure patient that he is not "going crazy" and that his symptoms are a typical reaction to the trauma he experienced. | (c) Patients experiencing flashbacks may fear they are losing contact with reality due to the vividness of the flashbacks. They may also be afraid they will be labeled as "crazy" if they report their symptoms. The nurse provides much needed emotional and psychological relief when explaining that this is a typical reaction. | (c) Verbalizes relief when reassured he is not "going crazy." |
| | (d) Assess for dissociative episodes. | (d) Dissociation is a common symptom of PTSD. | (d) Denies episodes of dissociation and has not exhibited any behavior indicating dissociation since being transferred to this unit. |

| Assessment Data:<br>O = Objective,<br>S = Subjective | Evidence-Based<br>Interventions: | Rationales: | Patient<br>Responses: |
|---|---|---|---|
| | (e) Use grounding techniques such as staying with the patient and reminding him that he is in a safe place, restating his location and who you are, and reorienting him to time/date when he is experiencing flashbacks or dissociation. | (e) Grounding techniques help the patient focus on reality and what is happening currently rather than on past traumatic events. | (e) Has not noted or reported any flashback or dissociation episodes at this time. |
| | (f) Teach coping and distracting strategies such as deep breathing, progressive relaxation exercises, guided imagery, listening to soft music, and physical exercise. | (f) Coping and distracting strategies can cause a physical, as well as psychological, relaxation response, which will lead to decreased autonomic sympathetic nervous system response. This can result in decreased anxiety and flashbacks. | (f) States willingness to try deep breathing, guided imagery, and physical exercise. |
| | (g) Assist patient to identify triggers for flashbacks and ways to avoid these triggers. | (g) Identifying triggers that stimulate flashbacks will enable patient to plan for ways to avoid triggers and as a result decrease the occurrence of flashbacks. | (g) Admits that until this admission he did not realize that watching the CNN reports on the current situation in Iraq would have caused him to react as he did. |
| | (h) Assess sleep pattern and encourage patient to develop a regular routine before going to bed. | (h) Patients with PTSD often have nightmares as well as flashbacks. Nightmares interrupt sleep, leaving the patient fatigued and less able to cope with anxiety or stress that may precede the occurrence of flashbacks. | (h) Awakens every 2 hours and moves restlessly during sleep, and reports having nightmares. Agrees to try a warm bath and listen to a relaxation tape of soft music before bed. |

*(continues)*

| Assessment Data:<br>O = Objective,<br>S = Subjective | Evidence-Based<br>Interventions: | Rationales: | Patient<br>Responses: |
|---|---|---|---|
| | (i) Provide spiritual support according to the patient's cultural and belief system. | (i) Flashbacks can be extremely spiritually distressing. Support can help decrease the negative effects of the flashback experiences. When a patient's cultural and belief system is respected, the intervention will be more therapeutic and help strengthen the trusting nurse/patient relationship. | (i) Asks to meet with the hospital chaplain. States that going to the beach makes him feel more peaceful. Agrees to try guided imagery of the beach. |

**Evaluation:** 1. Tolerates the presence of assigned nurses and other nursing staff. Cooperative with assessments and care. Becoming involved in treatment decisions.
2. Denies flashbacks or periods of dissociation and no behavior indicating this is noted. Reports having nightmares. Night shift notes that he awakens every 2 hours and moves about restlessly during periods of sleep. Continue care plan and evaluate every shift and prn if condition changes.

**Nursing Care Plan:** PTSD, uncontrolled Type II DM, HHS resolving.
**Nursing Diagnosis:** Risk for Other or Self-directed Violence r/t disturbances in sensory perception, stress, and anxiety s/t memories of military deployment to Iraq AEB flashbacks and nightmares, paranoia, carrying a gun, pushing neighbor down, barricading self in own dwelling, threatening to shoot police, and becoming physically combative in addition to threatening to harm others in the ambulance.
**Outcomes:** 1. Will refrain from attempting to hurt others or self throughout hospitalization. 2. Will verbalize intent to avoid triggers of flashbacks and nightmares whenever possible after discharge.

| Assessment Data: O = Objective, S = Subjective | Evidence-Based Interventions: | Rationales: | Patient Responses: |
|---|---|---|---|
| Carrying a gun (O) Paranoia (O) Misperceived neighbor's presence in the yard and accused him of helping enemy forces (S) Pushed neighbor down (O) Barricaded self in own dwelling and threatened to shoot police (O) Flashbacks (S) Nightmares (S) Signs and symptoms triggered by watching CNN coverage on television of the current situation in Iraq (S) Diagnosis of PTSD (O) Stopped attending weekly support group (S) While in ambulance being transported to the hospital became physically combative, started screaming, and verbally threatened to harm anyone who came near him (O) | 1(a) Begin to develop a rapport and a trusting relationship with the patient.

(b) Assess for risk of harming others and self. Obtain a verbal no harm to others or self contract with patient every shift and prn.

(c) Initiate and maintain safety checks every 15 minutes. | 1(a) Rapport and trust will help the nurse and other staff be more able to convince the patient that they want to help rather than harm him. It will help decrease the patient's anxiety level and in turn decrease the risk of agitating the patient.

(b) There is still high risk for the patient to attempt to harm others or himself due to his symptoms and the unpredictability of when flashbacks will occur. In addition, the patient has an IV and the tubing presents a potential means of harming others or himself. A behavior contract actively engages patients as active participants in their treatment and encourages personal responsibility for their behavior. It also demonstrates staff involvement. If a patient's condition changes, it may be necessary to obtain another contract earlier than the next scheduled shift.

(c) This measure ensures the patient's location is known by staff, which helps maintain the safety of others as well as himself. | 1(a) Tolerates the presence of the primary assigned nurse and other nursing staff.

(b) Denies thoughts or impulses to harm others or himself at this time. Denies flashbacks or periods of dissociation. Reports that he is having nightmares. Noted by night shift to awaken every 2 hours and move about restlessly during periods of sleep. Able to contract verbally not to harm others or himself. Continues to need IVFs and the tubing presents a potentially dangerous situation.

(c) Verbalizes understanding of the need for safety checks every 15 minutes. |

*(continues)*

| Assessment Data:<br>O = Objective,<br>S = Subjective | Evidence-Based<br>Interventions: | Rationales: | Patient<br>Responses: |
|---|---|---|---|
| | (d) Maintain an environment free from potentially harmful objects. | (d) This decreases opportunities for the patient to harm others or himself. | (d) Cooperates with unit rules regarding contraband and verbalizes understanding of safety needs. |
| | (e) Maintain a calm, soothing environment. | (e) A calm, soothing environment decreases the potential for the patient becoming overly anxious and agitated. It will also help decrease the chances of triggering a flashback episode. | (e) Seems hypervigilant and easily startled. Responds positively to calm, soothing environment. |
| | (f) Assess for flashbacks, dissociation, and nightmares. | (f) These are signs and symptoms of PTSD, and the patient will become increasingly anxious, agitated, and aggressive when experiencing these symptoms. Early recognition of these signs and symptoms will allow the nurse to intervene. | (f) Denies episodes of dissociation and has not exhibited any such behavior since being transferred to this unit. |
| | (g) Avoid touching the patient when he is experiencing flashbacks. | (g) A patient with PTSD is easily startled and very anxious. Touch can be very frightening and uncomfortable and may lead the patient to respond impulsively and aggressively from a self-defense standpoint. | (g) See (f) above. Seems hypervigilant and easily startled. Responds positively when care is explained prior to delivering it. |
| | (h) Assess for hypervigilence, increased muscle tension, and psychomotor agitation. | (h) These are signs and symptoms of increased anxiety and agitation. They are warning signs of impending violence. | (h) Is hypervigilant and easily startled. Exhibits less muscle tension when he is approached in a calm, non-threatening manner. Has received 1 prn dose of Zyprexa Zydis and 2 prn doses of Ativan since being transferred to this unit. |
| | (i) Reassure the patient about his safety. | (i) Reassuring the patient will help decrease his anxiety as well as the risk that he will act impulsively to protect himself. | (i) Accepts and expresses gratitude for verbal reassurances of safety. |

| Assessment Data:<br>O = Objective,<br>S = Subjective | Evidence-Based<br>Interventions: | Rationales: | Patient<br>Responses: |
|---|---|---|---|
|  | (j) Intervene as early as possible when noticing behavior that indicates the patient is experiencing flashbacks, dissociation, or nightmares.<br>(k) Avoid making verbal demands or physically cornering the patient.<br><br>(l) If patient begins to escalate, use simple, clear, firm statements when redirecting him to try to calm down. Suggest, rather than insist on, going to a quieter area on the unit or his own room. | (j) Early intervention decreases the risk of harm to the patient or others. It also allows for the use of the least restrictive intervention methods.<br>(k) This will help decrease the risk of agitating the patient and triggering aggressive responses.<br>(l) Complex directions and lengthy explanations will challenge the patient's ability to concentrate, which may result in increased agitation and aggression. The patient will be more able to understand and follow simple, clear, firm redirections. | (j) Accepts interventions by night shift, including deep breathing, soft music, guided imagery, and prn medication.<br><br>(k) Sensitive to subtle changes in his environment. Responds well to suggestions versus demands.<br>(l) Although hypervigilant and easily startled, cooperates with distraction techniques and prn medication when necessary. |
|  | (m) Give verbal praise for efforts made to control his behavior and impulses.<br>(n) Administer scheduled and prn medication as ordered. Assess for EPS and NMS. | (m) Verbal praise will help reinforce the same behavior for future situations.<br>(n) Medications may help the patient to maintain control by decreasing his PTSD signs and symptoms. The patient is ordered Geodon, which is less likely than traditional antipyschotics to cause EPS or NMS but may still do so. | (m) Accepts verbal praise.<br><br>(n) Accepts scheduled and prn medication when offered. |
|  | (o) Reorient patient to reality prn and help him to differentiate between flashbacks, nightmares, and reality.<br><br>(p) Teach adapative ways to cope with anxiety, impulses, and anger. | (o) This will help decrease the patient's misperceptions as well as impulsive, aggressive responses to what he thinks is happening.<br>(p) Adaptive coping will help decrease the patient's maladaptive, aggressive behavioral responses. | (o) Remains alert and oriented in all spheres. Denies episodes of dissociation and has not exhibited behavior indicating dissociation since being transferred to this unit.<br>(p) States willingness to try deep breathing, guided imagery, and physical exercise. Agrees to try to walk away from situations that cause him to be angry until more able to<br><br>*(continues)* |

| Assessment Data:<br>O = Objective,<br>S = Subjective | Evidence-Based<br>Interventions: | Rationales: | Patient<br>Responses: |
|---|---|---|---|
| | | | talk about what is bothering him. |
| | (q) Be sensitive to the patient's emotional and physical cues of needing to change the topic or postpone conversation. Offer to stay with the patient. | (q) Pressing the patient to continue will increase his anxiety and cause agitation that may lead to aggressive behavior. | (q) Declines to talk about Iraq experiences and changes the subject. |
| | (r) Teach patient the connections between trauma, triggers, and his responses. | (r) Patients do not always know the reasons behind their actions. This knowledge can increase their understanding and help decrease any guilt over previous actions. | (r) States he was not aware of any connections between what he experienced in Iraq, triggers, and his responses. |
| | (s) Assist patient to identify triggers of aggressive behavior and develop a plan to avoid these when possible. Include adaptive responses in plan. | (s) Identifying triggers will help the patient become more aware of what precedes his increased anxiety and impulsive, aggressive reactions. Adaptive responses will help decrease violent reactions if the patient cannot totally avoid the identified triggers. | (s) Admits that until this admission he did not realize that watching the CNN reports on the current situation in Iraq would have caused him to react as he did. Admits he did not realize that he had been going out in the yard at night. Does not remember accusing his neighbor of helping enemy forces or pushing him down. Does not remember barricading himself in his home. Collaborates with primary nurse and treatment team in planning treatment. Agrees to avoid violent TV programs and movies, to use new coping/distraction strategies that he is learning, and to return to the support group he had been attending. |

**Evaluation:** 1. Has refrained from harming others or himself.
2. Is collaborating with primary nurse and treatment team in planning both inpatient treatment and future outpatient treatment. Agrees to avoid violent TV programs and movies, to use new coping/distraction strategies that he is learning, and to return to the support group he had been attending. Continue care plan and evaluate every shift and prn if condition changes.

**Nursing Care Plan:** PTSD, uncontrolled Type II DM, HHS resolving.
**Nursing Diagnosis:** Imbalanced Nutrition: More Than Body Requirements r/t altered metabolism and stopping medication when experiencing flashbacks s/t uncontrolled Type II DM and HHS AEB blood glucose = 420, HgA1C = 8.5, and reportedly not taking Starlix/nateglinide 80 mg po tid before meals.
**Outcomes:** 1. Will be free from life-threatening complications of HHS throughout hospitalization. 2. Will experience blood glucose levels within a range of 70–110 within 72 hours of being transferred to the medical-psychiatric unit.

| Assessment Data:<br>O = Objective,<br>S = Subjective | Evidence-Based<br>Interventions: | Rationales: | Patient<br>Responses: |
|---|---|---|---|
| Blood glucose = 420 (O)<br>HgA1C = 8.5 (O)<br>Reportedly not taking Starlix/nateglinide when experiencing flashbacks (S)<br>Diagnoses of uncontrolled Type II DM and HHS (O) | 1(a) Maintain IVFs: 1000 cc D5W at 125 cc per hour as ordered. | 1(a) HHS patients have high serum levels of glucose, which results in osmotic dieresis and dehydration. If not corrected, it can lead to electrolyte imbalances, further dehydration, and hypovolemia. The most serious complications of HHS include seizures, coma, shock, and death (Lewis, Heitkemper, Dirkson, O'Brien, & Bucher, 2007, p. 1281). Therefore, it is important to keep the patient well hydrated. Also, when the serum glucose level reaches 250, the IVF solution is changed from 0.9% NS to D5W to prevent the serum glucose from falling too rapidly. | 1(a) Tolerates IVFs well. Has had no complications related to IV therapy. |
| | (b) Maintain I & O every shift. | (b) The nurse will need to assess the patient's I & O to help monitor the patient's fluid balance. | (b) Has normal intake and output. |
| | (c) Perform CBGs ac & hs as ordered. Administer regular insulin sliding scale with coverage starting at 151. | (c) Because the patient's serum glucose is still not controlled, he will require more frequent assessment and subcutaneous administration of insulin in addition to oral medication. | (c) Has CBGs ranging from 200 to 250. Receiving regular insulin as ordered. |
| | (d) Administer Starlix/nateglinide 80 mg po tid before meals. | (d) Starlix/nateglinide, a nonsulfonylurea hypoglycemic medication, stimulates insulin production by beta cells in the pancreas to help decrease serum glucose (McKenry, | (d) Accepts and physically tolerates Starlix/nateglinide. Verbalizes understanding of need to take medication regularly as ordered to maintain control of blood glucose.<br><br>*(continues)* |

| Assessment Data: O = Objective, S = Subjective | Evidence-Based Interventions: | Rationales: | Patient Responses: |
|---|---|---|---|
| | (e) Provide a 2000-calorie ADA diet as ordered. Include patient preferences when feasible. | Tessier, & Hogan, 2006, p. 880). (e) The patient will need an adequate amount of nutritious calories for his metabolic needs, without exceeding those requirements. Including his preferences when feasible will increase his adherence to the diet while in the hospital and after discharge. | (e) Verbalizes understanding of the need to adhere to specified diet. Expresses interest in learning to be able to vary the diet and include personal preferences when possible. |
| | (f) Explore with patient ways he can monitor himself related to taking medication (e.g., use a pillbox or a simple check-off system, or have a family member or friend check how much of his medication he is taking or has left in the bottle). | (f) The patient adheres to medication except when experiencing flashbacks. Other methods of ensuring that he takes his medication need to be explored. | (f) Agrees to ask some of the people in his support group to help him monitor his medication. |
| | (g) Request a dietician consult. | (g) The dietician will work with the patient to help increase adherence to the prescribed diet by helping him include as many of his preferred foods as possible and showing him healthy ways to cook foods. | (g) Agrees to meet with the dietician. |

**Evaluation:** 1. Remains free from life-threatening complication of HHS.
2. CBGs ranging from 200 to 250 at 48 hours from transfer to the medical-psychiatric unit. Receiving regular insulin on a sliding scale as ordered as well as regularly scheduled Starlix/nateglinide 80 mg po tid before meals. Continue care plan and evaluate in 24 hours and prn if condition changes.

# Question 7

   a. Recognize the signs and symptoms of PTSD: depression, anxiety, dissociation or dissociative amnesia, derealization, nightmares, or disturbing dreams, difficulty falling asleep, flashbacks, intrusive recollections of the event, avoidance of anything associated with the traumatic event, emotional numbing or absence of emotional responses, feelings of detachment, hyperarousal, poor concentration, and irritability or outbursts of anger. These symptoms do not mean the patient is "going crazy," but are instead psychological and biological reactions to the trauma that he experienced. The patient may also experience significant problems functioning in important areas of his life, including occupational and social areas. Early detection and treatment can decrease serious, lifelong consequences and help the patient achieve a better quality of life.

   b. Become familiar with the medications as well as psychotherapy that are used to treat PTSD. The medications ordered will depend on the symptoms the patient is experiencing. Klonopin/clonazepam and Ativan/lorazepam are antiseizure medications, specifically benzodiazepines, used to relieve anxiety. Klonopin/clonazepam has a longer half-life than Ativan/lorazepam, and therefore there is less risk of becoming dependent on the medication. Ativan/lorazepam has a shorter half-life and will be used only short term until there is time for a blood level of Klonopin/Clonazepam to be established. Common side effects include drowsiness, fatigue, dry mouth, incoordination, muscle weakness, dizziness, and blurred vision.

     Geodon/ziprasidone is a second generation or atypical antipsychotic medication used to treat flashbacks, dissociative episodes, or nightmares. Common side effects include sedation, fatigue, constipation, and weight gain. There is less risk for EPS or NMS with second generation or atypical antipsychotic medication, but the patient should still report any involuntary muscle movements, difficulty breathing or swallowing, high fever, increased sweating, rapid heart rate or palpitations, muscle rigidity, or mental confusion. There is less risk for increased serum glucose and cholesterol levels with Geodon/ziprasidone as compared to Clozaril/clozapine, Zyprexa/olanzapine, and Risperdal/risperidone.

   c. Stress the importance of taking medication exactly as prescribed to ensure maximum effectiveness and therapeutic blood level. No medication should be stopped without psychiatrist's or psychiatric nurse practitioner's knowledge to help avoid any potential withdrawal symptoms. (This would be less likely with Klonopin/clonazepam due to the long half-life.) It usually takes a few weeks to achieve the maximum benefit from medications.

d. Reinforce the avoidance of alcohol, illegal drugs, herbal preparations, and OTC medications, and the misuse of prescription medications. These will interfere with how well their medication works and may cause dangerous interactions.

e. Reinforce that Starlix/nateglinide is a hypoglycemic medication used to treat Type II DM. The medication helps stimulate the pancreas to produce more insulin. It is important to take the medication as ordered before meals so that there is more insulin available to the body when it is needed to metabolize any food eaten.

f. Reinforce signs and symptoms of both hyperglycemia and hypoglycemia. Include teaching the patient that infection, injury, and psychological or physical stress can increase blood glucose levels.

g. Assess patient's ability to perform his own CBGs.

h. Reinforce proper foot care and daily inspection of feet.

i. Relapse prevention: Continue to teach to avoid triggers such as viewing violent TV programs/movies. Provide information on adaptive coping and distraction strategies, including deep breathing, progressive relaxation exercises, guided imagery, listening to soft music, physical exercise, yoga, meditation, and aromatherapy with calming scents (e.g., lavender, chamomile, bergamot).

j. Reinforce the need to continue with CBT and systematic desensitization therapy to help decrease the negative impact of traumatic events that the patient experienced in Iraq.

k. Encourage patient to continue with spiritual practices.

l. Reinforce the importance of continuing to go to support groups.

m. Teach patient to listen to others when they say he is not acting like his usual self. This could be an important early relapse sign to be followed when possible by seeking help to prevent rehospitalization.

n. Advise patient to obtain a medical alert bracelet or card to carry in his wallet with his medications and conditions listed on it.

o. Suggest that the patient provide his next door neighbor with as much information as the patient is comfortable since the neighbor is close by and knows at least some of his problems.

# Question 8

Discharge referrals should include the following:

a. Veterans Affairs (VA) psychiatrist for continued assessment of condition and management of treatment, including psychotropic medications. The patient also has the right to seek healthcare services from a non-VA psychiatrist.

b. VA psychologist for individual and group psychotherapy, CBT, systematic desensitization therapy, and psychoeducation. The patient also has the right to seek healthcare services from a non-VA psychologist. These services may also be provided by a qualified APRN or social worker.

c. Medical physician for management of Type II DM.

d. Case management services to decrease chance of patient missing appointments or medications when experiencing flashbacks. Case management also helps ensure that the patient receives all the healthcare services he needs and is eligible for without duplicating services.

e. Assistance if needed for obtaining medications through VA or non-VA pharmacies.

f. Financial assistance if needed through social work or case management.

g. Assertive Community Treatment (ACT).

h. Support groups for PTSD and DM.

i. Involvement of family and friends to the degree that the patient is comfortable with.

# References

American Psychiatric Association. (2000). *Diagnostic and statistical manual of mental disorders* (4th ed.). Washington, DC: Author.

Bezchlibnyk-Butler, K. Z., & Jeffries, J. J. (2005). *Clinical handbook of psychotropic drugs* (15th ed.). Ashland, OH: Hogrefe & Huber.

Boyd, M. A. (2008). *Psychiatric nursing: Contemporary practice* (4th ed.). Philadelphia, PA: Wolters-Kluwer/Lippincott Williams & Wilkins.

Fischbach, F. (2004). *A manual of laboratory and diagnositic tests* (7th ed.). Philadelphia, PA: Lippincott Williams & Wilkins.

Fontaine, K. L., & Fletcher, J. S. (2003). *Mental health nursing* (5th ed.). Upper Saddle River, NJ: Pearson.

Fortinash, K. M., & Holoday Worret, P. A. (2007). *Psychiatric nursing care plans* (5th ed.). St. Louis, MO: Mosby, Elsevier.

Gahart, B. L., & Nazareno, A. R. (2003). *Intravenous medications: A handbook for nurses and allied health professions* (19th ed.). St. Louis, MO: Mosby.

Hodgson, B. B., & Kizior, R. J. (2005). *Saunders nursing drug handbook*. St. Louis, MO: Mosby.

Keltner, N. L., Schwecke, L. H., & Bostrom, C. E. (2007). *Psychiatric nursing* (5th ed.). St. Louis, MO: Mosby, Elsevier.

Kidd, P. S., & Wagner, K. D. (2001). *High acuity nursing* (3rd ed.). Upper Saddle River, NJ: Pearson.

Lewis, S. L., Heitkemper, M. M., & Dirksen, S. R. (2004). *Medical-Surgical nursing: Assessment strategies and management of clinical problems* (6th ed.). St. Louis, MO: Mosby.

Lewis, S. L., Heitkemper, M. M., Dirksen, S. R., O'Brien, P. G., & Bucher, L. (2007). *Medical-Surgical nursing: Assessment and management of clinical problems* (7th ed.). St. Louis, MO: Mosby, Elsevier.

McKenry, L., Tessier, E., & Hogan, M. (2006). *Mosby's pharmacology in nursing* (22nd ed.). St. Louis, MO: Mosby.

*Mosby's medical, nursing, and allied health dictionary* (6th ed.). (2002). St. Louis, MO: Mosby.

O'Brien, P. G., Kennedy, W. Z., & Ballard, K. A. (2008). *Psychiatric mental health nursing: An introduction to theory and practice.* Sudbury, MA: Jones and Bartlett.

Pagana, K. D., & Pagana, T. J. (2007). *Mosby's diagnostic and laboratory test reference* (8th ed.). St. Louis, MO: Mosby/Elsevier.

Townsend, M. C. (2008). *Essentials of psychiatric mental health nursing: Concepts of care in evidence-based practice* (4th ed.). Philadelphia, PA: F. A. Davis.

Varcarolis, E. M., Carson, V. B., & Shoemaker, N. C. (2006). *Foundations of psychiatric mental health nursing: A clinical approach* (6th ed.). St. Louis, MO: Saunders, Elsevier.

Videbeck, S. L. (2008). *Psychiatric-mental health nursing* (4th ed.). Philadelphia, PA: Wolters Kluwer/Lippincott Williams & Wilkins.

Wilder, S. S., & Sorenson, C. (2001). *Essentials of aggression management in health care.* Upper Saddle River, NJ: Prentice Hall.

# CHAPTER 8

# Sexual and Gender Identity Disorders: Gender Identity Disorder

## ANSWER KEY

## Question 1

The client states that he has always felt uncomfortable being around men and feels the most comfortable in the company of women. He also enjoys engaging in what would typically be described as "women's work." At age 12 he began secretly dressing in his younger sister's clothing and at age 16 he was discovered by his father when wearing a dress belonging to his younger sister. He is increasingly convinced that he should have been "born a woman" and "God must have goofed up with me." He asked his medical physician for a sex change operation.

## Question 2

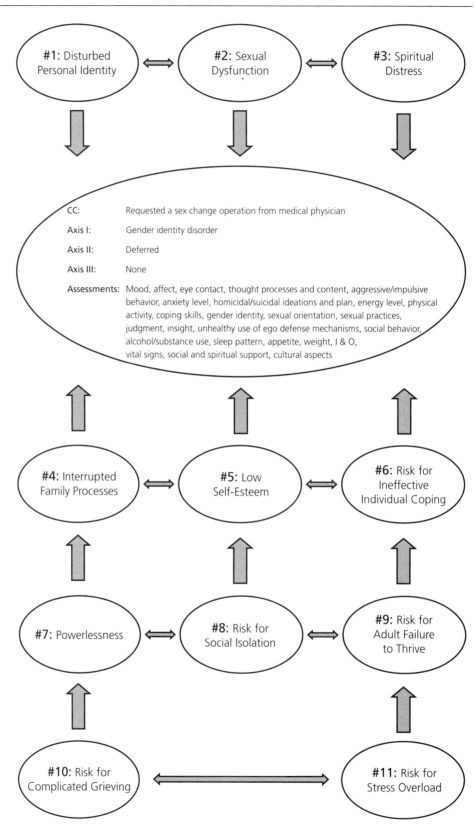

# Questions 3 and 4

**Nursing Care Plan:** Gender identity disorder.
**Nursing Diagnosis:** Disturbed Personal Identity r/t contradictory self-concept and body image AEB self-statements of being increasingly convinced that he should have been "born a woman" and "God must have goofed up with me."
**Outcomes:** 1. Will explore emotional contradictions in self concept and body image with genetic identity during the next 2 weeks of outpatient treatment.

| Assessment Data: O = Objective, S = Subjective | Evidence-Based Interventions: | Rationales: | Patient Responses:* |
|---|---|---|---|
| States always felt uncomfortable being around men (S) States feels the most comfortable in the company of women (S) Enjoys engaging in what would typically be described as "women's work" (S) At age 12 he began secretly dressing in his younger sister's clothing (S) His father discovered him at age 16 wearing a dress belonging to his younger sister and kicked him out of the house (S) States that he is increasingly convinced that he should have been "born a woman" and "God must have goofed up with me." (S) Requested a sex change operation (S) Wears gender neutral clothing (O) | 1(a) Begin to develop a rapport and a therapeutic nurse/patient alliance that is the beginning of the therapeutic nurse/patient relationship. (b) Maintain a nonjudgmental attitude when interacting with client. (c) Use therapeutic communication techniques to help client express feelings about how he perceived himself compared to his physical and secondary sexual characteristics. (d) Provide emotional support and verbal praise for attempts to verbalize feelings and thoughts. (e) Assist client to identify personal strengths. | 1(a) Developing a rapport with the patient will assist in gaining the patient's trust and cooperation in the future. According to Peplau the therapeutic nurse/patient relationship is the foundation that must be established to initiate future work in the healing process (Keltner, Schwecke, & Bostrom, 2007). (b) The client will be more able to trust the nurse and express feelings more openly when he perceives that he will be accepted rather than judged. (c) Therapeutic communication techniques are used to help patients express their thoughts and feelings as well as obtain information from them. (d) Emotional support and praise are very valuable when clients are expressing emotionally and psychologically sensitive topics. (e) The client's personal strengths will be used to | 1(a) Agrees to work with the nurse assigned to him. Asks appropriate questions. Verbalizes understanding of nurse's role as well as his own in the nurse/patient relationship. (b) Responds well to nonjudgmental attitude during interactions. (c) Opens up to nurse during therapeutic communication interactions. States that he truly believes that he is a female inside in spite of male physical characteristics. Admits that this makes him feel confused as to who he is as a person. (d) Accepts emotional support and verbal praise. (e) Worked with nurse to identify personal strengths such as |

*(continues)*

*Patient responses are examples of what students would look for to decide whether their planned interventions were successful, needed more time, or needed to be changed. Responses will vary depending on the patient.

| Assessment Data: O = Objective, S = Subjective | Evidence-Based Interventions: | Rationales: | Patient Responses: |
|---|---|---|---|
| | | help him cope more adaptively. | intelligence, caring, compassion, and physically attractive face. |
| | (f) Explore how client emotionally perceives his gender versus physical characteristics and possible reasons for the difference between his perception and reality. | (f) This approach will help the nurse obtain a clearer picture of what is happening to the client from his point of view. It may also help begin to identify what led to the client internally or emotionally perceiving himself as a woman. | (f) States that he feels he is a female even though his physical characteristics are male. Remembers even as a small child preferring to play with girls and disliking any rough sports. |
| | (g) Assess client's current knowledge of healthy sexuality and clarify misconceptions. | (g) A person's gender identity and genetic identity may be male even though the person may be interested in activities and interests stereotyped as female. This does not mean that the person should have been born a female instead. | (g) Because he prefers "female" activities and dress, states that he assumed that it may have meant he should have been born a female. |
| | (h) Encourage the use of journaling and various art modalities to express thoughts and feelings related to his personal identity, body image, and sexuality. | (h) Thoughts and feelings related to personal identity or self-concept are complex even when patients are not questioning their identity. These alternate methods of expression will help provide a clearer picture of how the client truly feels and what he is truly thinking. These issues can be shared with the client's outpatient treatment team and explored further in psychotherapy. | (h) States that he enjoys journaling. Painted two pictures of himself: one with a female body and the other with a male body. |

**Evaluation:** 1. Has begun to explore his emotional contradictions in self-concept and body image with his genetic identity. Continue care plan and evaluate in 1 week.

**Nursing Care Plan:** Gender identity disorder.
**Nursing Diagnosis:** Sexual Dysfunction r/t inability to maintain successful intimate relationships AEB admitting to having difficulty with satisfying sexual experiences because of his gender problems.
**Outcomes:** 1. Verbalize intent to try alternative satisfying activities in place of sexual activities while exploring treatment options, including a sex change operation as requested, during the next 2 weeks of outpatient treatment.

| Assessment Data: O = Objective, S = Subjective | Evidence-Based Interventions: | Rationales: | Patient Responses: |
|---|---|---|---|
| Difficulty with satisfying sexual experiences because of his gender problems (S) States that he is increasingly convinced that he should have been "born a woman" and "God must have goofed up with me." (S) | 1(a) Obtain a sexual history using a matter-of-fact, nonjudgmental approach. | 1(a) This will establish a baseline of information, clarify information already obtained, and help identify any additional problems not reported at this time. The information is emotionally sensitive and may be embarrassing for both the client and nurse. Using a matter-of-fact, nonjudgmental approach will help decrease any embarrassment for everyone involved. | 1(a) Cooperative with sexual history. Denies any feelings or thoughts that he is homosexual or bisexual. Denies any paraphilias. States he is romantically attracted to men, but "hates" his male genitals and wishes to have them removed. Perceives himself as the "female" in a relationship with a male. |
| | (b) Assess client's coping strategies. | (b) Adaptive coping strategies will be reinforced while maladaptive ones (e.g., substance abuse) will be discouraged. The nurse and other members of the treatment team will work with the client to replace maladaptive methods with adaptive ones. | (b) States that when he is upset he listens to soft music and walks in the local park. Agrees to continue using these coping strategies. |
| | (c) Explore alternative satisfying activities including hobbies, physical exercise, artistic expression, and activities requiring mental concentration. | (c) These alternatives will provide healthy distraction and adaptive methods of coping. | (c) States that he would like to learn to play chess and the guitar. |
| | (d) Assess for signs and symptoms of depression. | (d) Sexuality and sexual gratification are important aspects of the whole person. People who have difficulty getting their needs met may become depressed. A symptom of major depression is decreased libido. | (d) Denies signs and symptoms of major depression. Denies suicidal thoughts. States he has the desire to have a sexual relationship, but is having difficulty finding a suitable partner and being able to perform as the female he perceives himself to be. |

*(continues)*

| Assessment Data: O = Objective, S = Subjective | Evidence-Based Interventions: | Rationales: | Patient Responses: |
|---|---|---|---|
| | (e) Suggest a referral to a qualified sex therapist. | (e) An expert in sexual problems will be able to help the client deal with psychological issues related to sexual dysfunction. The client does not have any physical problems according to his medical physician. Even if the client does have a sex change operation, he will still need long-term counseling to deal with his new role and the physical changes in his body. | (e) Agrees to meet with a qualified sex therapist. |

**Evaluation:** 1. The client currently listens to soft music and walks in the local park. States that he would also like to learn to play chess and the guitar. Agrees to meet with a qualified sex therapist. Continue care plan and evaluate in 1 week.

**Nursing Care Plan:** Gender identity disorder.
**Nursing Diagnosis:** Spiritual Distress r/t difficulty connecting internal and external aspects of the self, disagreement with his higher power, and cultural differences AEB internal perception of being a female despite his male physical characteristics; states that he should have been "born a woman" and "God must have goofed up with me," and having to leave home at age 16.
**Outcomes:** 1. Will discuss spiritual concerns during the next 2 weeks of outpatient treatment.

| Assessment Data:<br>O = Objective,<br>S = Subjective | Evidence-Based Interventions: | Rationales: | Patient Responses: |
|---|---|---|---|
| States that he is increasingly convinced that he should have been "born a woman" and "God must have goofed up with me." (S)<br>States that he always felt uncomfortable being around men (S)<br>States that he feels the most comfortable in the company of women (S)<br>Enjoys engaging in what would typically be described as "women's work" (S)<br>Requested a sex change operation (S)<br>Wears gender neutral clothing (O)<br>His father discovered him at age 16 wearing a dress belonging to his younger sister and kicked him out of the house (S) | 1(a) Perform a spiritual assessment.<br><br><br>(b) Assess whether or not a spiritual belief system provides comfort and strength during times of stress or adds to the client's distress.<br><br><br>(c) Explore whether or not the client has a sense of meaning and purpose for his life. | 1(a) This will establish a baseline of information, clarify information already obtained, and be useful in planning client care.<br><br>(b) A client's spiritual belief system can offer invaluable support and comfort during times of stress if it positively enhances the client's sense of well-being. However, it can also have the opposite effect if it has a negative effect on the client's sense of meaning and purpose in the world.<br><br>(c) A sense of meaning and purpose for one's life is essential to optimal well-being. Without a sense of meaning or purpose, a person is at high risk to develop despair, powerlessness, and major | 1(a) Admits he has not been involved in any formal, organized religious activities "since I was kicked out of the house at age 16." States he still believes in a power greater than himself, but is ambivalent as to whether he feels loved and accepted by this higher power. Admits to occasionally praying, but he is "not sure if anyone is listening." His family of origin practiced Roman Catholicism, but he recently has been interested in some of the teachings of Buddha.<br>(b) States that he feels conflicted regarding the religious teachings of his childhood. If God is responsible for creation, "He goofed when he made me a man instead of a woman." Continues to believe in the theory of evolution and "some of the creation stuff." Cannot say for certain that he finds comfort or strength in his prior religious beliefs. Is seeking answers in other religious teachings.<br>(c) States that he is not totally certain he has a meaning or purpose for his life, but is seeking to discover it. |

*(continues)*

| Assessment Data:<br>O = Objective,<br>S = Subjective | Evidence-Based<br>Interventions: | Rationales: | Patient<br>Responses: |
|---|---|---|---|
| | (d) Assist the client to identify what gives him joy and helps him feel connected to others around him.<br><br>(e) Plan for support for spiritual practices and beliefs.<br><br><br><br><br><br>(f) Explore adaptive ways to cope with problems related to being accepted by his culture and family. | depression, and even to attempt suicide.<br>(d) Many things in life may cause joy and feelings of connectedness. A broader definition of spirituality encompasses these things.<br>(e) Support for spiritual practices and beliefs helps maintain healthy spiritual-ity and conveys that the nurse understands the importance of spirituality in the client's life.<br>(f) Adaptive ways of cop-ing will help decrease the risk of the client resorting to maladaptive or destructive ways of coping. | (d) States that most types of music give him joy, as does watching a beautiful sunset, and he feels connected to his current housemates.<br><br>(e) Accepts and is involved with planning continued support for current and future spiritual practices and beliefs.<br><br><br>(f) Acknowledges that he struggles with knowing he is not accepted by his family. States that his friends have become his "new family." Agrees that he needs to con-tinue working with his psy-chotherapist on these issues. Collaborated with nurse on a list of positive affirmations to use on a daily basis. |

**Evaluation:** 1. Conflicted regarding the religious teachings of his childhood and not certain that he finds comfort or strength in his prior religious beliefs. Seeking answers in other religious teachings and seeking to discover meaning and purpose for his life.
2. Able to identify what gives him joy in life and he feels connected to his current housemates.
3. Acknowledges that he struggles with knowing he is not accepted by his family of origin, but his current friends have become his "new family." Continue care plan and evaluate in 1 week.

# References

American Psychiatric Association. (2000). *Diagnostic and statistical manual of mental disorders* (4th ed.). Text revision. Washington, DC: Author.

Fortinash, K. M., & Holoday Worret, P. A. (2007). *Psychiatric nursing care plans* (5th ed.). St. Louis, MO: Mosby, Elsevier.

Keltner, N. L., Schwecke, L. H., & Bostrom, C. E. (2007). *Psychiatric nursing* (5th ed.). St. Louis, MO: Mosby, Elsevier.

O'Brien, P. G., Kennedy, W. Z., & Ballard, K. A. (2008). *Psychiatric mental health nursing: An introduction to theory and practice.* Sudbury, MA: Jones and Bartlett.

Stuart, G. W., & Laraia, M. T. (2005). *Principles and practice of psychiatric nursing* (8th ed.). St. Louis, MO: Mosby, Elsevier.

Townsend, M. C. (2008). *Essentials of psychiatric mental health nursing: Concepts of care in evidence based practice* (4th ed.). Philadelphia, PA: F. A. Davis.

Varcarolis, E. M., Carson, V. B., & Shoemaker, N. C. (2006). *Foundations of psychiatric mental health nursing: A clinical approach* (6th ed.). St. Louis, MO: Saunders, Elsevier.

# Web Sites

American Psychological Association: www.apa.org

Gender Identity Disorder & Transgenderism: www.genderpsychology.org

Information About Gender Identity Disorders: www.fags.org/healthtopics/21/Gender-identity_disorder.htm

# Cognitive and Medical Disorders: Alzheimer's Dementia, Coronary Artery Disease, and Atrial Fibrillation

## ANSWER KEY

## Question 1

Agnosia, apraxia, amnesia, and some aphasia; wandering behavior prior to coming to the hospital and during the admission intake interview, disorientation, self-care deficits and sundowning behavior over the past 4 months at the personal care home, and memory impairment and difficulty concentrating.

## Question 2

Hold the next scheduled dose of Coumadin/warfarin and notify the physician. Have vitamin K/Aquamephyton available if needed. Assess patient for signs and symptoms of hemorrhage including intercranial bleeding. For patients not requiring anticoagulant therapy, a PT result within the range of 11–13 is considered to be normal. A different control or reference range is used for patients requiring anticoagulant therapy and will depend on the individual laboratory. The laboratory's control or reference range must be known in order to correctly interpret the PT results. Typically the therapeutic range of the PT for a patient on anticoagulant therapy is 1.5 to 2.5 times the control or reference range. Additionally, the INR is also monitored in patients requiring anticoagulant therapy. INR values greater than 3.5 increase patients' risk of intercranial hemorrhage (McKenry, Tessier, & Hogan, 2006, pp. 607, 610). Both the PT and INR results for this patient are abnormally high, placing the patient at risk for hemorrhage.

# Question 3

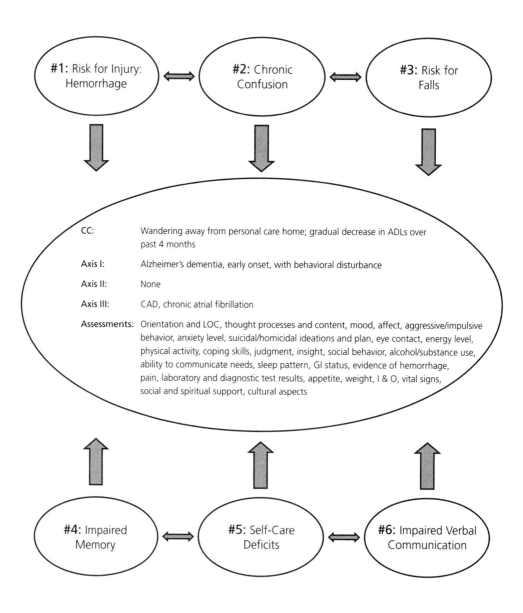

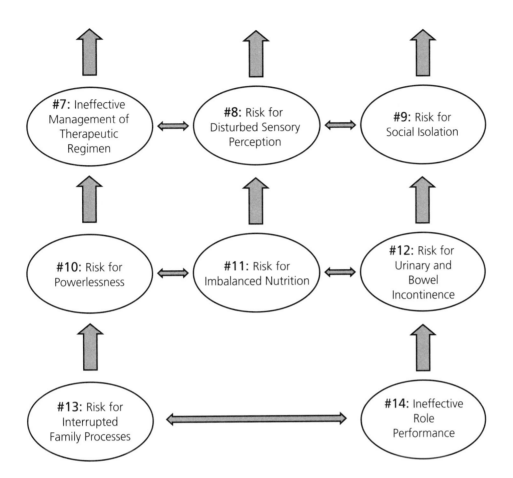

# Questions 4 and 5

**Nursing Care Plan:** Alzheimer's dementia, early onset, with behavioral disturbance.
**Nursing Diagnosis:** Risk for Injury: Hemorrhage r/t adverse effects of medication s/t anticoagulant therapy AEB PT = 60, INR = 3.8, and order for Coumadin/warfarin 5 mg po every day at 5 p.m.
**Outcomes:** 1. Will remain free from hemorrhage and ensuing shock throughout hospitalization.

| Assessment Data: O = Objective, S = Subjective | Evidence-Based Interventions: | Rationales: | Patient Responses:* |
|---|---|---|---|
| Coumadin/warfarin 5 mg po every day at 5 p.m. (O) PT = 60 (control range 11–22) (O) INR = 3.8 (2–3 normal range) (O) | 1(a) Hold next scheduled dose of Coumadin and notify physician. | 1(a) Continuing to administer Coumadin will cause further increases in the PT and INR values, putting the patient at even greater risk of hemorrhage. | 1(a) Patient's daughter as well as the patient verbalize understanding of reasons for holding Coumadin. |
| | (b) Assess for signs and symptoms of hemorrhage including bleeding; decreased LOC or orientation; increasing mental confusion, anxiety; hypotension; tachycardia; tachypnea; cool, clammy, pale skin; abdominal pain; agitation; amber or bloody urine; tarry stools. | (b) Recognizing and reporting signs and symptoms of hemorrhage as early as possible is imperative to avoid life-threatening complications or death. | (b) Patient's daughter as well as the patient verbalize understanding of close observation and daughter agrees to immediately report any bleeding or changes in the patient's condition that they notice. No changes noted in LOC, orientation, mental state, or level of anxiety. No agitation noted. No change in frequency of wandering. Patient's vital signs remain WNL. Patient's skin warm, dry, and pink in color; denies abdominal pain. Patient's urine clear yellow, but has not had a BM. |
| | (c) Administer vitamin K if ordered. | (c) Vitamin K reverses the effects of Coumadin. | (c) No order to administer vitamin K has been given at this time, but it is available if needed. |
| | (d) Limit laboratory tests and needle sticks as much as possible. | (d) This will help decrease the chance of further bleeding. | (d) The patient and his daughter are aware that all laboratory staff and nursing personal have been alerted. |
| | (e) Provide soft toothbrush and electric razor. | (e) These toiletry items are less likely to cause bleeding when performing ADL. | (e) The patient and his daughter agree to use toiletry items as instructed. |

*Patient responses are examples of what students would look for to decide whether their planned interventions were successful, needed more time, or needed to be changed. Responses will vary depending on the patient.

**Evaluation:** 1. Remains free from hemorrhage and ensuing shock. Continue care plan and evaluate in 8 hours and prn if condition changes.

**Nursing Care Plan:** Alzheimer's dementia, early onset, with behavioral disturbance.
**Nursing Diagnosis:** Chronic Confusion r/t changes in cognitive functioning s/t Alzheimer's dementia AEB orientation to self and place only, wandering away from personal care home, and sundowning behavior over the past 4 months.
**Outcomes:** 1. Will participate in the milieu to the full extent he is able throughout hospitalization.

| Assessment Data:<br>O = Objective,<br>S = Subjective | Evidence-Based<br>Interventions: | Rationales: | Patient<br>Responses: |
|---|---|---|---|
| Oriented to self and place only (O)<br>Wandering away from personal care home (S)<br>Sundowning behavior over the past 4 months (S) | 1(a) Assign the same nurses and other staff to the patient when possible.<br><br>(b) Provide a calm, consistent milieu. | 1(a) This will help provide consistency of care for the patient and help reinforce the trusting relationship.<br>(b) This helps the patient know what to expect and decreases irritating stimuli that in turn can help decrease confusion and anxiety. Patients with any type of dementia react negatively to changes in their routine and environment. | 1(a) Responds positively when working with the same nurses and other assigned staff.<br><br>(b) Remains calm. |
|  | (c) Use a calm, nonthreatening approach and avoid sudden movements. | (c) These types of behaviors from nurses and staff members will help decrease the patient's anxiety and confusion. This approach will also decrease the likelihood of causing the patient to feel threatened and become agitated. | (c) Responds well to a calm, nonthreatening approach. Very cooperative. Becomes more confused and anxious when other patients around him move suddenly. |
|  | (d) Explain all care and procedures before beginning. Speak slowly and use clear, concise statements. | (d) This approach will help ensure the patient's cooperation, increase his level of understanding, decrease the chance of startling him, or increasing his anxiety level. It will also decrease the possibility of escalating behavior if he feels threatened. | (d) Cooperates with all care offered. |
|  | (e) If the patient requires eyeglasses or hearing aids, be sure these are available and work properly. | (e) There are normal changes in vision and hearing due to the aging process that can cause confusion in a "normal" patient let alone someone who also has Alzheimer's dementia. | (e) Wears eyeglasses to read only. Needs to be reminded to use them. |
|  | (f) Reorient to time every shift and prn using memory aids such as large | (f) Memory aids are helpful when reorienting patients. | (f) Has difficulty remembering the time, date, or season of the year. *(continues)* |

| Assessment Data:<br>O = Objective,<br>S = Subjective | Evidence-Based<br>Interventions: | Rationales: | Patient<br>Responses: |
|---|---|---|---|
| | calendars and clocks with large print numbers.<br>(g) Perform a Mini Mental Status Exam (MMSE) or Folstein Mini Mental State Exam. | (g) This will provide not only a baseline of the patient's cognition, but also can be used over time to help evaluate the patient's progress. Education level and any physical disabilities must be taken into account when scoring the results. A score of 24–30 indicates no cognitive impairment. | (g) Scores 19 out of 30 on the MMSE. |
| | (h) Avoid changing the type and placement of furniture on the unit. | (h) Again, changes of any type are not tolerated well by patients with any type of dementia. Changes lead to increased confusion, anxiety, and agitation. | (h) Has increased confusion when housekeeping moves furniture to clean the floor. |
| | (i) Provide ample space free from clutter for the patient to wander. | (i) Curtailing the patient's wandering activities will only increase his anxiety level and confusion. This can lead to agitated behavior. | (i) Calm during periods of wandering. If he encounters an obstacle in his path, he becomes anxious and more confused. |
| | (j) Remind patient of program groups and activities. Assist patient as needed to attend. Place program schedule in common area of unit where it is easily visible to all patients. | (j) Confused patients will have more difficulty remembering when groups and other activities are scheduled. They may also forget where the group or activity is being held and need assistance to attend. | (j) Attends scheduled programs and activities if reminded to do so. |
| | (k) Assign a staff member to stay with the patient if needed and avoid physical restraints whenever possible. | (k) Restraining a patient with any type of dementia leads to increased confusion, anxiety, and agitation as well as increased risk for physical harm. Having someone sit with the patient helps provide safety and security without unnecessary legal or ethical restriction of their behavior. | (k) Responds well to having a staff member stay with him prn. |

**Evaluation:** 1. Participates in the milieu to the extent he is able with reminders of when programs, groups, and activities are scheduled. Continue care plan and evaluate in 48 hours and prn if condition changes.

**Nursing Care Plan:** Alzheimer's dementia, early onset, with behavioral disturbance.
**Nursing Diagnosis:** Risk for Falls r/t increased susceptibility s/t confusion, Alzheimer's dementia, and chronic atrial fibrillation AEB increased frequency of wandering from personal care home, oriented to self and place only, and score of 19 out of 30 on MMSE.
**Outcomes:** 1. Will remain free from falls throughout hospitalization.

| Assessment Data:<br>O = Objective,<br>S = Subjective | Evidence-Based Interventions: | Rationales: | Patient Responses: |
|---|---|---|---|
| Increased frequency of wandering from personal care home (S)<br>Oriented to self and place only (O)<br>Score of 19 out of 30 on MMSE (O) | 1(a) Orient patient to surroundings upon admission and reorient prn. | 1(a) When the patient is more familiar with objects in his environment, he will be less likely to run into them, trip, or fall. Since he does have problems with confusion, he will need more frequent reorientation to his surroundings. | 1(a) Needs to be reoriented to surroundings at least once per shift. |
| | (b) Turn bed monitor on and keep bed in low position. | (b) The bed monitor has an alarm that will ring when the patient gets out of bed, alerting nursing staff to check even more frequently on the patient. | (b) Agrees to have bed monitor turned on and verbalizes understanding of why this is important for his safety. |
| | (c) Maintain clutter-free environment in patient room and throughout the unit common areas. | (c) A cluttered environment increases the risk that the patient will trip or fall. | (c) At first displayed increased anxiety when some of his belongings were placed in the closet in his room. Became less anxious when reasons for reducing clutter that might increase his risk of falling was explained to him. |
| | (d) Assist to ambulate when necessary. | (d) If the patient is unsteady on his feet, he is at increased risk for falling. Assisting him to ambulate can help prevent falls. | (d) At this time the patient states he does not require assistance to ambulate, and this is validated. Staff will continue to monitor him closely. |
| | (e) Be sure patient is wearing properly fitting, supportive, non-skid footwear when ambulating.<br>(f) Maintain proper lighting in patient room and on the unit. | (e) Ill-fitting, nonsupportive, or slippery footwear contributes to falls.<br><br>(f) Proper lighting is necessary for the patient to be able to see clearly and decrease his risk for falling. | (e) Wears properly fitting, supportive, nonskid footwear when ambulating to the bathroom and anywhere on the unit.<br>(f) Patient agrees that lighting is suitable for his needs. |

**Evaluation:** 1. Remains free from falls. Continue care plan and evaluate in 24 hours and prn if condition changes.

# Question 6

The following Alzheimer's caregiver support groups can provide information or support:

Alzheimer's Association: www.alz.org

National Institute on Aging at the National Institutes of Health: www.nia .nih.gov

# References

American Psychiatric Association. (2000). *Diagnostic and statistical manual of mental disorders* (4th ed.). Text Revision. Washington, DC: Author.

Bezchlibnyk-Butler, K. Z., & Jeffries, J. J. (2005). *Clinical handbook of psychotropic drugs* (15th ed.). Ashland, OH: Hogrefe & Huber.

Carpenito-Moyat, L. J. (2008). *Nursing diagnosis: Application to clinical practice* (12th ed.). Philadelphia, PA: WoltersKluwer Lippincott Williams & Wilkins.

Fischbach, F. (2004). *A manual of laboratory and diagnositic tests* (7th ed.). Philadelphia, PA: Lippincott Williams & Wilkins.

Keltner, N. L., Schwecke, L. H., & Bostrom, C. E. (2007). *Psychiatric nursing* (5th ed.). St. Louis, MO: Mosby, Elsevier.

Lewis, S. L., Heitkemper, M. M., & Dirksen, S. R. (2004). *Medical-surgical nursing: Assessment strategies and management of clinical problems* (6th ed.). St. Louis, MO: Mosby.

Lewis, S. L., Heitkemper, M. M., Dirksen, S. R., O'Brien, P. G., & Bucher, L. (2007). *Medical-surgical nursing: Assessment and management of clinical problems* (7th ed.). St. Louis, MO: Mosby/Elsevier.

McKenry, L., Tessier, E., & Hogan, M. (2006). *Mosby's pharmacology in nursing* (22nd ed.). St. Louis, MO: Mosby.

*Mosby's medical, nursing, and allied health dictionary* (6th ed.). (2002). St. Louis, MO: Mosby.

O'Brien, P. G., Kennedy, W. Z., & Ballard, K. A. (2008). *Psychiatric mental health nursing: An introduction to theory and practice.* Sudbury, MA: Jones and Bartlett.

# Web Sites

Alzheimer's Association: www.alz.org

National Institute on Aging: www.nia.nih.gov

# CHAPTER 10

# Psychiatric Emergencies

## *Domestic Violence and Sexual Assault*

## ANSWER KEY

## Question 1

The patient's current and past injuries do not match the reasons given; they are more severe than should result from the reasons given. X-rays of the patient's right arm show a spiral fracture of the humerus, which would not be sustained from tripping over children's toys. She also has several bruises in various stages of healing on her extremities. She describes herself as clumsy. The patient also is fearful in her husband's presence. Her affect is anxious, she displays poor eye contact, and she flinches when he stands close to her. She is visibly more relaxed after he leaves the area. Also, the husband becomes argumentative when asked to leave the area as if there may be something to hide.

## Question 2

A sexual assault nurse examiner (SANE) will examine the victim and collect evidence of the rape from the victim herself and her belongings. Evidence must be collected using specific methods to be used as evidence in a court of law. A rape kit is usually available that contains supplies typically used in evidence collection. Traditionally the victim is asked to refrain from changing clothes or bathing before being examined so as to preserve as much of the evidence of possible. Some evidence may still be present even though the victim has changed her clothes and bathed before seeking treatment. In addition to physical examination, specimens are collected, with some to be tested for sexually transmitted diseases. Medications are prescribed prophylactically with the approval of the physician. Evidence may be collected up to 96 hours, and in some states 120 hours, after the rape occurred. Pictures are taken with the patient's written consent because by the time a case goes to court injuries may be healed.

The SANE acts as an objective presenter of evidence in court helping to strengthen the victim's case against the perpetrator. Follow-up care is scheduled before the victim leaves the ER. Evidence collection is completely documented. If there is a situation where there are dependent children in need of care, the social worker is notified to evaluate the situation and provide necessary services.

The sexual assault advocate, or in some areas rape counselor, provides much needed emotional support during this emotionally devastating time. This person may provide comfort measures, offer to call someone, and help with other basic needs at this time. Victims who live alone are usually advised to ask someone they trust to stay with them rather than be alone. Both the sexual assault advocate and the SANE will reinforce that the victim did whatever they needed to survive the situation and is not to be blamed for what happened. Appropriate documentation must be done in the victim's chart including who was contacted regarding the situation and their response.

# Question 3

Legal and ethical responsibilities of the nurse include following individual state and facility reporting laws. All facilities have specific reporting forms to be used. Any pictures taken must have the victim's written consent for authorization. The victim can legally refuse to have pictures taken and refuse to press legal charges. The nurse would provide privacy and empathy, and she would reinforce that the victim did whatever they needed to survive the situation and is not to be blamed for what happened. The nurse should assess the victim for suicidal thoughts, plans, and previous attempts. If a SANE or sexual assault advocate is not available in the area, the nurse in the ER will assist the physician during the examination, provide emotional support and empathy, provide comfort measures, offer to call someone, and help with other basic needs.

Follow-up care is scheduled before the victim leaves the ER. If there is a situation where there are dependent children in need of care, the social worker is notified to evaluate the situation and provide necessary services. The care and safety of dependent children is a concern and responsibility whether the situation involves only sexual assault, only domestic violence, or both situations. Appropriate documentation must be done in the victim's chart including who was contacted regarding the situation and their response.

# Question 4

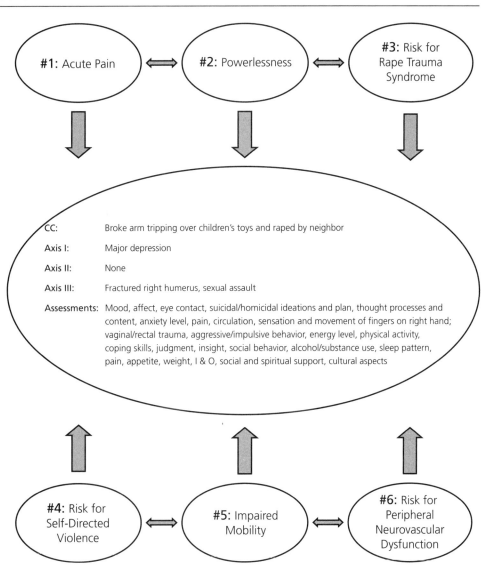

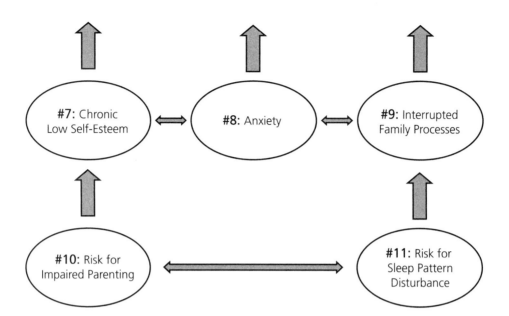

# Questions 5 and 6

**Nursing Care Plan:** Fractured right humerus, sexual assault, and major depression.
**Nursing Diagnosis:** Acute Pain r/t trauma s/t fractured humerus AEB guarding her arm and wincing with any movement.
**Outcomes:** 1. Will obtain satisfactory management of pain as rated at less than 3 on a scale of 0–10 (0 = none, 10 = extreme).

| Assessment Data:<br>O = Objective,<br>S = Subjective | Evidence-Based Interventions: | Rationales: | Patient Responses:* |
|---|---|---|---|
| Guards her arm (O)<br>Winces with any movement (O)<br>Spiral fracture noted on X-ray (O) | 1(a) Perform baseline pain assessment.<br><br>(b) Assess circulation, sensation, and movement of areas distal to the fracture.<br><br><br><br><br><br><br>(c) Medicate as ordered for pain.<br>(d) Maintain proper alignment and positioning of right extremity. (If a sling, immobilizing device, or cast has been applied, standard care would then be performed according to what has been applied.)<br>(e) Teach the patient distraction techniques including deep breathing and guided imagery. | 1(a) Information obtained will be used to assess the effectiveness of pain management.<br>(b) There is a risk of edema secondary to trauma causing enough pressure to decrease circulation and cause nerve damage. Abnormalities need to be identified and reported immediately so that appropriate intervention can decrease complications.<br>(c) Analgesic medication will offer relief from pain.<br>(d) The extremity must be in proper alignment to heal without deformity and promote normal circulation. Proper positioning will also help decrease pain.<br><br>(e) Distraction techniques will help decrease pain perception. | 1(a) Rates pain an "8" on a scale of 0–10 (0 = none, 10 = extreme).<br><br>(b) Capillary refill less than 3 seconds; normal sensation and movement.<br><br><br><br><br><br><br>(c) Accepted medication offered.<br>(d) Maintains proper alignment and positioning. Verbalizes understanding of why this is important.<br><br><br><br>(e) States that the deep breathing exercises are helpful. |

*Patient responses are examples of what students would look for to decide whether their planned interventions were successful, needed more time, or needed to be changed. Responses will vary depending on the patient.

**Evaluation:** 1. One hour after receiving medication and performing deep-breathing exercises rates pain a "2" on a scale of 0–10 (0 = none, 10 = extreme). Continue care plan and evaluate before patient is discharged or hospitalized.

**Nursing Care Plan:** Fractured right humerus, sexual assault, and major depression.
**Nursing Diagnosis:** Powerlessness r/t maladaptive coping and decisional conflict AEB remaining in domestic abuse situation; anxious affect, poor eye contact, and flinches when the husband stands close to her; recent sexual assault and history of major depression.
**Outcomes:** 1. Will accept information on domestic abuse shelters and safety plan.

| Assessment Data:<br>O = Objective,<br>S = Subjective | Evidence-Based<br>Interventions: | Rationales: | Patient<br>Responses: |
| --- | --- | --- | --- |
| Remains in domestic abuse situation (O)<br>Anxious affect, poor eye contact, and flinches when husband stands close to her (O)<br>Recent sexual assault (S) | 1(a) Interview patient in a private area without husband present.<br><br>(b) Using a nonjudgmental approach, share observations of patient's behavior when husband stood close to her. | 1(a) The patient will be more likely to provide information without the perpetrator present.<br>(b) This type of approach will help ensure that the patient will listen to the nurse's objective information. This lets her know that other people notice something is wrong. It may stimulate her to respond and provide even more information. She will be more likely to accept assistance from someone she perceives as helpful versus judgmental. | 1(a) Visibly more relaxed when the husband is not present.<br><br>(b) Quiet, poor eye contact, shoulders slumped when observations shared. |
| | (c) Use therapeutic communication techniques to encourage patient to verbalize feelings and thoughts without forcing her to do so.<br>(d) Offer information on domestic abuse shelters and formulating a personal safety plan. | (c) Therapeutic communication techniques, including open-ended questions, can assist patients to communicate feelings and thoughts.<br>(d) Knowledge of resources can decrease the patient's sense of powerlessness. Patients in these situations do not always accept information offered, but the offer of information lets them know that help is available when they choose to seek it and empowers them to start taking some control over their situation. Some patients take information, but do not immediately act upon it. They may do so at a later time. Information | (c) Admits that there has been more tension between her husband and herself. States that he has been working longer hours than usual. Does not admit to being abused.<br>(d) Accepts information and says she will think about it. |

| Assessment Data: O = Objective, S = Subjective | Evidence-Based Interventions: | Rationales: | Patient Responses: |
|---|---|---|---|
| | | materials should be small enough that they can be hidden in the lining of shoes or clothing so that the perpetrator does not find it and fear the patient is planning on leaving. If the perpetrator suspects the patient may be leaving him, it may cause escalated violence toward the patient. | |

**Evaluation:** 1. Accepted information offered. Stated that she would think about it, but did not indicate that she would act upon it. Continue care plan and evaluate before patient is discharged or hospitalized.

**Nursing Care Plan:** Sexual assault, fractured right humerus, and major depression.
**Nursing Diagnosis:** Risk for Rape Trauma Syndrome r/t sexual assault AEB verbalizations of sexual assault by neighbor and signs of vaginal trauma.
**Outcomes:** 1. Will accept needed care and treatment from nurse and other healthcare professionals in the ER. 2. Will have a plan for meeting immediate needs following the incident before discharge from the ER or hospitalization for further care.

| Assessment Data: O = Objective, S = Subjective | Evidence-Based Interventions: | Rationales: | Patient Responses: |
|---|---|---|---|
| Verbalizations of sexual assault by neighbor (S) Vaginal trauma (O) | 1(a) Begin to develop a rapport and a therapeutic nurse/patient alliance that is the beginning of the therapeutic nurse/patient relationship. | 1(a) Developing a rapport with the patient will assist in gaining the patient's trust and cooperation and help start the healing process. | 1(a) Accepts the nurse's presence. States that she feels safe with the nurse. |
| | (b) Provide acceptance and empathy while reinforcing that the patient did what she needed to do to survive the situation and is not to blame for the rape. | (b) This approach will continue to build trust between the nurse and patient and validate her worth as a human being. | (b) States that she can't help thinking she must have done something to provoke the attack. |
| | (c) Provide privacy for assessment and examination. | (c) The examination and information that will be shared is very emotionally sensitive. | (c) Grateful for privacy provided. |
| | (d) Use active listening and encourage the patient to talk about what happened but avoid probing for information. | (d) Active listening is very therapeutic and is helpful in the healing process. This can help decrease the patient's feeling of being totally alone. Also, accurate information will be needed to complete mandatory reporting responsibilities and provide legal documentation if the patient chooses to press legal charges at a later date. Probing for information can increase emotional pain and is not therapeutic. | (d) States that she appreciates someone listening to her and believing her. Frequently becomes tearful when talking about what happened. |
| | (e) Offer to make telephone calls to anyone the patient thinks would be supportive or helpful to her at this time. | (e) Some patients have family members or close friends they think would support them at a time like this. Others do not and will need even more emotional support from the nurse. | (e) States that she will think about who she would like to call. |

| Assessment Data:<br>O = Objective,<br>S = Subjective | Evidence-Based<br>Interventions: | Rationales: | Patient<br>Responses: |
|---|---|---|---|
| | (f) Explain all assessment, examinations, and procedures in advance and in simple, direct language. | (f) This approach can help decrease some of the patient's anxiety. This is an emotionally stressful time making it difficult for the patient to focus. Explanations that are too lengthy or complex will be more difficult for the patient to understand and cause unnecessary confusion. | (f) Thanks the nurse and states, "Well at least I know what to expect next." |
| | (g) Contact the SANE and sexual assault advocate as ordered and available. | (g) The SANE will collect evidence using proper collection methods. The sexual assault advocate will provide resources for the patient and stay with the patient during any assessments and examinations if the patient so desires. If a SANE or sexual assault advocate is not available, the nurse will aid the physician in the collection of evidence and properly document the collection. | (g) After SANE nurse and sexual assault advocate contacted, patient thanks the nurse for explaining who they were and what would happen next. |
| | (h) Provide follow-up written instructions and referrals for care after discharge. Explain that if she starts experiencing symptoms of rape-truama syndrome or suicidal thoughts to seek help right away. | (h) Written instructions and information will reinforce what is said verbally. The patient will have difficulty retaining what is said verbally due to her psychological and emotional state. Written instructions and information help increase patient adherence to follow-up care. | (h) Verbalizes understanding of instructions and information. States that she plans to have prescriptions filled and to take medication as ordered. |
| | 2(a) Assess basic immediate needs for safety, shelter, food, and clothing. | 2(a) The patient may have many unmet basic needs especially if she cannot return to her current living situation. | 2(a) States that she plans to return home with her husband. Denies any needs at this time. |
| | (b) Determine whether the patient's young children are being cared for by someone while both parents are in the ER. | (b) The location and situation of dependent children must be established for their safety and well-being. | (b) States that her mother-in-law is watching the children. |

*(continues)*

| Assessment Data: O = Objective, S = Subjective | Evidence-Based Interventions: | Rationales: | Patient Responses: |
|---|---|---|---|
| | (c) Contact the social worker to determine whether children are in a safe situation and to obtain needed resources for shelter, food, and clothing as needed. | (c) The social worker will be able to go, or contact an agency to go, to the dependent children's location if necessary to determine if the children are in the care of a safe, responsible person. If they are not, steps will be taken to at least temporarily place the children in a safe place. | (c) Declines offer of social services, but is aware that the social worker was notified of the situation. |

**Evaluation:** 1. Accepts care and treatment from the nurse and other healthcare professionals. Plans on returning home with her husband. Denies any immediate needs and declines offer of social services even though she is aware that the social worker was contacted. Continue care plan and evaluate before patient is discharged or hospitalized.

# References

American Psychiatric Association. (2000). *Diagnostic and statistical manual of mental disorders* (4th ed.). Text Revision. Washington, DC: Author.

Keltner, N. L., Schwecke, L. H., & Bostrom, C. E. (2007). *Psychiatric nursing* (5th ed.). St. Louis, MO: Mosby, Elsevier.

Lewis, S. L., Heitkemper, M. M., Dirksen, S. R., O'Brien, P. G., & Bucher, L. (2007). *Medical-surgical nursing: Assessment and management of clinical problems*, (7th ed.). St. Louis, MO: Mosby/Elsevier.

*Mosby's medical, nursing, and allied health dictionary* (6th ed.). (2002). St. Louis, MO: Mosby.

O'Brien, P. G., Kennedy, W. Z., & Ballard, K. A. (2008). *Psychiatric mental health nursing: An introduction to theory and practice.* Sudbury, MA: Jones and Bartlett.

Stuller Place, P.O. Box 53967, Lafayette, LA, 90505. Telephone: (337) 269-1557.

Townsend, M. C. (2008). *Essentials of psychiatric mental health nursing* (4th ed.). Philadelphia, PA: F. A. Davis.

Varcarolis, E. M., Carson, V. B., & Shoemaker, N. C. (2006). *Foundations of psychiatric mental health nursing: A clinical approach* (6th ed.). St. Louis, MO: Saunders, Elsevier.

Varcarolis, E. M. (2006). *Manual of psychiatric nursing care plans* (3rd ed.). St. Louis, MO: Saunders, Elsevier.

# Web Sites

Domestic Violence Safety Plan: www.hsdcfs.utah.gov/violence_safety_plan.htm

Family Violence and Sexual Assault Institute: www.fvsai.org

National Coalition Against Domestic Violence: www.ncadv.org

Stuller Place Support Services for the Sexually Abused: www.stullerplace.com

# Overdose: Mood Stabilizers, Benzodiazepine, and Muscle Relaxants

## ANSWER KEY

## Question 1

    a. Activated charcoal and gastric lavage

    b. EKG/ECG and telemetry monitoring

    c. Oxygen and mechanical ventilation if needed

    d. Monitor neurologic status

    e. IVFs

    f. Hemodialysis if needed

    g. Romazicon/flumazenil 0.2 mg IVP over 15 seconds

May repeat Romazicon/flumazenil 0.3–0.5 mg IVP given over 30 seconds at 60-second intervals until effective or max dose of 3 mg has been given. If resedation occurs, continue with the same repeat dose instructions (Romazicon effects wear off before the effects of the benzodiazepines do). Romazicon decreases the effect of other seizure medications; if patient has a previous diagnosis of seizure d/o, the risk of seizures may increase.

## Question 2

The treatment for Lithium overdose would be as follows:

    a. IVFs to prevent dehydration

    b. Kayexalate or GoLYTELY substituted for activated charcoal and gastric lavage (activated charcoal not effective in this case)

    c. EKG/ECG and telemetry monitoring

    d. Hemodialysis if needed; may need to repeat d/t $LiCO_3$ levels increasing as medication moves from tissues into bloodstream

    e. Lithium levels and electrolytes to monitor progress

The treatment for Depakote overdose would be as follows:

a. IVFs

b. Neurologic status monitoring

c. CBC with differential, including platelets

d. PT and INR

e. Liver function tests: AST/SGOT and ALT/SGPT

# Question 3

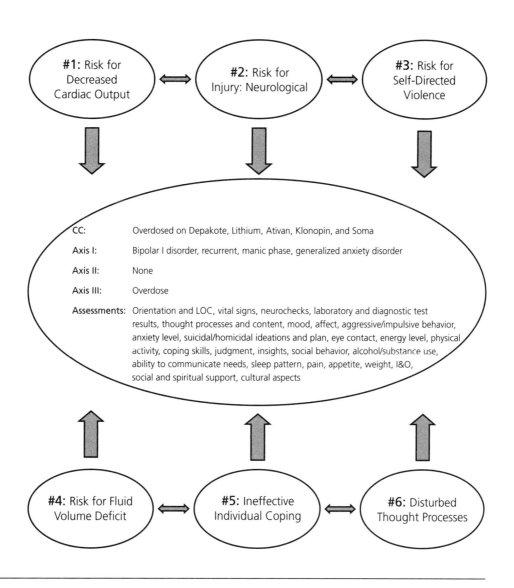

CC:          Overdosed on Depakote, Lithium, Ativan, Klonopin, and Soma

Axis I:       Bipolar I disorder, recurrent, manic phase, generalized anxiety disorder

Axis II:      None

Axis III:     Overdose

Assessments: Orientation and LOC, vital signs, neurochecks, laboratory and diagnostic test results, thought processes and content, mood, affect, aggressive/impulsive behavior, anxiety level, suicidal/homicidal ideations and plan, eye contact, energy level, physical activity, coping skills, judgment, insights, social behavior, alcohol/substance use, ability to communicate needs, sleep pattern, pain, appetite, weight, I&O, social and spiritual support, cultural aspects

**#1:** Risk for Decreased Cardiac Output

**#2:** Risk for Injury: Neurological

**#3:** Risk for Self-Directed Violence

**#4:** Risk for Fluid Volume Deficit

**#5:** Ineffective Individual Coping

**#6:** Disturbed Thought Processes

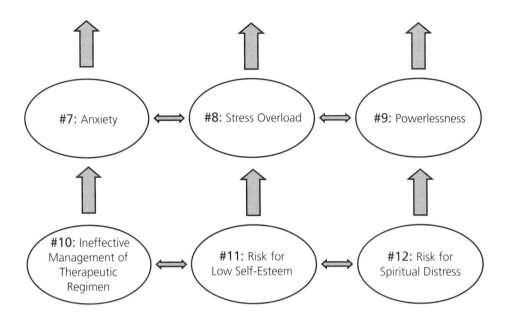

# Questions 4 and 5

**Nursing Care Plan:** Overdose, bipolar I disorder, recurrent, manic phase, and generalized anxiety disorder.
**Nursing Diagnosis:** Risk for Decreased Cardiac Output r/t potential for dysrhythmias and dehydration s/t overdose AEB overdose on multiple prescription medications, including Lithium, Depakote, and Soma.
**Outcomes:** 1. Will maintain normal cardiac output.

| Assessment Data:<br>O = Objective,<br>S = Subjective | Evidence-Based<br>Interventions: | Rationales: | Patient<br>Responses:* |
|---|---|---|---|
| Overdosed on multiple prescription medications including Lithium, Depakote, and Soma (O) | 1(a) Perform baseline cardiac and respiratory assessment, and obtain vital signs and pulse oximetry upon initial contact with patient, every hour and prn. | 1(a) Information obtained with these baseline assessments will be used to help determine initial treatment, the patient's progress, and additional changes to treatment when necessary. Early deterioration in the patient's condition will be more readily noted if frequent assessments are performed and results communicated to the physician. | 1(a) Shows abnormal results, including apical pulse = 106 and respiratory rate = 22. |
| | (b) Monitor EKG/ECG result and maintain telemetry. | (b) EKG/ECG result and telemetry monitoring will help determine the presence and type of dysrhythmia. | (b) EKG/ECG and telemetry show sinus tachycardia. |
| | (c) Initiate and maintain IVFs as ordered. | (c) IVFs will help maintain cardiac output and help prevent dehydration. If the patient becomes dehydrated, her cardiac output will also decrease and potential electrolyte imbalances may occur, which could also lead to dysrhythmias. | (c) Tolerates IV start fairly well. Verbalizes understanding of need for IVFs. |
| | (d) Monitor LOC every hour and prn. | (d) As cardiac output falls, the patient's level of oxygen will decrease as well, causing decreased LOC. | (d) Drowsy, but responds to verbal commands. |
| | | | *(continues)* |

*Patient responses are examples of what students would look for to decide whether their planned interventions were successful, needed more time, or needed to be changed. Responses will vary depending on the patient.

| Assessment Data:<br>O = Objective,<br>S = Subjective | Evidence-Based<br>Interventions: | Rationales: | Patient<br>Responses: |
|---|---|---|---|
| | (e) Medicate as ordered/per facility protocol (will depend on the type of dysrhythmia that occurs). | (e) Different types of medication are used depending upon the type of dysrhythmia that occurs. | (e) Requires no medications for dysrhythmia at this time. |
| | (f) Monitor I & O every 8 hours. | (f) When cardiac output falls, there is decreased blood flow to the kidneys, resulting in decreased urine output. | (f) Tolerated placement of indwelling Foley catheter. Draining clear, yellow urine. Output = 1000 cc in 8 hours. |
| | (g) Place patient in high Fowler's position. | (g) Placing the patient in this position increases venous return blood flow to the heart and helps decrease oxygen requirements. | (g) Verbalizes understanding of need to be in high Fowler's position. |
| | (h) Provide adequate rest and assist with ADLs. | (h) Bedrest and assistance with ADLs will decrease the body's oxygen requirements. | (h) Cooperates with bedrest. Accepts assistance with ADLs. |

**Evaluation:** 1. At this time cardiac output WNL. Continue care plan and evaluate in 8 hours and prn if condition changes.

**Nursing Care Plan:** Overdose, bipolar I disorder, recurrent, manic phase, and generalized anxiety disorder.
**Nursing Diagnosis:** Risk for Injury: Neurological r/t effects of overdose AEB overdose on multiple prescription medications including Depakote, Ativan, and Klonopin.
**Outcomes:** Will maintain normal neurological functioning.

| Assessment Data:<br>O = Objective,<br>S = Subjective | Evidence-Based Interventions: | Rationales: | Patient Responses: |
|---|---|---|---|
| Overdosed on multiple prescription medications including Depakote, Ativan, and Klonopin (O) | 1(a) Perform baseline neurological assessment, including cranial nerves and LOC, upon initial contact with patient, every hour and prn. | 1(a) Information obtained with these baseline assessments will be used to help determine initial treatment, the patient's progress, and additional changes to treatment when necessary. Early deterioration in the patient's condition will be more readily noted if frequent assessments are performed and results communicated to the physician. Abnormal neurological assessments may indicate increased intercranial pressure, possibly d/t cerebral edema, which could lead to coma and death. | 1(a) Drowsy, but responds to verbal commands. Neurological assessments otherwise WNL. |
| | (b) Perform neurochecks every hour. (More invasive neurological monitoring may be done if increased intercranial pressure is suspected, but is beyond the scope of this text.) | (b) This will help the nurse monitor the patient's progress. | (b) Neurochecks WNL. Verbalizes understanding of need for frequent assessments and is cooperative. |

**Evaluation:** 1. At this time the patient is drowsy, but responds to verbal commands; otherwise normal neurological assessment. Continue care plan and evaluate in 8 hours and prn if condition changes.

**Nursing Care Plan:** Overdose, bipolar I disorder, recurrent, manic phase, and generalized anxiety disorder.
**Nursing Diagnosis:** Risk for Self-Directed Violence r/t impulsivity, anxiety, and ineffective coping s/t Bipolar I Disorder, manic phase, and generalized anxiety disorder AEB overdose following manic behavior for 2 days and an argument with roommate.
**Outcomes:** Will remain free from impulsive behavior throughout hospitalization.

| Assessment Data: O = Objective, S = Subjective | Evidence-Based Interventions: | Rationales: | Patient Responses: |
|---|---|---|---|
| Manic behavior for 2 days (S) Arguments with roommate (S) Prescribed lithium and Depakote for bipolar I disorder (O) Prescribed Ativan and Klonopin for GAD (O) Discovered by roommate to have overdosed (S) | 1(a) Begin to develop a rapport and a therapeutic nurse/patient alliance that is the beginning of the therapeutic nurse/patient relationship. | 1(a) Developing a rapport with the patient will assist in gaining the patient's trust and cooperation in the future. According to Peplau, the therapeutic nurse/patient relationship is the foundation that must be established to initiate future work in the healing process (Keltner, Schwecke, & Bostrom, 2007). | 1(a) Tearfully accepts the nurse's offer of help. Agrees to work with the nurse during hospitalization. |
| | (b) Perform a suicide risk assessment and obtain a verbal no harm to self or others contract with patient during the initial intake assessment process, every shift, and prn throughout hospitalization. | (b) Patients with bipolar diagnoses are high risk for committing suicide due to extreme impulsivity in the manic phase or the severity of depression in the depressed phase. A behavior contract actively engages patients in their treatment and encourages personal responsibility for their behavior. It also demonstrates staff involvement. The patient's condition may change, making it necessary to obtain another contract earlier than the next scheduled shift. | (b) Has exhibited impulsive behavior and has had a suicide attempt, which puts her at high risk for another attempt. At this time she is able to verbally contract to refrain from harming herself. |
| | (c) Use therapeutic communication to explore other ways the patient could have dealt with the arguments with her roommate. | (c) During times of crisis, patients are more open to hearing alternatives. Crisis times can be teachable moments. | (c) States that she is ashamed of her actions and agrees that she could have called the on-call therapist who works with her psychiatrist or another friend to talk to. Also admits that she occasionally does not take her medication so that she can go out drinking with friends. |

| Assessment Data:<br>O = Objective,<br>S = Subjective | Evidence-Based<br>Interventions: | Rationales: | Patient<br>Responses: |
|---|---|---|---|
| | (d) Instruct to come to staff if she feels she may do something impulsive.<br><br>(e) Review signs and symptoms of relapse with patient while stressing the need to seek help before her symptoms get more out of control.<br>(f) Maintain 1:1 or COs at this time. | (d) The patient needs to be able to come to staff when feeling as if she will do something impulsive.<br>(e) Early intervention can lead to decreased need for hospitalization or life-threatening consequences of out-of-control behavior.<br><br>(f) The patient is drowsy, but responds to verbal commands. There is still a risk that she will attempt to harm herself or leave the ER when the staff are busy with other patients. Therefore, it is still necessary to monitor her closely. | (d) Verbally contracts to come to staff when she feels as if she will do something impulsive.<br>(e) Verbalizes at least four signs and symptoms of relapse. Verbalizes understanding of the benefits of seeking help early in the relapse phase.<br>(f) Verbalizes understanding for remaining on 1:1 or COs. Cooperates with staff. |
| | (g) Maintain an environment free from potentially harmful objects. | (g) This is more difficult to do in a nonroutine psychiatric setting, but is even more important because there are more potentially dangerous objects available to the patient. | (g) Asks why her personal belongings were secured in a locked area, but is cooperative. |

**Evaluation:** 1. No impulsive behavior noted and agrees to come to staff if she feels she will do something impulsive. Remains free from self-harm. Continue care plan and evaluate in 8 hours and prn if condition changes.

# References

American Psychiatric Association. (2000). *Diagnostic and statistical manual of mental disorders* (4th ed.). Text Revision. Washington, DC: Author.

Antai-Otong, D. (2004). *Psychiatric emergencies: How to accurately assess and manage the patient in crisis.* Eau Claire, WI: PESI Healthcare.

Bezchlibnyk-Butler, K. Z., & Jeffries, J. J. (2005). *Clinical handbook of psychotropic drugs* (15th ed.). Ashland, OH: Hogrefe & Huber.

Carpenito-Moyat, L. J. (2008). *Nursing diagnosis: Application to clinical practice* (12th ed.). Philadelphia, PA: WoltersKluwer Lippincott Williams & Wilkins.

Fischbach, F. (2004). *A manual of laboratory and diagnositic tests* (7th ed.). Philadelphia, PA: Lippincott Williams & Wilkins.

Keltner, N. L., & Folks, D. G. (2005). *Psychiatric drugs* (4th ed.). St. Louis, MO: Elsevier/Mosby.

Keltner, N. L., Schwecke, L. H., & Bostrom, C. E. (2007). *Psychiatric nursing* (5th ed.). St. Louis, MO: Mosby, Elsevier.

Lewis, S. M., Heitkemper, M. M., & Dirksen, S. R. (2004). *Medical-surgical nursing: Assessment and management of clinical problems* (6th ed.). St. Louis, MO: Mosby.

Lewis, S. L., Heitkemper, M. M., Dirksen, S. R., O'Brien, P. G., & Bucher, L. (2007). *Medical-surgical nursing: Assessment and management of clinical problems* (7th ed.). St. Louis, MO: Mosby/Elsevier.

Lieberman, J. A., & Tasman, A. (2006). *Handbook of psychiatric drugs.* West Sussex, England: Wiley.

McKenrey, L., Tessier, E., & Hogan, M. (2006). *Mosby's pharmacology in nursing* (22nd ed.). St. Louis, MO: Mosby.

O'Brien, P. G., Kennedy, W. Z., & Ballard, K. A. (2008). *Psychiatric mental health nursing: An introduction to theory and practice.* Sudbury, MA: Jones and Bartlett.

Sadock, B. J., & Sadock, V. A. (2003). *Kaplan and Sadock's synopsis of psychiatry: Behavioral sciences/clinical psychiatry* (9th ed.). Philadelphia: Lippincott Williams & Wilkins.

# Adverse Medication Effects:
## Serotonin Syndrome

## ANSWER KEY

# Question 1

a. Prozac/Serafem/fluoxetine
Zoloft/sertraline
Paxil/paroxetine
Celexa/citalopram
Luvox/fluvoximine
Lexapro/escitalopram

b. Effexor/venlafaxine
Cymbalta/duloxetine

c. Nardil/phenylzine
Marplan/isocarboxazid
Parnate/tranylcypromine
Eldepryl/selegiline (patch)

# Question 2

Fever of 103°F, shaking chills, difficulty walking, and muscle rigidity.

a. Restlessness and agitation; altered mental status including confusion, disorientation, or hypomania; hyperreflexia; tremor; seizures; fluctuating blood pressure; tachycardia; increased respirations; shivering or shaking chills; coma; headache; nausea; abdominal cramping or diarrhea.

# Question 3

    a. Discontinue medication.

    b. Antipyretics such as Tylenol or Aspirin (if not contraindicated) for hyperthermia and a cooling blanket if antipyretics insufficient to control elevated temperature.

    c. Klonopin/clonazepam 0.25 PO bid and may increase up to 4 mg/day; Valium/diazepam 5 mg PO, IM, or IVP; Ativan/lorazepam 1–2 mg PO, IM, or IVP for seizure activity.

    d. Periaction/cyproheptadine 4 mg PO tid for headache.

    e. Cogentin/benztropine 1 to 2 mg IM, IVP, or PO for muscle rigidity.

    f. Propranolol/inderol 10 mg qid or 40 mg PO bid to control blood pressure.

    g. Dantrium/dantrolene sodium 1 mg/kg IVP for severe muscle rigidity or twitching and hyperthermia. May repeat dose up to a maximum dose of 10 mg.

    h. Mechanical ventilation as needed.

# Questions 4 and 5

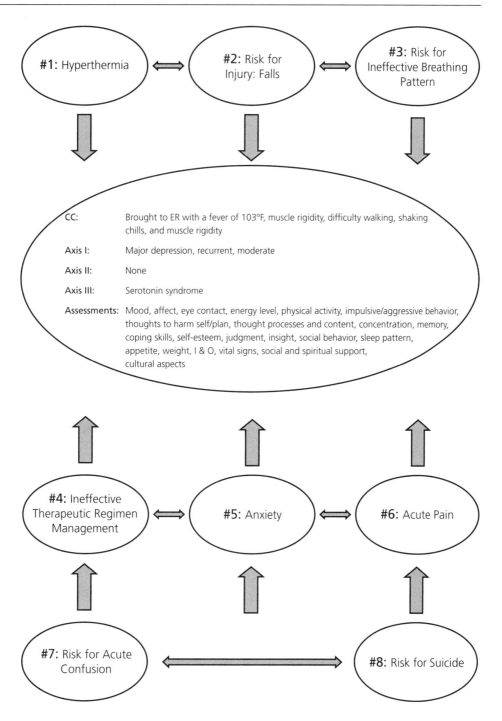

CC:    Brought to ER with a fever of 103°F, muscle rigidity, difficulty walking, shaking chills, and muscle rigidity

Axis I:    Major depression, recurrent, moderate

Axis II:    None

Axis III:    Serotonin syndrome

Assessments: Mood, affect, eye contact, energy level, physical activity, impulsive/aggressive behavior, thoughts to harm self/plan, thought processes and content, concentration, memory, coping skills, self-esteem, judgment, insight, social behavior, sleep pattern, appetite, weight, I & O, vital signs, social and spiritual support, cultural aspects

#1: Hyperthermia

#2: Risk for Injury: Falls

#3: Risk for Ineffective Breathing Pattern

#4: Ineffective Therapeutic Regimen Management

#5: Anxiety

#6: Acute Pain

#7: Risk for Acute Confusion

#8: Risk for Suicide

**Nursing Care Plan:** Serotonin syndrome; major depression, recurrent, moderate.
**Nursing Diagnosis:** Hyperthermia r/t adverse effects of antidepressant medication s/t serotonin syndrome AEB self-report of taking Saint-John's-wort and Zoloft, oral temperature = 103°F, and shaking chills.
**Outcomes** (include time frames): 1. Will experience an oral temperature less than 100°F in 24 hours.

| Assessment Data:<br>O = Objective,<br>S = Subjective | Evidence-Based Interventions: | Rationales: | Patient Responses:* |
|---|---|---|---|
| Oral temperature = 103°F (O)<br>Shaking chills (O)<br>Reports taking Saint-John's-wort and Zoloft (S) | 1(a) Vital signs every 1 hour for 4 hours, then every 2 hours for 4 hours, then every 4 hours for 72 hours. | 1(a) The patient's condition is unstable and the vital signs may become even more unstable. Shaking chills may be a prodromal sign prior to the body temperature increases. The patient must be monitored very closely, and worsening of her condition must be reported immediately to the psychiatrist/physician. If this occurs, more orders may be given or the patient may be transferred to a higher level of care (ICU). Nursing care will need to be adapted to the patient's change in condition. Also, frequent vital signs will help the nurse assess improvement in the patient's condition and make changes in care based upon this. | 1(a) Oral temperature = 103°F, pulse regular, rate = 100, respirations even, regular = 22, blood pressure lying = 148/94. |
| | (b) Start and maintain IV 0.9% normal saline at 125 cc per hour. | (b) Adequate fluid is needed to help regulate body temperature. An elevated body temperature is accompanied by increased metabolic rate and fluid requirements. At least 2000 ml of fluid should be provided in a 24-hour period to meet normal needs. The patient has increased fluid needs related to increased body temperature and meta- | (b) Tolerates IV being started fairly well. Verbalizes understanding of need and purpose for IV fluids. |

*Patient responses are examples of what students would look for to decide whether their planned interventions were successful, needed more time, or needed to be changed. Responses will vary depending on the patient.

| Assessment Data: O = Objective, S = Subjective | Evidence-Based Interventions: | Rationales: | Patient Responses: |
|---|---|---|---|
| | | bolic rate. Also, the patient may not be able to drink enough oral fluids to meet the body's increased requirements. | |
| | (c) Administer Tylenol 650 mg po as ordered. Administer Dantrium if oral temperature is greater than 104°F. | (c) Antipyretics will help decreased the patient's temperature as well. Dantrium, a muscle relaxant, is used in the treatment of hyperthermia as well as muscle hyperrigidity that occurs in serotonin syndrome. | (c) Verbalizes understanding of why she is receiving Tylenol. |
| | (d) Apply cooling blanket for oral temperature greater than 104°F. | (d) It is imperative that the patient's temperature be returned to normal. Temperatures greater than 104°F can cause seizure, delirium, or damage to body cells. Temperatures greater than 105.8°F can cause damage to brain cells in the hypothalamus, thus affecting the temperature control center of the brain (Lewis, Heitkemper, & Dirksen, 2004, p. 219). | (d) Accepts teaching and potential need for cooling blanket. Verbalizes understanding of teaching. |
| | (e) Encourage patient to drink at least 100 ml every 1–2 hours while awake. | (e) Oral fluids help decrease fever and meet increased body requirements, and they are a more normal route of delivering fluid. As soon as the patient can drink enough oral fluids, the IV may be changed to a saline lock in case it is needed to administer emergency medications. The saline lock will be removed as soon as possible to prevent possible complications such as infection. | (e) Agrees to drink at least 100 ml of fluid every 1–2 hours while awake. |

*(continues)*

| Assessment Data: O = Objective, S = Subjective | Evidence-Based Interventions: | Rationales: | Patient Responses: |
|---|---|---|---|
| | (f) Monitor intake and output every 8 hours. | (f) Monitoring I & O every shift will give the nurse more accurate information about the patient's fluid status. This information will be included when making decisions regarding the patient's needs. | (f) Intake for 8 hours = 1400 ml; output for 8 hours = 1200 ml. Understands she needs to drink more fluids and agrees to try to do this. More oral fluids provided. |
| | (g) Assist patient with meal choices and teach to avoid beverages such as coffee, tea, and grapefruit juice. Provide patient preferences when able. | (g) Coffee, tea, and grapefruit juice act as diuretics and will increase fluid loss, which will be counterproductive to the patient's care. Providing preferences will increase patient cooperation. | (g) Verbalizes understanding and accepts guidance. Prefers apple juice. Agrees to try decaffeinated coffee or tea. |
| | (h) Assist with bathing more frequently; change bed linens frequently. | (h) Because the patient will be diaphoretic, these measures promote comfort. Changing bed linens frequently also prevents shivering, which can lead to an increase in body temperature. | (h) Expresses gratitude for assistance with bathing and linen changes. States that she feels more comfortable. |
| | (i) Avoid layering heavy blankets. | (i) Layering heavy blankets will increase body temperature. Also, if a cooling blanket is used, heavy blankets will counteract the therapeutic effect. | (i) States that she is comfortable with sheet and one light blanket on bed. Oral temperature = 102.8°F. |
| | (j) Perform mental status exam, assess for suicide risk, and obtain verbal no self-harm contract every 8 hours and prn. | (j) Patient's physical condition is unstable, but she is at risk for suicide related to the diagnosis of recurrent major depression, needing to stop antidepressant medication, and the accessibility of IV tubing. Also, the cooling blanket apparatus may have coils and tubing that would present a safety risk for this patient. The patient may be too physically ill to act upon suicidal thoughts at this time, but as her physical condition | (j) Alert and oriented in all spheres. Reports mood as "good" and rates depression a "2" on a scale of 0 to 10 (0 = none; 10 = severe). Affect is appropriate to situation, speech is logical and goal-directed; no behavior or speech indicating delusions or hallucinations and patient denies these; recent and remote memory intact; appearance slightly disheveled; no aggressive or impulsive behavior noted and patient denies feelings of both. Denies current suicidal ideations and |

| Assessment Data:<br>O = Objective,<br>S = Subjective | Evidence-Based<br>Interventions: | Rationales: | Patient<br>Responses: |
|---|---|---|---|
| | (k) Monitor every 15 minutes and prn. | improves she would have more energy and decreased antidepressant medication levels, both of which could lead to her carrying through with an attempt.<br>(k) Frequent monitoring of the patient's location and activity helps ensure her safety while being less restrictive than placing her on a 1:1 or constant observation (CO). [See also rationale for (j).] | she is able to verbally contract to not harm self. Agrees to report any suicidal ideations. Remains free from self-harm.<br><br>(k) Remains in own room lying on bed; resting quietly. |

**Evaluation:** 1. Oral temperature = 102.8°F. No need for cooling blanket at this time. Continue plan and evaluate in 24 hours.

**Nursing Care Plan:** Serotonin syndrome; major depression, recurrent, moderate.
**Nursing Diagnosis:** Risk for Injury: Falls r/t adverse effects of antidepressant medication s/t serotonin syndrome AEB self-report of taking Saint-John's-wort and Zoloft, difficulty walking, and muscle rigidity.
**Outcomes:** 1. Will remain free from injury throughout hospitalization.

| Assessment Data: O = Objective, S = Subjective | Evidence-Based Interventions: | Rationales: | Patient Responses: |
|---|---|---|---|
| Reports difficulty walking (S) Reports muscle rigidity (S) Noted to have unsteady gait (O) Moderate amount of muscle rigidity (O) Reports taking Saint-John's-wort and Zoloft (S) | 1(a) Institute and maintain fall precautions including side rails on bed; make sure bed alarm is on and working properly. | 1(a) Instituting and maintaining fall precautions and side rails help decrease the risk of falls. Bed alarms help alert the staff that the patient is getting out of bed. All equipment must be checked periodically to ensure it is working properly. | 1(a) Agrees to adhere to fall precautions. States that she feels "safe" knowing about these precautions. |
| | (b) Assess level of muscle rigidity and pain every 4 hours. | (b) A baseline of the patient's condition must be obtained to use when assessing for improvement or worsening of her condition as well as the effectiveness of medication. | (b) Moderate amount of muscle rigidity noted. |
| | (c) Administer Cogentin as ordered. Assess for side effects and adverse effects including blurred vision, dry mouth, mental confusion, delirium or psychosis, urinary retention, and constipation. If Cogentin not effective and muscle rigidity increases, administer Dantrium 1m/kg IVP as ordered and transfer to ICU as ordered. | (c) Cogentin is an anticholinergic medication used in this case to treat muscle rigidity secondary to serotonin syndrome. It is also frequently used to treat certain side effects of antipsychotic medications (dystonia). It is imperative to assess the patient for new onset confusion or delirium secondary to Cogentin or an increase in confusion or delirium already present related to serotonin syndrome. Blurred vision will increase her risk of falling. Urinary retention and constipation can lead to serious medical complications including possible kidney damage or paralytic ileus if not recognized and treated promptly. Dry | (c) Verbalizes understanding of reason why she is receiving Cogentin and possible side effects or adverse effects. Agrees to report any side effects or adverse effects. |

| Assessment Data: O = Objective, S = Subjective | Evidence-Based Interventions: | Rationales: | Patient Responses: |
|---|---|---|---|
| | | mouth can be relieved by increasing water intake, offering ice chips, and more frequent oral care. Dantrium, a muscle relaxant, is used in the treatment of muscle hyperrigidity, as well as hyperthermia, that occurs in serotonin syndrome. | |
| | (d) Orient to surroundings. | (d) Orienting the patient to her surroundings will help decrease the risk of stumbling into objects that would increase her risk of falling when combined with her unsteady gait. Also, patients experiencing serotonin syndrome can be confused or disoriented and this can lead to increased risk for falling. | (d) Expresses appreciation for being oriented to the unit and her room. |
| | (e) Provide assistance and instruct patient to ask for assistance when getting out of bed, going to the bathroom, or walking. Provide cordless call bell at bedside. | (e) These measures will decrease the patient's risk of falling. A cordless call bell will provide the patient a way of contacting the staff for assistance while not introducing another cord that the patient could use to harm herself if she experiences suicidal thoughts. | (e) Agrees to ask for assistance and verbalizes understanding of how important this is to her safety. |
| | (f) Assess for and teach patient signs and symptoms of hypotension/ orthostatic hypotension. Teach patient to report these and to change positions slowly. Take BP lying, sitting, and standing if patient reports or is noted to have signs and symptoms of orthostatic hypotension. | (f) The patient is receiving Inderol 10 mg po qid and has an unsteady gait causing an increased risk for falls. | (f) Denies signs and symptoms of hypotension/orthostatic hypotension and no signs or symptoms noted. BP lying = 148/94, pulse = 100, respirations = 22. |

*(continues)*

| Assessment Data:<br>O = Objective,<br>S = Subjective | Evidence-Based<br>Interventions: | Rationales: | Patient<br>Responses: |
|---|---|---|---|
| | (g) Provide adequate lighting in all areas of unit. If patient wears eyeglasses or contact lenses, be sure that they are clean and patient is wearing them before getting out of bed.<br>(h) Be sure patient is wearing supportive, non-skid footwear when getting out of bed. | (g) Increasing and maintaining the patient's ability to see clearly will decrease her risk of stumbling or falling.<br><br>(h) Supportive, non-skid footwear is important in promoting the patient's balance and traction, and will prevent falls. | (g) Does not wear eyeglasses. Reports that she is able to see well with the amount of lighting provided.<br><br>(h) Calls family member to bring more appropriate footwear. Provided with hospital slippers with non-skid bottoms until family member visits. |

**Evaluation:** 1. Remains free from injury related to falls. Continue plan and evaluate in 24 hours.

**Nursing Care Plan:** Serotonin syndrome; major depression, recurrent, moderate.
**Nursing Diagnosis:** Risk for Ineffective Breathing Pattern r/t adverse effects of antidepressant medication s/t serotonin syndrome AEB self-report of taking Saint-John's-wort and Zoloft.
**Outcomes:** 1. Will demonstrate regular, even, unlabored respirations with rate between 12 and 20 throughout hospitalization.

| Assessment Data: O = Objective, S = Subjective | Evidence-Based Interventions: | Rationales: | Patient Responses: |
|---|---|---|---|
| Reports taking Saint-John's-wort and Zoloft (S) Reports muscle rigidity (S) Respirations even, regular, unlabored, rate = 22 (O) Pulse = 100 (O) Oral temperature = 104.8°F (O) Moderate amount of muscle rigidity (O) | 1(a) Assess lung sounds, respirations, and pulse oximetry upon admission and every hour until pulse oximetry at least 96%. | 1(a) A baseline of the patient's condition must be obtained to use when assessing for improvement or worsening of her condition as well as the effectiveness of medication. If muscle rigidity is affecting her ability to breathe, improvement should be seen after the administration of Cogentin. | 1(a) Normal lung sounds in all fields both anterior and posterior; respirations remain even, regular, unlabored, rate = 22 pulse oximetry = 97%. Pulse rate remains regular, rate = 100. |
| | (b) Assess for nostril flaring and use of accessory muscles to breathe. | (b) Nostril flaring or use of accessory neck, shoulder, or intercostal muscles indicate that the patient is having difficulty breathing and needs more intense intervention to promote adequate oxygenation. | (b) No nostril flaring or use of accessory muscles noted. |
| | (c) Assess mental status and skin color. | (c) A patient who is having difficulty maintaining adequate oxygenation will demonstrate altered mental status and pale or cyanotic skin color. The patient will need to have oxygen administered. | (c) Alert and oriented in all spheres. Reports mood as "good" and rates depression a "2" on a scale of 0 to 10 (0 = none; 10 = severe). Affect is appropriate to situation, speech is logical and goal-directed; no behavior or speech indicating delusions or hallucinations and patient denies these; recent and remote memory intact; appearance slightly disheveled. No aggressive or impulsive behavior noted and patient denies feelings of both. |
| | (d) Promote calm, relaxing atmosphere and environment. | (d) A calm, relaxing atmosphere and environment help decrease patient anxiety. | (d) Admits to feeling anxious, but also states that she feels safe being in the hospital and with the nursing staff. |

*(continues)*

| Assessment Data: O = Objective, S = Subjective | Evidence-Based Interventions: | Rationales: | Patient Responses: |
|---|---|---|---|
| | (e) Provide emotional support and assist patient to verbalize feelings related to situation. | (e) Any hospital admission can be anxiety provoking. Even small changes in the ability to breathe can be frightening for the patient. Needing to be closely monitored and being taught the potential seriousness of the situation can increase the patient's anxiety. Providing emotional support and assisting patients to verbalize feelings can decrease their anxiety and help promote the relaxation response leading to decreased muscle rigidity and easier breathing. | (e) Responds positively to emotional support offered. Talks about initially being afraid that something was wrong, but unsure of what to do. |
| | (f) Notify psychiatrist/ physician if lung sounds, respirations, pulse oximetry, mental status, or muscle rigidity worsen. Administer Dantrium 1 mg/kg IVP as well as oxygen, and prepare to transfer to ICU as ordered. | (f) Dantrium, a muscle relaxant, is used in the treatment of hyperthermia as well as hyperrigidity that occurs in serotonin syndrome (and also NMS). The patient's ability to breathe on her own is being compromised by muscle hyperrigidity and must be augmented by the administration of oxygen as well as Dantrium. | (f) Not necessary to administer Dantrium at this time. Continue to closely monitor and assess patient condition. |

**Evaluation:** 1. Respiratory rate remains at 22, but there are no other abnormal respiratory signs or symptoms. Continue plan and evaluate in 8 hours.

# References

American Psychiatric Association. (2000). *Diagnostic and statistical manual of mental disorders* (4th ed.). Text Revision. Washington, DC: Author.

Carpenito-Moyat, L. J. (2008). *Nursing diagnosis: Application to clinical practice* (12th ed.). Philadelphia, PA: WoltersKluwer Lippincott Williams & Wilkins.

Fontaine, K. L., & Fletcher, J. S. (2003). *Mental health nursing* (5th ed.). Upper Saddle River, NJ: Prentice Hall.

Keltner, N. L., Schwecke, L. H., & Bostrom, C. E. (2007). *Psychiatric nursing* (5th ed.). St. Louis, MO: Mosby, Elsevier.

Lewis, S. M., Heitkemper, M. M., & Dirksen, S. R. (2004). *Medical-surgical nursing: Assessment strategies and management of clinical problems* (6th ed.). St. Louis, MO: Mosby.

McKenrey, L., Tessier, E., & Hogan, M. (2006). *Mosby's pharmacology in nursing* (22nd ed.). St. Louis, MO: Mosby.

O'Brien, P. G., Kennedy, W. Z., & Ballard, K. A. (2008). *Psychiatric mental health nursing: An introduction to theory and practice.* Sudbury, MA: Jones and Bartlett.

Stuart, G. W., & Laraia, M. T. (2005). *Principles and practice of psychiatric nursing* (8th ed.). St. Louis, MO: Mosby, Elsevier.

Townsend, M. C. (2008). *Essentials of psychiatric mental health nursing: Concepts of care in evidence-based practice.* Philadelphia, PA: F. A. Davis.

# *Adverse Medication Effects: Neuroleptic Malignant Syndrome*

## ANSWER KEY

## Question 1

Thorazine/chlorpromazine, Haldol/haloperidol, Prolixin/fluphenazine, Mellaril/thioridazine, Navane/thiothixene, Stelazine/trifluoperizine, Trilafon/perphenazine, Loxitane/loxipine, Moban/molidone, Orap/pimozide

## Question 2

Clozaril/clozapine, Risperdal/risperidone, Zyprexa/olanzapine, Seroquel/quetiapine, Geodon/ziprasidone, Abilify/aripiprazle, Invega/paliperidone

## Question 3

Haldol/haloperidal

## Question 4

Muscle rigidity, +3 deep tendon reflexes, difficulty breathing, mental confusion, CPK = 1000; WBCs = 15, ALT/SGPT = 100, AST/SGOT = 80, GFR = 120, Creatinine = 0.8, BUN = 20, oral temperature = 105°F, pulse = 100, respirations = 24, blood pressure = 160/96, and diaphoresis.

# Question 5

  a. Discontinuation of antipsychotics/neuroleptics

  b. Intravenous fluids

  c. Cooling blanket

  d. Dantrolene/Dantrium 1 mg/kg IVP; may repeat up to 10 mg/kg. Change to po dosing 4–8 mg/day in 4 divided doses × 3 days *or* dantrolene/Dantrium 1–3 mg/kg/day IVP in 4 divided doses; max 10 mg/kg/day; then oral maintenance dose ranges from 50–200 mg/day

  e. Bromocriptine/Parlodel may be ordered as an alternative to dantrolene. Bromocriptine/Parlodel 2.5–10 mg tid po initially; if no improvement in 24 hours, increase to max dose of 20 mg po qid.

  f. Bromocriptine/Parlodel 1.25–2.5 mg/day for milder cases

  g. Oxygen prn

  h. Mechanical ventilation may be needed.

  i. Benzodiazepines may be added to treat anxiety.

# Questions 6 and 7

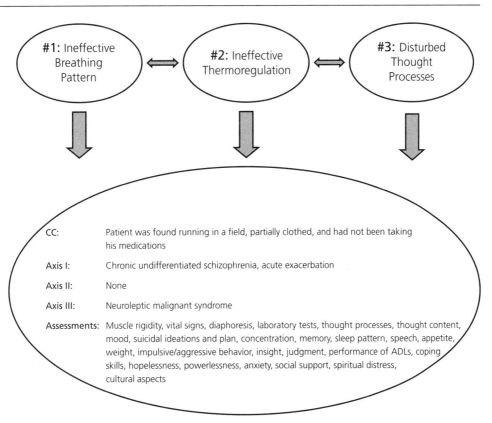

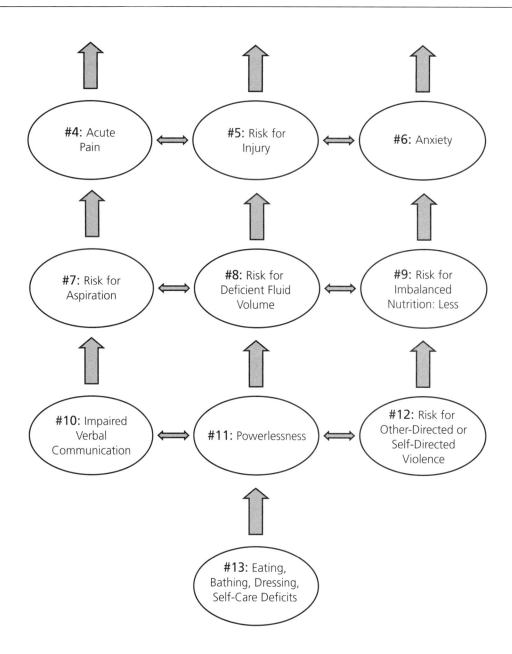

# Questions 8 and 9

\*It is assumed that the patient is on a medical-psychiatric unit. If the unit offers only psychiatric/mental healthcare, the patient would be transferred to a medical-surgical or ICU setting. If the patient came into the ER with these symptoms, treatment would be initiated in the ER.

**Nursing Care Plan:** Neuroleptic malignant syndrome, chronic undifferentiated schizophrenia.
**Nursing Diagnosis:** Ineffective Breathing Pattern r/t adverse effects of antipsychotic medication AEB irregular respiratory rate of 24, complaining of difficulty breathing, and muscle rigidity.
**Outcomes** (include time frames): 1. Will demonstrate respiratory rate within range of 12 to 20 per minute, pulse oximetry of at least 93% on room air, and decreased muscle rigidity in 1 hour.

| Assessment Data: O = Objective, S = Subjective | Evidence-Based Interventions: | Rationales: | Patient Responses:* |
|---|---|---|---|
| Pulse oximetry = 89% on room air (O)<br>Respirations 24 and irregular (O)<br>Pulse = 100 (O)<br>BP = 160/96 (O)<br>Muscle rigidity (O)<br>Complains of difficulty breathing (S)<br>States that he is having difficulty remembering where his room is (S) | 1(a) Administer oxygen as ordered. | 1(a) A pulse oximetry of 89%, irregular respirations of 24, muscle rigidity, and complaint of difficulty breathing show that the patient is experiencing an oxygen deficit that must be corrected immediately to prevent further physical deterioration and respiratory arrest. | 1(a) Pulse oximetry reading is 93% on 2 liters of oxygen via nasal cannula. |
| | (b) Assess lung sounds, pulse oximetry, respiratory rate and quality, for nostril flaring and use of accessory muscles, muscle rigidity, and mental status every 15 minutes and prn. | (b) The patient requires close monitoring of these parameters to determine if his condition is improving, worsening, or remaining the same. Nostril flaring and use of accessory neck, shoulder, or intercostal muscles indicate the patient is having difficulty breathing and needs more intense intervention to promote adequate oxygenation. | (b) Lung sounds diminished bilaterally in posterior bases; pulse oximetry 93% on 2 liters of oxygen, respiratory rate 22; continues to have significant muscle rigidity and is oriented to person and place only. Delusional thinking remains at the same level since admission without increasing. |
| | (c) Start IV and administer Dantrolene/Dantrium as ordered and repeat if necessary according to protocol ordered. | (c) Dantrolene/Dantrium, a muscle relaxant, is needed IVP and IVFs will provide adequate hydration. The patient is having difficulty breathing and requires IV | (c) Muscle rigidity starting to decrease 5 minutes after administration of Dantrolene/Dantrium. DTRs remain +3.<br><br>*(continues)* |

*Patient responses are examples of what students would look for to decide whether their planned interventions were successful, needed more time, or needed to be changed. Responses will vary depending on the patient.

| Assessment Data: O = Objective, S = Subjective | Evidence-Based Interventions: | Rationales: | Patient Responses: |
|---|---|---|---|
| | (d) Discontinue Haldol/haloperidol. | medication versus po to prevent a potential respiratory arrest. (d) Haldol/haloperidol is an antipsychotic/neuroleptic medication and is the cause of the patient's symptoms of NMS. | (d) No worsening of symptoms noted and patient denies any worsening of symptoms. |
| | (e) Place on 1:1 or constant observation (CO); explain reason for this measure as well as what is happening using simple statements. | (e) Patient is in danger of respiratory arrest. He is also anxious and afraid because of the symptoms he is experiencing. These factors can also increase the psychotic disturbances already present related to schizophrenia. Simple statements are better understood when people are frightened and/or psychotic. | (e) At this time agrees to be on 1:1 or constant observation (CO). Verbalizes understanding of precautions and states that he feels safe with a staff member present. |
| | (f) Encourage patient to rest and stay calm. | (f) Activity and anxiety increase oxygen use. The patient needs to conserve oxygen. | (f) Lies quietly on bed in own room with staff member in attendance. |
| | (g) Maintain a calm, soothing environment and dim the lights while leaving enough light to assess patient and maintain orientation. Soft music may be used if patient is able to tolerate it. | (g) These measures help decrease the patient's anxiety and increase relaxation, which in turn affects oxygen use and muscle tension. | (g) States that he feels more relaxed. Small improvement in muscle rigidity. |
| | (h) Reorient patient to person, place, time, and situation when assessing mental status. | (h) Reorienting the patient helps maintain his present level of orientation and increase his ability to become more oriented. | (h) Remains oriented to person and place only. |
| | (i) Offer emotional support and therapeutic use of self. | (i) Difficulty breathing, mental confusion, elevated vital signs, and muscle rigidity can be very frightening. The patient needs much emotional support and assurance of safety while experiencing these symptoms. | (i) Appreciates emotional support offered. Asks to not be left alone. |

| Assessment Data:<br>O = Objective,<br>S = Subjective | Evidence-Based<br>Interventions: | Rationales: | Patient<br>Responses: |
|---|---|---|---|
| | (j) If physical condition deteriorates, prepare for transfer to ICU setting. Notify nurse manager of possible need to transfer patient. | (j) Patients with NMS may need mechanical ventilation and cardiac monitoring. | (j) Shows gradual improvement but needs constant monitoring; there is still potential for a transfer to the ICU setting. |

**Evaluation:** 1. Some improvement noted in pulse oximetry, respiratory rate, and muscle rigidity. However, patient required constant monitoring due to unpredictable respiratory status and diminished lung sounds in bilateral posterior bases. Continue care plan and evaluate every shift and prn if condition changes.

**Nursing Care Plan:** Neuroleptic malignant syndrome, chronic undifferentiated schizophrenia.
**Nursing Diagnosis:** Ineffective Thermoregulation r/t adverse effects of antipsychotic medication AEB oral temperature = 105°F and diaphoresis.
**Outcomes** (include time frames): 1. Will experience temperature within range of 98.6 to 99°F in 24 hours.

| Assessment Data: O = Objective, S = Subjective | Evidence-Based Interventions: | Rationales: | Patient Responses: |
|---|---|---|---|
| Oral temperature = 105°F (O) Diaphoresis (O) States that he is having difficulty remembering where his room is (S) | 1(a) Start IV fluids as ordered. | 1(a) Fluids are needed to decrease body temperature. The patient is at risk for aspiration with irregular, rapid respirations and mental disorientation. Also, IVFs can be given at a more rapid rate than oral fluids to achieve a decrease in core body temperature. | 1(a) Tolerates start of IV fairly well. Verbalizes understanding of reason for IVFs. |
| | (b) Apply cooling blanket. | (b) A cooling blanket is used to decrease body core temperature when IVFs or oral fluids may not be enough to achieve desired results. Because the patient has elevated liver enzymes, the psychiatrist/physician will not order Tylenol/ acetaminophen. Later on, Aspirin/acetylsalicylic acid or Motrin/ibuprofen may be ordered, especially if the patient's temperature does not decrease significantly with the cooling blanket. With a temperature of 105°F, it is critical to return the body to a normal core temperature as soon as possible to prevent potential brain tissue damage. | (b) Questions reason for cooling blanket, but allows nurse to apply it after explaining why it is necessary. |
| | (c) Assess temperature every hour and prn. | (c) The patient's temperature requires close monitoring to determine if there is any improvement or worsening of his condition. Temperatures greater than 104°F can cause | (c) Has an oral temperature of 104°F 1 hour after initiation of IVFs and cooling blanket. |

| Assessment Data: O = Objective, S = Subjective | Evidence-Based Interventions: | Rationales: | Patient Responses: |
|---|---|---|---|
| | | seizure, delirium, or damage to body cells. Temperatures greater than 105.8°F can cause damage to brain cells in the hypothalamus, thus affecting the temperature control center of the brain (Lewis, Heitkemper, & Dirksen, 2004, p. 219). | |
| | (d) Provide tepid sponge baths and fresh bed linens prn. | (d) This may not be necessary to decrease temperature since a cooling blanket is being used. However, it would be helpful as a comfort measure due to diaphoresis. Tepid water is effective, prevents chilling, and is more comfortable than using cold water. | (d) States that he felt more comfortable after being bathed and having bed linens changed. |
| | (e) Administer antipyretics, or other temperature-lowering medications, if ordered. | (e) Antipyretics will help reduce the body core temperature. However, the patient has elevated liver enzymes so the psychiatrist/physician will not order Tylenol/ acetaminophen. Dantrium is used to treat hyperthermia as well as muscle hyper-rigidity. Later on, Aspirin/acetylsalicylic acid or Motrin/ibuprofen may be ordered, especially if the patient's temperature does not decrease significantly with the cooling blanket, IV fluids, and Dantrium. | (e) No antipyretic medications are ordered at this time. Receiving Dantrium and cooling blanket is in place. |
| | (f) As soon as patient's respirations are regular, offer oral fluids every hour. | (f) Increasing fluids are an essential part of treatment for fever. IVFs are very effective, but having an IV increases the patient's risk for infection. However, due to the patient's difficulty | (f) Requires IVFs at this time; tolerates them fairly well. |

*(continues)*

| Assessment Data: O = Objective, S = Subjective | Evidence-Based Interventions: | Rationales: | Patient Responses: |
|---|---|---|---|
| | | breathing and severe muscle rigidity there is an increased risk of aspiration. Therefore, it is better to maintain IVFs at this time. | |

**Evaluation:** 1. Oral temperature = 104°F. Continues to require IVFs and cooling blanket. Continue care plan and evaluate in 8 hours and prn.

**Nursing Care Plan:** Neuroleptic malignant syndrome, chronic undifferentiated schizophrenia.
**Nursing Diagnosis:** Disturbed Thought Processes r/t neurobiochemical alterations s/t adverse antipsychotic medications and chronic undifferentiated schizophrenia AEB reporting difficulty remembering where his room is on the unit and delusions of being from outer space and having a force field around him.
**Outcomes** (include time frames): 1. Will demonstrate orientation in all spheres in 36 hours. 2. Will refrain from acting on delusional thinking (e.g., someone invading his "force field") in 72 hours.

| Assessment Data: O = Objective, S = Subjective | Evidence-Based Interventions: | Rationales: | Patient Responses: |
|---|---|---|---|
| States having difficulty remembering where his room is (S) Bizzare delusional thinking including being from another planet and having a force field around him (S) Found by police running around in a field only partially clothed (O) Struck CNA in ER for presumably disrupting his force field when attempting to place him in a hospital gown (O) Not taking prescribed medications prior to being brought to the ER (S) Received IM Haldol/haloperidol as part of a medication cocktail and later an oral dose of Haldol/haloperidol in the ER. | 1(a) Reorient to all spheres every 4 hours and prn. | 1(a) Reorienting the patient helps maintain his present level of orientation and increase his ability to become more oriented. | 1(a) Oriented to person and place only at this time. |
| | (b) Assess oxygen status: LOC, increased confusion, lung sounds, pulse oximetry, respiratory rate and quality, and muscle rigidity every 4 hours when stabilized. (See previous care plan "Ineffective Breathing Pattern" for initial frequency.) | (b) Decreased oxygenation is demonstrated by decreased LOC, mental confusion, abnormal lung sounds, decreased pulse oximetry results, increased/decreased respiratory rate and quality, and thoracic muscle rigidity. | (b) Remains oriented to person and place only. Delusional thinking remains intact. Lung sounds are diminished bilaterally in posterior bases; pulse oximetry = 93% on 2 liters of oxygen, respiratory rate 22, small improvement in muscle rigidity. |
| | (c) Provide physical reminders of room location (name on door and arrow stickers in the direction of his room from the dining room, dayroom, and nurse's station). Help patient locate room as needed. | (c) Reminders help the patient locate his room, decrease his confusion, and increase his independence. Assistance in a nonjudgmental manner may be needed until the mental confusion clears. | (c) Able to recognize name on door and able to follow arrows with assistance. |
| | 2(a) Perform mental status exam every shift and prn, including assessment for command auditory hallucinations and paranoia. | 2(a) This will establish a baseline of information, help you evaluate whether his psychosis is improving, worsening, or remaining the same. Treatment and nursing interventions will be adjusted depending on many factors, including the results of the mental status exam. | 2(a) Bizzare delusions of being from another planet and having a force field around him persist. Denies paranoia and hallucinations of any type, including command auditory hallucinations. |
| | (b) Continue therapeutic use of self to strengthen therapeutic nurse/patient alliance. | (b) This promotes and strengthens trust between the patient and nurse. Paranoid patients have great difficulty trusting anyone, which makes it | (b) At this time accepts the presence of the nurse and other staff members. |

*(continues)*

| Assessment Data: O = Objective, S = Subjective | Evidence-Based Interventions: | Rationales: | Patient Responses: |
|---|---|---|---|
| | | difficult for them to obtain treatment, accept any help offered, and make significant positive progress toward healing. | |
| | (c) Ask patient for permission to touch him if need to provide physical care. | (c) Asking permission warns the patient ahead of time that he will be touched, decreases his anxiety and fear, and decreases the potential of the patient physically striking out to protect himself. | (c) At this time accepts physical care needed if told ahead of time what will be done. |
| | (d) Use short, simple directions and explanations of care. | (d) Simple words, directions, and explanations increase patients' ability to understand and follow, especially when they are experiencing competing internal stimuli such as delusional thinking, hallucinations, have cognitive deficits or problems with correct perception. Patients diagnosed with schizophrenia have "concrete" versus abstract thinking and interpret what is said literally, which also makes it necessary to communicate with them in simple, direct language. | (d) Verbalizes understanding of requests and explanations. |
| | (e) Continually assess patient for increasing irritability or intolerance to presence of nurse or staff members. | (e) These are signs that the patient's behavior is escalating and may signal impending physical escalation or striking out. | (e) At this time seems calm and relaxed. |
| | (f) Decrease environmental stimuli (e.g., number of people in area, noise, light). | (f) Many times patients experience increased frequency of psychotic symptoms in noisy, chaotic environments. This intervention helps decrease the risk of triggering the patient's psychotic symptoms as well as agitation or aggressive behavior. | (f) Continues to be calm and relaxed. Noted to be sensitive to changes in environment. |

| Assessment Data: O = Objective, S = Subjective | Evidence-Based Interventions: | Rationales: | Patient Responses: |
|---|---|---|---|
| | (g) Use a calm, matter-of-fact tone of voice, consistent manner, and open, relaxed body posture when interacting with this patient. Refrain from arguing with patient about delusions and hallucinations. | (g) Strong feelings—whether positive or negative—are transmitted as energy. Patients with any type of psychiatric illness are very sensitive to specific and general environmental changes including how they are approached, voice tone, and any nonverbal communication including body language by any healthcare professional. They may feel threatened or intimidated. The use of a calm, matter-of-fact tone of voice, and open, relaxed body posture transmits a therapeutic feeling of calmness and safety to the patient and helps him feel more calm and safe. This helps decrease the risk of escalating his behavior or triggering agitation. Also, because the patient believes his delusions and hallucinations are real, arguing with him to the contrary is not therapeutic and will cause only increased risk of escalating his behavior, triggering agitation or even physical aggression. It may erode his trust in you. | (g) Responds positively to calm, matter-of-fact verbal voice tone and open, relaxed body posture. |
| | (h) Maintain consistency in nurse and other staff members assigned to work with this patient. | (h) Consistency promotes the establishment of rapport and trust between the patient and nurse/staff members. It also increases the patient's feelings of safety. Nurses and staff members who work consistently with a patient will | (h) Is comfortable with consistent nurse/staff member assignments, but becomes anxious when he sees a staff member who has had scheduled days off and is meeting the patient for the first time. |

*(continues)*

| Assessment Data: O = Objective, S = Subjective | Evidence-Based Interventions: | Rationales: | Patient Responses: |
|---|---|---|---|
| | | be able to notice subtle changes in the patient's condition that are valuable in providing and evaluating care. | |

**Evaluation:** 1. Remains oriented to person and place only. Able to use reminders with assistance.
2. Bizarre delusional thinking persists, but no physical striking out behaviors. Continue plan and evaluate in 24 hours and prn.

# References

American Psychiatric Association. (2000). *Diagnostic and statistical manual of mental disorders* (4th ed.). Text Revision. Washington, DC: Author.

Antai-Otong, D. (2004). *Psychiatric emergencies: How to accurately assess and manage the patient in crisis.* Eau Claire, WI: PESI HealthCare.

Carpenito-Moyat, L. J. (2008). *Nursing diagnosis: Application to clinical practice* (12th ed.). Philadelphia, PA: WoltersKluwer Lippincott Williams & Wilkins.

Fischbach, F. (2004). *A manual of laboratory and diagnositic tests* (7th ed.). Philadelphia, PA: Lippincott Williams & Wilkins.

Fontaine, K. L. (2009). *Mental health nursing* (6th ed.). Upper Saddle River, NJ: Prentice Hall.

Fontaine, K. L., & Fletcher, J. S. (2003). *Mental health nursing* (5th ed.). Upper Saddle River, NJ: Prentice Hall.

Fortinash, K. M., & Holoday Worret, P. A. (2007). *Psychiatric nursing care plans* (5th ed.). St. Louis, MO: Mosby, Elsevier.

Keltner, N. L., Schwecke, L. H., & Bostrom, C. E. (2007). *Psychiatric nursing* (5th ed.). St. Louis, MO: Mosby, Elsevier.

Lewis, S. M., Heitkemper, M. M., & Dirksen, S. R. (2004). *Medical-surgical nursing: Assessment strategies and management of clinical problems* (6th ed.). St. Louis, MO: Mosby.

McKenrey, L., Tessier, E., & Hogan, M. (2006). *Mosby's pharmacology in nursing* (22nd ed.). St. Louis, MO: Mosby.

O'Brien, P. G., Kennedy, W. Z., & Ballard, K. A. (2008). *Psychiatric mental health nursing: An introduction to theory and practice.* Sudbury, MA: Jones and Bartlett.

Varcarolis, E. M. (2006). *Manual of psychiatric nursing care plans* (3rd ed.). St. Louis, MO: Saunders, Elsevier.

Zarrouf, F. A., & Bhanot, V. (2007, August). Neuroleptic malignant syndrome: Don't let your guard down yet. *Current Psychiatry, 6*(8), 89–95.

# *Adverse Medication Effects: Hypertensive Crisis*

## ANSWER KEY

## Question 1

Stiff neck and severe, throbbing occipital headache that began suddenly at the end of the meal; pulse = 108, and blood pressure = 190/104.

    a.  The following foods should be avoided:

        Aged, smoked, or processed meats; other unrefrigerated meats, liver, and game that has been hung

        Pickled herring, dried salted fish

        Improperly stored fish or poultry

        Mature or aged cheeses

        Tap/draft beer, alcohol-free beer

        Chianti or sherry

        Broad bean pods

        Soups in packets

        Sauerkraut

        Soy sauce, soybean condiments, tofu

        Ripe avocados

        Bananas

        Concentrated yeast extracts

        Caffeinated beverages in large amounts

    b.  Restrict to no more than 2 oz. per day of the following foods:

        Yogurt

        Sour cream

        Chocolate

        Cottage cheese

        Mild Swiss or American cheese

        Wine

# Question 2

    a. Stopping medication

    b. Starting Apresoline/hydralazine 10–40 mg IV (or IM); repeat if necessary (check BP & pulse q 5 min until stable); Regitine/phentolamine may also be used as well as diuretics

    c. Monitoring temperature and respirations

    d. Cooling blanket if hyperthermia

    e. Supportive care

# Questions 3 and 4

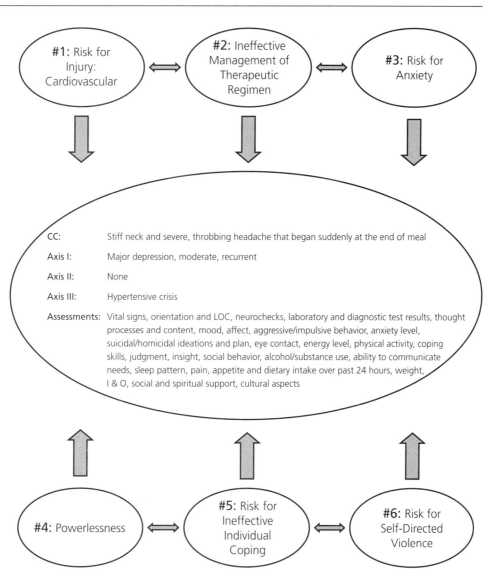

# Questions 5 and 6

**Nursing Care Plan:** Hypertensive crisis, major depression, moderate, recurrent.
**Nursing Diagnosis:** Risk for Injury: Cardiovascular r/t adverse medication effects s/t MAOIs AEB stiff neck and severe, throbbing headache that began suddenly at the end of meal; currently prescribed Nardil/phenelzine, BP = 190/104, and pulse = 108.
**Outcomes:** 1. Will begin to experience a decrease in symptoms within 2 hours of presenting for treatment.

| Assessment Data:<br>O = Objective,<br>S = Subjective | Evidence-Based<br>Interventions: | Rationales: | Patient<br>Responses:* |
|---|---|---|---|
| Stiff neck and severe, throbbing occipital headache that began suddenly at end of meal (S)<br>Dining in a restaurant prior to the start of symptoms (S)<br>Currently prescribed Nardil (O)<br>BP = 190/104 (O)<br>Pulse = 108 (O)<br>Respirations = 22 (O) | 1(a) Perform baseline cardiac assessment, respiratory assessment including pulse oximetry every hour and prn. | 1(a) Information obtained with these baseline assessments will be used to help determine initial treatment, the patient's progress, and additional changes to treatment when necessary. Early deterioration in the patient's condition will be more readily noted if frequent assessments are performed and results communicated to the physician. | 1(a) BP = 190/104, pulse = 108, respirations = 22; denies chest pain or discomfort; all remaining assessments WNL. |
| | (b) Assess LOC and orientation every hour and prn. | (b) If the patient is experiencing an oxygen deficit s/t circulatory collapse or neurological impairment s/t increased intracranial pressure, he will exhibit decreased LOC and disorientation. | (b) Remains alert and oriented in all spheres. Anxious but grateful for care he is receiving. |
| | (c) Obtain vital signs every 15 minutes for 1 hour. If stable, then every 30 minutes for 1 hour. | (c) Frequent vital signs will help determine if the patient's blood pressure and pulse are improving, staying the same, or worsening. The nurse will also be able to monitor the effectiveness of medication administered. | (c) See (a) above. Temperature remains at 99.8°F. |
| | (d) Initiate and maintain IV access as ordered. | (d) IV access will be needed to medicate the patient and in case a code situation develops. | (d) Tolerates venipuncture well. Verbalizes understanding of reason for IV access. |

*Patient responses are examples of what students would look for to decide whether their planned interventions were successful, needed more time, or needed to be changed. Responses will vary depending on the patient.

| Assessment Data: O = Objective, S = Subjective | Evidence-Based Interventions: | Rationales: | Patient Responses: |
|---|---|---|---|
| | (e) Hold Nardil and medicate as ordered for BP = 190/104.

(f) Observe for edema of feet and lower legs. | (e) As the BP begins to improve, the pulse should also. Holding the Nardil will also help decrease the patient's pulse.
(f) Edema of the feet and lower legs is a side effect of Apresoline. The patient may need to have his legs elevated or wear TED hose. | (e) BP = 160/95, pulse = 96 when taken 15 minutes after administration of medication. Verbalizes understanding of medication administered.
(f) Noted at this time. Continue to observe closely. |

**Evaluation:** 1. Beginning to respond to treatment. BP = 160/95, pulse = 96 when taken 15 minutes after administration of medication. Continue care plan and evaluate in 2 hours and prn if condition changes.

**Nursing Care Plan:** Hypertensive crisis, major depression, moderate, recurrent.
**Nursing Diagnosis:** Ineffective Management of Therapeutic Regimen r/t limited knowledge of tyramine content of restaurant food items s/t dietary restrictions while taking MAOIs AEB symptoms occurring suddenly at end of meal.
**Outcomes:** 1. Will verbalize increased knowledge and understanding of how to handle dining out, or ordering food to be delivered, by discharge.

| Assessment Data:<br>O = Objective,<br>S = Subjective | Evidence-Based Interventions: | Rationales: | Patient Responses: |
|---|---|---|---|
| Dining in a restaurant prior to the start of symptoms (S)<br>Stiff neck and severe, throbbing occipital headache that began suddenly at the end of the meal (S)<br>Currently prescribed Nardil (O) | 1(a) Assess patient's current knowledge of dietary substances that contain tyramine and the interaction between tyramine and MAOI medications. | 1(a) There is much information available regarding medications and any type of treatment. The amount of information can be overwhelming for most patients. It may take several sessions of working with patients to be sure they truly understand all the information. Printed materials are helpful, especially with shorter inpatient stays that leave less time to care for and teach patients everything they need to know. Patients may not fully understand the seriousness of medication-food interactions until they experience such an interaction. | 1(a) Has a fair knowledge of information, but admits that he misplaced the printed information he received when he was first prescribed Nardil. |
| | (b) Clarify misconceptions. | (b) Patients may verbalize understanding, but still have misconceptions. When discussing information further with patients, their misconceptions become more apparent. | (b) Open to receiving printed materials to replace those he misplaced. Needed clarification of food substances he can use in moderation. |
| | (c) Use nonjudgmental approach when interacting with patient. | (c) Patients may become defensive when very anxious and overwhelmed by a situation. A nonjudgmental approach shows that the nurse is not blaming or shaming patients in any way for their actions. Patients may be more likely to report information and ask questions when | (c) Responds positively to a nonjudgmental approach. Stated that he was afraid we would think he had purposely eaten something he wasn't supposed to or was trying to "get away with something." |

| Assessment Data: O = Objective, S = Subjective | Evidence-Based Interventions: | Rationales: | Patient Responses: |
|---|---|---|---|
| | (d) Encourage patient to ask for more detailed information regarding food substances when dining out, or ordering food to be delivered, without compromising his confidentiality. | feeling accepted rather than judged. Having a clearer picture helps the nurse and the entire treatment team provide more specific diagnosis and treatment in the patient's best interest.<br><br>(d) It can be difficult to determine the content of food substances prepared elsewhere. The patient can learn to be more assertive and ask about the content with an explanation of having an allergy or that he takes medication, but he does not have to divulge the type of medication he takes. | (d) Agreed that he could ask for more information. Likes the idea of saying he has an "allergy" rather than admitting to a stranger that he is taking medication. |

**Evaluation:** 1. Verbalizes increased knowledge and understanding of how to handle dining out, or ordering food to be delivered, by discharge. Continue to reinforce information provided until discharge.

**Nursing Care Plan:** Hypertensive crisis, major depression, moderate, recurrent.
**Nursing Diagnosis:** Risk for Anxiety r/t fear of unknown causes of symptoms AEB sudden, unexpected onset of symptoms and seeking treatment in ER.
**Outcomes:** 1. Will verbalize what he can control in the situation by discharge.

| Assessment Data:<br>O = Objective,<br>S = Subjective | Evidence-Based<br>Interventions: | Rationales: | Patient<br>Responses |
|---|---|---|---|
| Sudden, unexpected onset of symptoms (S)<br>BP = 190/104 (O)<br>Pulse = 108 (O)<br>Respirations = 22 (O) | 1(a) Use calm approach and simple statements when interacting with patient. | 1(a) If a patient perceives that the nurse is calm, he will in turn feel more calm. When patients are anxious, they may be too overwhelmed to focus on what is being said to them and retain less information. | 1(a) Responds positively to calm approach. Understands simple requests and information provided. |
| | (b) Decrease environmental stimuli. | (b) Environmental stimuli can increase a patient's anxiety. Decreasing them will promote a more relaxing environment and help decrease the patient's anxiety. | (b) Less anxious after curtain drawn between bay areas in ER and informed he would be moved to a room soon. |
| | (c) Explore what the patient fears the most about the situation. | (c) Once fears and anxieties are more specifically identified, work can begin to deal with them. | (c) States that he was afraid he was "going to have a stroke." |
| | (d) Assist patient to identify what he can and cannot control about the situation. | (d) Once patients identify what they can control about a situation, they can then deal more effectively with the situation. They can also learn to "let go" and not waste energy on what they cannot control. | (d) Admits that he can control whether or not he seeks treatment and adheres to the treatment offered. Also states that he can be more careful in the future regarding the contents of food items when dining out. |
| | (e) Teach relaxation and distraction techniques such as deep breathing, progressive relaxation exercises, and simple guided imagery. | (e) Relaxation and distraction techniques will help decrease the patient's anxiety and promote relaxation. They will also help decrease the autonomic nervous system response that is adding to the adverse physiologic effects from Nardil and from food substances containing tyramine. | (e) Makes an effort to learn deep breathing, progressive relaxation exercises, and guided imagery. States that he has heard about some of these techniques but never tried them because he wasn't sure if they would work or not. |

**Evaluation:** 1. Able to verbalize what he can control in this situation. Verbalized fear of having a stroke. Continue to work with patient on relaxation and distraction techniques. Evaluate plan before discharge.

# References

Bezchlibnyk-Butler, K. Z., & Jeffries, J. J. (2005). *Clinical handbook of psychotropic drugs* (15th ed.). Ashland, OH: Hogrefe & Huber.

Fontaine, K. L., & Fletcher, J. S. (2003). *Mental health nursing* (5th ed.). Upper Saddle River, NJ: Pearson.

Keltner, N. L., Schwecke, L. H., & Bostrom, C. E. (2007). *Psychiatric nursing* (5th ed.). St. Louis, MO: Mosby, Elsevier.

McKenrey, L., Tessier, E., & Hogan, M. (2006). *Mosby's pharmacology in nursing* (22nd ed.). St. Louis, MO: Mosby.

*Mosby's medical, nursing, and allied health dictionary* (6th ed.). (2002). St. Louis, MO: Mosby.

Sadock, B. J., & Sadock, V. A. (2003). *Kaplan and Sadock's synopsis of psychiatry: Behavioral sciences/clinical psychiatry* (9th ed.). Philadelphia, PA: Lippincott Williams & Wilkins.

# Therapeutic Communication Techniques

**Actively listening:** Maintaining eye contact, nodding head, and leaning toward the patient.

**Agreeing:** Agreeing with patients can help diffuse their anger. There may be a grain of truth in what angry nonpsychotic patients say.

> PATIENT: I hate this place! It feels like I'm in jail!
>
> NURSE: I can see how you would feel that way. Let's go to a quieter area and talk about how you can be more comfortable here.

**Clarifying:** "Let's see if I heard you correctly."

**Encouraging comparison:** "How have you handled difficult situations in the past?"

**Encouraging decision making:** "What can you do the next time you find yourself in a difficult situation?"

**Exploring:** "Tell me more about your sister." "What do think holds you back from being more social?"

**Focusing:** "Let's go back to what you were saying about your marriage problems."

**Focusing on feeling content:** Acknowledging feelings can be useful when working with a patient experiencing delusions:

> PATIENT: People are trying to kill me! Don't you see them?
>
> NURSE: It must be very frightening to feel that way.

**Interpreting:** "You sound anxious." "It sounds as if this is a difficult topic for you to talk about."

**Limit setting:** Set limits when working with an aggressive patient: "I will come back to talk with you when you calm down."

**Placing events in sequence:** "Did you start using cocaine before or after you started feeling depressed?"; "When did you first become aware you were having problems with your memory?"

**Reinforcing reality:** Reinforce reality when working with a patient experiencing hallucinations:

> PATIENT: The voices are really loud today.
>
> NURSE: The only voices I hear are your voice and mine.

**Silence:** Silence can be very therapeutic. Try sitting quietly with patients and allow them time to collect their thoughts or think about what they wish to say.

**Suggesting collaboration:** "Let's see if we can work together to solve your problem."

**Transitioning gently:** "I understand that what you are saying is important, but right now we need to talk about the reason you came to the hospital. We can spend some time talking about this other matter later."

**Voicing doubt:** "Is there any other explanation for that person's behavior?" "How else could you interpret her response?"

# References

Keltner, N. L., Schwecke, L. H., & Bostrom, C. E. (2007). *Psychiatric nursing* (5th ed.). St. Louis, MO: Mosby, Elsevier.

O'Brien, P. G., Kennedy, W. Z., & Ballard, K. A. (2008). *Psychiatric mental health nursing: An introduction to theory and practice.* Sudbury, MA: Jones and Bartlett.

# Assessment Tools

## Abnormal Involuntary Movement Scale (AIMS)

Name: _____ Date: _____

*Instructions:* Complete the examination procedure before making ratings. Rate the highest severity of movement for each movement observed. Circle the number corresponding to the severity of movement observed. Ask the patient being assessed to remove any gum or candy from their mouth before beginning.

*Rating scale:* 0 = none/normal, 1 = minimal, may be extreme normal; 2 = mild, 3 = moderate, 4 = severe

## Facial and Oral Movements

1. Muscles of facial expression (e.g., movements of eyebrows, forehead, periorbital area, cheeks; include blinking, smiling, frowning, grimacing).    0   1   2   3   4

2. Lips and perioral area (e.g., smacking, pouting, puckering).    0   1   2   3   4

3. Jaw (e.g., chewing, clenching, biting, mouth opening, lateral movements).    0   1   2   3   4

4. Tongue (rate only an increase in movements both in and out of the mouth, not an inability to sustain movement).    0   1   2   3   4

## Extremity Movements

5. Upper, including arms, wrists, hands, fingers. Include choreic movements (e.g., rapid, purposeless, irregular, spontaneous) and athetoid movements (e.g., slow, irregular, serpentine, complex). Do not include tremor (e.g., regular, repetitive, rhythmic).   0   1   2   3   4

6. Lower, including legs, knees, ankles, toes (e.g., foot tapping, lateral knee movement, heel dropping, foot squirming, inversion and eversion of foot).   0   1   2   3   4

## Trunk Movements

7. Neck, shoulders, hip (e.g., twisting, rocking, squirming, pelvic gyrations).   0   1   2   3   4

## Global Judgments

8. Severity of abnormal movements.   0   1   2   3   4

9. Incapacitation due to abnormal movements.   0   1   2   3   4

10. Patient's awareness of abnormal movements.   0   1   2   3   4

## Dental Status

Any current problems with teeth? With dentures?   Yes   No

Does the patient usually wear dentures?   Yes   No

## Hamilton Rating Scale for Depression (HAM-D)

*Instructions:* Please enter the score for *each* item.

| Item | Legend | Score |
|---|---|---|
| 1. Depressed mood | 0 = Absent<br>1 = Feeling states indicated only on questioning<br>2 = Feeling states reported spontaneously, verbally<br>3 = Feeling states reported nonverbally<br>4 = Feelings states reported verbally and nonverbally | |
| 2. Feelings of guilt | 0 = Absent<br>1 = Self-reproach; feels has let other people down<br>2 = Rumination over past mistakes or misdeeds<br>3 = Views present illness as a punishment; delusions of guilt<br>4 = Hears accusatory or denunciatory voices and/or experiences threatening visual hallucinations | |
| 3. Suicide | 0 = Absent thoughts or attempts<br>1 = Feels life is not worth living<br>2 = Wishes to be dead<br>3 = Suicidal ideas or gestures<br>4 = Suicide attempts | |
| 4. Insomnia—early | 0 = No difficulty falling asleep<br>1 = Complains of occasional difficulty falling asleep (i.e., more than 30 minutes)<br>2 = Complains of nightly difficulty falling asleep | |
| 5. Insomnia—middle | 0 = No difficulty<br>1 = Complains of restlessness during the night<br>2 = Awakens during the night; gets out of bed (other than to use the bathroom) | |
| 6. Insomnia—late | 0 = No difficulty<br>1 = Awakens in the early hours of the morning, but able to go back to sleep<br>2 = Unable to fall asleep again if gets out of bed | |
| 7. Work and activities | 0 = No difficulty<br>1 = Thoughts and feelings of fatigue, weakness, or incapacity related to work, activities, or hobbies<br>2 = Loss of interest in work, activities, or hobbies<br>3 = Decrease in actual time spent in productive work or activity<br>4 = Stopped working because of present illness | |
| 8. Psychomotor retardation | 0 = Normal rate of speech and thought<br>1 = Slight retardation during interview<br>2 = Obvious retardation during interview<br>3 = Difficult to interview<br>4 = Complete stupor | |

*(continues)*

| Item | Legend | Score |
|---|---|---|
| 9. Psychomotor agitation | 0 = None<br>1 = Fidgets<br>2 = Plays with hands, hair, etc.<br>3 = Difficulty sitting still, moves about<br>4 = Hand wringing, hair pulling, biting lips, biting finger nails | |
| 10. Anxiety, psychic | 0 = No difficulty<br>1 = Subjective report of irritability and tension<br>2 = Worries about minor matters<br>3 = Apprehensive affect or attitude in speech<br>4 = Expresses fears spontaneously without being questioned | |
| 11. Anxiety, somatic | 0 = Absent<br>1 = Mild<br>2 = Moderate<br>3 = Severe<br>4 = Incapacitating | |
| 12. Somatic, GI | 0 = None<br>1 = Loss of appetite, but does eat<br>2 = Difficulty eating; uses medication for GI symptoms | |
| 13. Somatic, general | 0 = None<br>1 = Reports heavy sensation of extremities, head, or back; complains of headaches, backaches, muscle aches, low energy, fatigue<br>2 = More specific symptoms | |
| 14. Genital symptoms | 0 = Absent<br>1 = Mild<br>2 = Severe | |
| 15. Hypochondriasis | 0 = Not present<br>1 = Self-absorption (bodily)<br>2 = Preoccupation with health<br>3 = Frequent complaints, requests for help<br>4 = Hypochondriacal delusions | |
| 16. Weight loss (subjective report) | 0 = No weight loss<br>1 = Probable weight loss associated with present illness<br>2 = Definite weight loss | |
| 17. Insight | 0 = Aware of being depressed and ill<br>1 = Aware of illness, but attributes cause to something else, such as being overworked or having a physical illness<br>2 = Denies any illness | |
| | | Total Score: |

### Young Mania Rating Scale (YMRS)

*Instructions:* Please enter the score for *each* item. The purpose of the rating is to rate the severity of the symptom. The presence of only one is needed to qualify for that rating. Whole or half points may be given.

| Item | Legend | Score |
|---|---|---|
| 1. Elevated mood | 0 = Absent<br>1 = Mildly<br>2 = Subjective elevation, optimistic, cheerful, self-confident; appropriate to content<br>3 = Elevated, humorous; inappropriate to content<br>4 = Euphoric, singing; inappropriate laughter | |
| 2. Increased motor activity energy | 0 = Absent<br>1 = Subjective increase<br>2 = Animated, increased gestures<br>3 = Excessive energy, restless, hyperactive at times; able to be calmed down<br>4 = Motor excitement, continuous hyperactivity; unable to be calmed down | |
| 3. Sexual interest | 0 = Normal, not increased<br>1 = Mildly increased<br>2 = Subjective increase<br>3 = Spontaneously verbalizes sexual content, elaborates on sexual matters, reports self to be hypersexual<br>4 = Overt sexual acts toward interviewer or others present | |
| 4. Sleep | 0 = No decrease in sleep<br>1 = Decreased sleep up to 1 hour<br>2 = Decreased sleep of more than 1 hour<br>3 = Decreased need for sleep<br>4 = Denies need for sleep | |
| 5. Irritability | 0 = Absent<br>2 = Subjectively increased<br>4 = Irritable at times during interview; recent episodes of annoyance or anger noted by others<br>6 = Frequently irritable during interview<br>8 = Hostile, uncooperative; unable to be interviewed | |
| 6. Speech (rate and amount) | 0 = No increase<br>2 = Feels talkative<br>4 = Increased rate or amount at times<br>6 = Consistent increase in rate and amount, difficult to interrupt<br>8 = Continuous, pressured, unable to be interrupted | |

*(continues)*

| Item | Legend | Score |
|---|---|---|
| 7. Language—thought disorder | 0 = Absent<br>1 = Circumstantial, mild distractibility, quick thoughts<br>2 = Distractible; changes topics frequently; racing thoughts; loses goal of thought<br>3 = Flight of ideas; tangentiality; difficult to follow; rhyming, echolalia<br>4 = Incoherent | |
| 8. Content | 0 = Normal<br>2 = Questionable plans, new interests<br>4 = Special projects; hyperreligious<br>6 = Grandiose or paranoid ideas; ideas of reference<br>8 = Delusions; hallucinations | |
| 9. Disruptive—aggressive behavior | 0 = Absent, cooperative<br>2 = Sarcastic; guarded; loud at times<br>4 = Demanding; makes threats<br>6 = Threatens interviewer; shouting; difficult to interview<br>8 = Assaultive; destructive; unable to be interviewed | |
| 10. Appearance | 0 = Appropriate dress and grooming<br>1 = Minimally unkempt<br>2 = Poorly groomed; moderately disheveled; overdressed<br>3 = Disheveled; partly clothed; inappropriate/garish make-up<br>4 = Completely unkempt; bizarre clothing | |
| 11. Insight | 0 = Admits illness; agrees need for treatment<br>1 = Admits to possibly being ill<br>2 = Admits behavior has changed, but denies illness<br>3 = Admits possible behavior change, but denies illness<br>4 = Denies any behavior change | |

# Cage Questionnaire:
# Screening for Alcohol Abuse

## Questions

1. Have you ever felt you should cut down on your drinking?    Yes    No
2. Have people annoyed you by criticizing your drinking?    Yes    No
3. Have you ever felt bad or guilty about your drinking?    Yes    No
4. Have you ever had a drink first thing in the morning to steady your nerves or to get rid of a hangover?    Yes    No

## Interpretation

Answering *Yes* to two questions: strong indication for alcohol abuse.

Answering *Yes* to three or more questions: confirms alcoholism.

## References

Mullen, J., Endicott, J., Hirschfeld, R. M., Yonkers, K., Tarcum, S., & Bullinger, A. L. (Eds.). (2004). *Manual of rating scales: For the assessment of mood disorders*. Wilmington, DE: Astrazeneca Pharmaceuticals.

O'Brien, F. G., Kennedy, W. Z., & Ballard, K. A. (2008). *Psychiatric mental health nursing: An introduction to theory and practice*. Sudbury, MA: Jones and Bartlett.

## Web Site

Comprehensive Risk Counseling & Services, Screening for Alcohol Abuse–CAGE Questionnaire: www.cdc.gov/hiv/topics/prev_prog/ CRCS/resources/CRCS_Manual/pdf/O-Cage_11102005.pdf

# Glossary

**Abstinence:** Totally refraining from the use of any alcohol or other substances.

**Abuse:** Actions or behaviors intended to harm or injure another person.

**Addiction:** Relying upon a substance either physically, psychologically, or both.

**Affect:** The observable components of an emotion (objective); facial expression.

**Aggression:** Forceful, verbal and physical action that is the motor counterpart of anger, rage, or hostility.

**Agnosia:** The inability to recognize familiar objects in the absence of reduced alertness.

**Akasthesia:** Motor restlessness demonstrated as difficulty sitting still or staying in one position for any length of time; pacing, fidgeting, shifting weight frequently from one foot to another, tapping one foot, or inability to sit still in a chair. Patients with this condition frequently make statements about feeling as if they are going to "jump out of" their "skin."

**Akinesia:** Decrease in motor movement or muscle weakness; complaints of fatigue or tiring easily with physical activity.

**Alogia:** Literally "without speech"; very limited speech, without elaboration.

**Aloofness:** An attitude or manner of disinterest or disdain; desire to remain separate or apart from others.

**Amnesia:** A cognitive disorder involving loss of memory.

**Anger:** Feelings of an expression of anxiety that is aroused by a real or perceived threat to one's possessions, values, or significant others.

**Anorexia nervosa (AN):** The extreme pursuit of a thin body accompanied by a profoundly disturbed body image.

**Antipsychotics:** Medications that reduce or relieve psychotic symptoms such as delusional thinking, hallucinations, or other cognitive misperceptions. Also referred to as *Neuroleptics*.

**Anxiety:** General uneasiness or apprehension that occurs in anticipation of a threat or danger to self. More vague than fear, which is more specific. When anxiety interferes with effectiveness in everyday living or ability to function normally, it is diagnosed as pathological.

**Apathetic/Apathy:** Lack of feeling, emotions, interest, or concerns.

**Aphasia:** A disorder of speech or language affecting expressive or receptive functioning or both.

**Appropriate:** Emotional tone that is in harmony with accompanying idea, thought, or verbalized words. Acceptable.

**Apraxia:** The loss of ability to perform motor skills or purposeful acts.

**Assault:** Actions or behaviors, including verbal threats, that pose an immediate threat of physical harm to another person.

**Assertive Community Treatment (ACT):** Comprehensive, multidisciplinary services delivered to the patient in the community wherever the patient needs the support. Services are available 24 hours a day, 7 days a week.

**Atrial fibrillation:** Loss of effective atrial contraction due to multiple, uncoordinated electrical impulses. Commonly occurs in patients with underlying cardiac disease.

**Atypical antipsychotics:** See *antipsychotics*. Atypical antipsychotics, also referred to as second generation antipsychotics (SGAs), are the newest medications developed for the treatment of psychotic disorders such as schizophrenia. They are also used to treat mood disorders.

**Battering:** A repeated pattern of the use of threats or violence to establish control and power through fear and intimidation.

**Binge eating:** Recurrent episodes of eating large amounts of food in a small amount of time *without* engaging in purging activities, but there is still a feeling of being out of control.

**Bipolar disorder:** A mood disorder consisting of two phases: depressed phase and manic phase.

**Blackouts:** An early sign of alcoholism. Blackouts are a form of amnesia for events that occurred during the drinking period when a person may function "normally."

**Blunted affect:** A disturbance manifested by severe reduction in the intensity of affect.

**Body mass index (BMI):** A formula used to determine if a person is obese. It is only one measure of obesity.

**Boundaries:** Psychological, emotional, social, or physical limits that help define and protect a person's identity or sense of self. Healthy boundaries allow a person to choose an appropriate degree of interaction. Boundaries that are inflexible, rigid, enmeshed, unclear, or too permeable are unhealthy.

**Bright affect:** Happy and cheerful.

**Bulimia nervosa (BN):** A disorder involving recurrent episodes of binge-eating followed by purging accompanied by feeling out of control. Includes overvaluation of body weight and shape and low self-esteem.

**Catatonia:** Decreased reactivity or unresponsiveness to one's environment.

**Circumstantiality:** Pattern of speech that is indirect and delayed in reaching its goal because of irrelevant details or parenthetical remarks. The speaker does not lose the point, as is characteristic of loosening of associations, and clauses remain logically connected, but to the listener it seems that the end will never be reached. The speaker does eventually get back to the beginning topic.

**Clang association:** A type of thinking in which the sound of a word rather than its meanings gives the direction to subsequent associations.

**Codependency:** *Excessive* focus on the needs of another to the detriment or harm of the person not using substances; dysfunctional behavior patterns.

**Cognition:** Thinking, knowing, perceiving.

**Cognitive behavioral therapy (CBT):** A form of psychotherapy used to identify and modify a patient's unrealistic, maladaptive thoughts and behavior that results from thoughts.

**Cognitive distortion:** Errors that occur in thinking or perceiving leading a person to arrive at false conclusions. The person makes decisions, experiences emotions, and behaves in ways based upon these errors and false conclusions. These errors do not meet criteria for delusional thinking or hallucinations.

**Compensatory behaviors:** Behaviors or methods used to counteract an undesireable event, situation, or condition.

**Concrete:** Focused thinking on facts and details, a literal interpretation of messages, and an inability to generate or think abstractly/hypothetically.

**Confabulation:** Making up plausible (possibly believable) information to cover up for memory problems.

**Contraband:** An object or material that can be used to harm oneself or others. Includes illegal drugs and alcohol.

**Countertransference:** A nurse or other staff member's unconscious displacement of feelings for significant people in his or her past onto the patient in the current therapeutic relationship.

**Cravings:** Nearly irresistible urges to obtain and use any psychoactive substance including alcohol.

**Delirium:** Temporary, rapidly developing, potentially reversible mental disorder affecting cognition. May be caused by several different reasons including acute changes in medical-surgical conditions, infections, toxic metabolic syndromes, inability to clear medications from the body resulting in toxic serum levels, or infections. If left untreated may result in permanent brain damage or even death.

**Delirium tremens (DTs):** Withdrawal signs and symptoms including grand mal seizures occurring in a person who drinks heavily and then stops drinking. If untreated, can be fatal.

**Delusion:** A fixed, false belief that is firmly maintained and is not shared by others and is contradicted by society or any facts to the contrary. Distorted or exaggerated thoughts. There are many different types of delusions.

**Dementia:** Chronic, usually progressive, cognitive disorder associated with changes in brain structure and functioning. Dementia may be the result of a variety of causes.

**Denial:** A frequently used unconscious ego defense mechanism involving refusal to believe events are happening or the existence of intolerable situations and circumstances. When used as a coping mechanism over long periods of time, it can become unhealthy and destructive.

**Depersonalization:** Feeling of strangeness or unreality related to one's own body, body parts, thoughts, the self, or the environment. Depersonalized individuals feel as if they are outside their bodies and observing themselves; they feel as if they are robots, yet are aware they are not.

**Depression:** Feelings of sadness, despair, unhappiness.

**Derealization:** Feelings of detachment or separation from one's personal environment. Also, a distortion of spatial relationships between objects in the environment may occur causing people to feel their environment is unfamiliar or different in some way.

A false perception that their environment has changed making objects appear larger or smaller to them. Some people may say they feel as if they are in a movie and things around them seem unreal.

**Desensitization:** Systematic desensitization; a therapy used to treat anxiety disorders including PTSD and phobias. The person is gradually exposed to increasingly greater stressful triggers or situations with the result of eventually extinguishing the emotional responses.

**Detachment:** Interpersonal (between people) and intrapersonal (within the person) dissociation from emotional or affective expression of emotions. The person appears emotionally cold, distant, or aloof.

**Detoxification:** "Detox"; converting substances into less harmful forms that can be more readily metabolized and excreted; medical intervention with related medication while maintaining physiological stability.

**Dialectical Behavioral Therapy (DBT):** A type of long-term psychotherapy developed by M. Linehan specifically for the treatment of patients diagnosed with borderline personality disorder. This therapy combines CBT with the concept of mindfulness. Patients are also taught techniques including impulse control, self-soothing, and how to appropriately ask for what they need.

**Dichotomous thinking:** Specific type of cognitive distortion where a person views people, behavior, situations or events in an "all or none" context or way of thinking.

**Disorganization:** Confused and/or illogical thoughts.

**Dissociation:** An unconscious defense mechanism in which the person temporarily experiences an altered state of consciousness and may engage in behaviors without conscious awareness. Dissociative symptoms involve changes in consciousness, motor function, and even identity to protect the self from painful emotions or psychological conflicts including anxiety, physical or psychological trauma, or abuse. Dissociative amnesia involves memory loss for an acute precipitating event.

**Domestic violence:** When one partner acts violently toward an intimate partner. The victim is socially isolated, has limited freedom, and limited access to financial resources making it difficult to leave the perpetrator.

**Dual diagnosis:** Term used most often for people diagnosed with a substance abuse or dependence diagnosis and another Axis I diagnosis (e.g., major depression, bipolar disorders, or schizophrenia). This term may also be used for people diagnosed with mental retardation (Axis II) who also have been diagnosed with Axis I disorders such as major depression, bipolar disorders, or schizophrenia.

**Dysphoria:** The opposite of euphoria or euphoric; depressed mood.

**Dystonia or dystonic reactions:** Muscle spasms or uncoordinated spastic muscle movements involving the face, tongue, extraocular muscles (e.g., oculogyric crisis), trachea/larynx (i.e. laryngospasm), esophagus, neck (e.g., torticollis), thorax/respiratory muscles (e.g., respiratory problems), trunk (e.g., opisthotonus or arching of the back), or pelvis (e.g., swaying or difficulty walking).

**Ego defense mechanisms:** Unconscious mental processes theorized by Freud as one explanation for human behavior used to relieve intense emotional states such as anxiety attributed to increased conflict or tension between the superego and the id component of personality.

**Ego-dystonia:** Behaviors and thoughts that disagree with a person's desires and values.

**Ego-syntonia:** Behaviors and thoughts that agree with a person's desires and values.

**Emotional numbing:** Decreased ability to appreciate and enjoy previously enjoyable activities; feeling of detachment from others and difficulty with intimacy.

**Empowerment:** A process by which a person gains self-confidence and improved self-esteem to actively engage in and control his or her own environment.

**Enmeshment:** Blurred or unhealthy boundaries where parents are overinvolved in their childrens' lives to the point of interfering with the development of their natural tendencies; "sameness" and obedience are rewarded and autonomy or individuality are not valued and may be discouraged.

**Euphoria:** A false sense of elation or well-being; pathological elevation of mood.

**Fear:** Apprehension or uneasiness occurring as a response to a specific event, person, or other trigger. It occurs in anticipation of a threat or danger to the self. Anxiety is similar, but is a response to a more vague, general perceived threat.

**Flashback:** Re-experiencing a traumatic event emotionally, cognitively, psychologically, and physically. Flashbacks can occur at any time and are not able to be controlled by the person experiencing them.

**Flat affect:** Absence or near absence of any sign of affective expression.

**Flight of ideas (FOI):** A nearly continuous flow of accelerated speech with abrupt changes from one topic to another, usually based on understandable associations, distracting stimuli, or playing on words. More reality-based than "loose associations" (e.g., "How are you doing, kid, no kidding around, I'm going home . . . home is where the heart is, the heart of the matter is I want out and that ain't hay . . . hey Doc . . . get me out of this place.").

**Flooding:** A more extreme form of desensitization therapy where the person is exposed to or confronted with the actual or similar stressful triggers/situations for an extended period of time. The goal is to extinguish the person's emotional responses.

**Gender identity:** Internal sense or perception of oneself as a male, female, or existing somewhere on a continuum.

**Gender role:** Role expectations of values, behaviors, emotional responses, thinking, and occupations attributed by a culture according to gender.

**Genetic identity:** A person's gender by chromosomes.

**Global Assessment of Functioning (GAF):** A score given after assessment of a person's overall functioning including the areas of occupational, psychological, and social functioning. A range of 1–100 is used. 1 = serious suicidal act clearly expecting to die and 100 = superior functioning in a wide range of activities; no mental health problems.

**Grandiose thinking:** Delusion consisting of perception of importance, special powers, or religious significance that is not in line with reality.

**Guarded behavior or verbal response:** Cautious; careful; restrained.

**Guilt:** Deserving blame or punishment for having committed an offense or having done something wrong.

**Helplessness:** A person's belief that neither he nor anyone else can help him.

**Hopelessness:** A person's belief that people, situations, or events will never change for the better.

**Hostility:** Anger and resentment characterized by destructive behavior.

**Hyperarousal:** Increased or exaggerated state of alertness; hypervigilance; visually scanning the environment for potential danger; exaggerated startle response emotionally and physically.

**Ideas of reference:** Incorrect interpretation of casual incidents and external events as having direct reference to oneself. Misinterpreting the behavior of others (e.g., thinking the newspaper headline has special significance for them; radio or TV personalities are speaking directly to them sometimes in "code").

**Ideations:** Thoughts.

**Illogical thinking:** Drawing erroneous conclusions or being subject to internal contradictions; irrational thoughts.

**Incest:** Intimate sexual behavior or intercourse between members of the same family.

**Intoxication:** The accumulation of poisonous levels of a substance including alcohol in the body as a result of decreased rate of metabolism and clearance.

**Irritable mood:** Easily annoyed or provoked; impatient; fretful, get upset easily.

**Labile mood:** Subject to frequent and/or unpredictable changes in mood, affect, or behavior.

**Loose association:** Thinking in which there is no apparent relationship between thoughts evidenced when speaking (e.g., "The thing is the ozone level is going away and people aren't told about it. Do you know why my bed is so soft? God bless America.").

**Manipulation:** Negative use of unhealthy behaviors or actions by a person to obtain needs. Positive uses of manipulation include changes in the therapeutic milieu to reinforce healthy behavior.

**Mindfulness:** Consciously being aware or present in the moment; focusing one's attention to the moment. An important concept used in spiritual meditation practices of ancient religions, cultural, and health practices. Also used in DBT and complementary-alternative health practices.

**Monoamine oxidase inhibitors (MAOI):** A classification of antidepressant medications.

**Mood:** Internal sensations of an emotion (subjective); the state of mind exhibited through emotions and feelings.

**Mute speech:** Refraining from producing speech or vocal sound.

**Neologism:** A newly invented word or condensed combination of several words coined by a person to express a highly complex idea.

**Neuroleptic malignant syndrome (NMS):** A potentially fatal adverse reaction to neuroleptic (antipsychotic) medication.

**Neuroleptics:** Medications that reduce or relieve psychotic symptoms such as delusional thinking, hallucinations, or other cognitive misperceptions. Also referred to as *Antipsychotics*.

**Nihilism:** The delusion of nonexistence of the self or part of the self, or of some object in the external reality.

**Obsession:** Recurrent thought, image, or impulse that is experienced as intrusive and inappropriate and that causes marked anxiety or distress.

**Oculogyric crisis:** See *Dystonia or dystonic reactions.*

**Opisthotonus:** See *Dystonia or dystonic reactions.*

**Organized thoughts:** Logical thoughts.

**Overdose:** Physical state when poisonous or excessive levels of a substance overwhelm the body's ability to metabolize and eliminate the substance/chemical.

**Paranoia:** Suspiciousness that is not based in reality.

**Perception:** Awareness of environmental stimuli from all senses and meaning attributed to those stimuli.

**Perpetrator:** A person who engages in the abuse of, violence toward, or battering of another person; the abuser.

**Persecutory thoughts:** Delusion consisting of paranoid perception that others are "out to get me" or punishing the person.

**Perseveration:** Uncontrollable repetition of a particular response, such as a word, phrase, or gesture, despite the absence or cessation of a stimulus, usually caused by brain injury or other organic disorder.

**Personality:** A combination of genetic and environmental influences that contributes to a person's attitudes and behavior patterns.

**Personality traits:** Stable or repeated patterns of feelings, thoughts, and behaviors that develop as individuals adapt to their environment. Includes how a they view both themselves and others.

**Phobia:** Persistent fear of an object or a situation.

**Poor concentration:** Inability to focus one's thought.

**Poverty of speech:** Inability to speak or to have very limited speech because of decreased *mental* processing, confusion, aphasia, or alogia.

**Preoccupation:** Occupied with or absorbed in one's thoughts.

**Pressured or rapid pressured speech:** The words seem as if they are being pushed out of the person's mouth; may be described as a "push" of speech; sounds almost as if they are stuttering in their attempt to get the words out of their mouth.

**Projection:** An ego defense mechanism commonly used by patients with borderline personality disorder. These individuals blame someone else for their problems or place their own desires on someone else (e.g., sexual desires, jealousy, anger) and accuse others of feeling or acting that way.

**Pseudoparkinsonism:** Signs and symptoms similar to those seen in Parkinson's disease in a person not diagnosed with that disease. Includes slow motor movements, tremors, muscle rigidity, cogwheel rigidity, stooped posture, shuffling gait, facial masking or flattened affect, and pill rolling finger movements.

**Psychomotor agitation:** A speeding up of motor movements (restlessness, difficulty sitting still) and cognition seen in depressed patients or patients in a manic phase of bipolar disorders.

**Psychomotor retardation:** A slowing down of motor movements and cognition seen in depressed patients.

**Rape:** Forced sexual, intimate behavior that is not mutually consented to. Sexual assault.

**Rational emotive behavior therapy (REBT):** Behavioral psychotherapy used to identify irrational beliefs and to challenge as well as change them. The therapist confronts, and teaches the patient to confront, illogical thoughts and beliefs, at times using a more confrontational approach than with CBT.

**Recovery:** As related to domestic violence, sexual assault. A process through which individuals work through helplessness and vulnerability to reorganize their lives and move from victim to survivor.

**Recovery:** As related to substance abuse. Current behavior or actions in a dynamic, life-long process of working toward and maintaining sobriety or drug-free living.

**Relapse:** A return to drinking or using drugs after a period of abstinence. Also refers to the return of signs and symptoms of psychiatric illness after a period of improvement or stability.

**Restricted affect:** Emotions are kept within limits; emotions are limited.

**Sad affect:** Unhappy.

**Schizophrenia:** A psychiatric disorder characterized by significant disorganization of thinking (cognition), behavior, impaired reality testing (delusions, hallucinations), and decreased general functioning. Signs and symptoms last at least 6 months. Subtypes include paranoid, disorganized, undifferentiated, catatonic, and residual.

**Self-harm:** Negative consequences for the physical and/or mental well-being of a person.

**Self-harm behaviors:** An activity that has negative consequences for a person's physical or mental well-being.

**Self-mutilation:** An activity involving a range of physically harmful behaviors including biting, pinching, scratching, choking, burning, or cutting oneself. These behaviors are different from suicide attempts because the person purposely engages in self-mutilation not to end their life, but as a maladaptive coping response.

**Sexual orientation:** The gender to which people are erotically, physically, or romantically attracted.

**Somatic:** Related to the *body*. Some patients who are depressed or anxious experience physical symptoms such as headaches, lower back pain, or GI distress.

**Splitting:** A behavioral phenomenon that occurs frequently in patients diagnosed with borderline personality disorder involving a specific type of cognitive distortion known as dichotomous thinking. A patient will attempt to divide one nurse or staff member against another over various issues including unit policies and what patients are allowed to do.

**Substance abuse:** The use of a substance including alcohol over at least a 1-year period as an unhealthy coping strategy that results in problems in major areas of life: failure to meet responsibilities or obligations; legal problems; recurrent social or interpersonal problems; recurrent problems at work or school; or continued use of substances during physically hazardous situations. There are no signs or symptoms of physical withdrawal, tolerance, or psychological dependence.

**Substance dependence:** Excessive, continued use of a substance including alcohol over at least a 1-year period as an unhealthy coping strategy regardless of health consequences or significant impairment in major areas of life including failure to meet responsibilities or obligations; legal problems; recurrent social or interpersonal problems; or recurrent problems at work or school. Additionally there is a preoccupation with obtaining and compulsion to use the substances, including giving up time with family or friends to do so; development of tolerance; physical and/or psychological withdrawal when abstaining from use; and ineffective attempts to stop or decrease use on one's own.

**Sundowning:** Increasing confusion that occurs in dementia usually in the early evening as the light in the sky lessens. May occur in some patients as early as midafternoon.

**Synergism:** The combined effect or result of two separate treatment modalities or approaches used together that is greater than either one used separately. Enhanced or greater effect when combining substances (e.g., barbiturates/benzodiazepines and alcohol, opiates and alcohol), which can be deadly.

**Tangential thoughts:** The veering of thoughts or speech from a main idea without ever getting back to it.

**Tardive dyskinesia:** Abnormal or purposeless muscle movements of the extremities, trunk, face, jaw, or oral-buccal muscles causing rocking or twisting motions, pelvic thrusting or gyrations, tremors, tongue darting or writhing, spastic facial movements, frowning, blinking, blowing, teeth grinding, lip smacking, or chewing movements as if the patient has food or gum in their mouth. This type of extrapyramidal symptoms (EPS) may be irreversible.

**Thought broadcasting:** The belief that others can "hear" one's thoughts (as if over a public address or broadcasting system) or read one's mind.

**Thought content:** What a person is thinking about; topic of conversation.

**Thought insertion:** The belief that others are "putting" thoughts "into" one's mind.

**Thought process:** The way a person thinks.

**Thought withdrawal:** The belief that others are "removing" or "stealing" one's thoughts.

**Tolerance:** The need for markedly increased amounts of a substance to achieve desired effect or experiencing a markedly diminished effect with continued use of same amount.

**Torticollis:** See *Dystonia or dystonic reactions.*

**Toxic substance:** Poisonous.

**Transference:** A patient's unconscious displacement of feelings for significant people in his or her past onto the nurse or other staff member in the current therapeutic relationship.

**Transgender:** Gender identity that varies significantly from a person's chromosomal sex.

**Transsexual:** Identifying with the opposite gender; seeking to live in the gender role of the opposite sex.

**Trauma:** An injury that may be emotional, psychological, or physical or a combination of these.

**Trigger:** Anything (situations, events, people, geographic locations, activities, odors, sights, etc.) that increases risk of drinking or using substances; increases risk or probability of relapse. This word is also used when assessing emotional responses in other disorders, including anxiety disorders, PTSD, and phobias.

**Tyramine:** An amino acid that causes the release of norepinephrine and epinephrine.

**Victim:** A person of any age who is violated by acts of harassment, disorderly conduct, reckless endangerment, entrapment, and attempted or actual assault of any type including sexual assault.

**Wernicke-Korsakoff syndrome:** In some sources referred to as Wernicke's encephalopathy and Korsakoff's syndrome. A group of signs and symptoms resulting from poor nutrition (specifically thiamine deficiency) frequently seen in alcoholics. Wernicke's encephalopathy includes signs and symptoms of confusion, ataxia, and abnormal eye movements/nystagmus whereas Korsakoff's syndrome includes severe short- and long-term memory impairment.

**Word salad:** A mixture of words and phrases that lack comprehensive meaning or logical coherence; commonly seen in schizophrenia.

**Withdrawal:** A substance-specific process or syndrome that follows the cessation of or reduction in intake of psychoactive drugs or alcohol on which an individual has physical, cognitive, behavioral, or affective dependence.

# References

American Psychiatric Association. (2000). *Diagnostic and statistical manual of mental disorders* (4th ed.). Text Revision. Washington, DC: Author.

American Psychological Association. (2007). *APA dictionary of psychology.* Washington, DC: Author.

Fontaine K. L., & Fletcher, J. S. (2003). *Mental health nursing* (5th ed.). Upper Saddle Ridge, NJ: Prentice Hall/Pearson.

Fortinash, K. M., & Holoway-Worret, P. A. (2003). *Psychiatric nursing care plans* (4th ed.). St. Louis, MO: Mosby.

Keltner, N. L., Schwecke, L. H., & Bostrom, C. E. (2007). *Psychiatric nursing* (5th ed.). St. Louis, MO: Mosby, Elsevier.

McCance, K. L., & Huether, S. E. (2002). *Pathophysiology: The biological basis for disease in adults and children* (4th ed.). St. Louis, MO: Mosby.

Miller-Keane. (2003). *Encyclopedia and dictionary of medicine, nursing, and allied health* (7th ed.).

*Mosby's medical, nursing, and allied health dictionary* (6th ed.). (2002). St. Louis, MO: Mosby.

O'Brien, P. G., Kennedy, W. Z., & Ballard, K. A. (2008). *Psychiatric mental health nursing: An introduction to theory and practice.* Sudbury, MA: Jones and Bartlett.

Sadock, B. J., & Sadock, V. A. (2005). *Kaplan and Sadock's comprehensive textbook of psychiatry* (8th ed., Vol. I). Philadelphia, PA: Lippincott Williams & Wilkins.

Sadock, B. J., & Sadock, V. A. (2003). *Kaplan and Sadock's synopsis of psychiatry: Behavioral sciences/clinical psychiatry* (9th ed.). Philadelphia, PA: Lippincott Williams & Wilkins.

Varcarolis, E. M., Carson, V. B., & Shoemaker, N. C. (2006). *Foundations of psychiatric mental health nursing: A clinical approach* (6th ed.). St. Louis, MO: Saunders, Elsevier.

# Index